FUNDAMENTALS
of HEALTHCARE FINANCE

FUNDAMENTALS
of HEALTHCARE FINANCE

LOUIS C. GAPENSKI

WITH EDITORIAL REVIEWS BY ROD MCADAMS, KRISTIN REITER, AND DEBRA TENNYSON

AUPHA

Health Administration Press, Chicago
Association of University Programs in Health Administration, VA

Your board, staff, or clients may also benefit from this book's insight. For more information on quantity discounts, contact the Health Administration Press Marketing Manager at (312) 424-9470.

This publication is intended to provide accurate and authoritative information in regard to the subject matter covered. It is sold, or otherwise provided, with the understanding that the publisher is not engaged in rendering professional services. If professional advice or other expert assistance is required, the services of a competent professional should be sought.

The statements and opinions contained in this book are strictly those of the author(s) and do not represent the official positions of the American College of Healthcare Executives, of the Foundation of the American College of Healthcare Executives, or of the Association of University Programs in Health Administration.

13   12   11   10   09   5   4   3   2   1

Library of Congress Cataloging-in-Publication Data

Gapenski, Louis C.
   Fundamentals of healthcare finance / Louis C. Gapenski.
     p. cm.
   Includes index.
   ISBN 978-1-56793-315-4 (alk. paper)
   1. Medical economics. I. Title.
   RA410.G37 2009
   338.4'33621—dc22

                    2009001019

The paper used in this publication meets the minimum requirements of American National Standard for Information Sciences—Permanence of Paper for Printed Library Materials, ANSI Z39.48-1984.°™

Found an error or typo? We want to know! Please e-mail it to hap1@ache.org, and put "Book Error" in the subject line.

Project manager/editor: Jane Calayag; Acquisitions editor: Janet Davis; Layout and cover designer: Scott Miller

Health Administration Press
A division of the Foundation
  of the American College of
  Healthcare Executives
One North Franklin Street
Suite 1700
Chicago, IL 60606
(312) 424-2800

Association of University Programs
  in Health Administration
2000 14th Street North
Suite 780
Arlington, VA 22201
(703) 894-0940

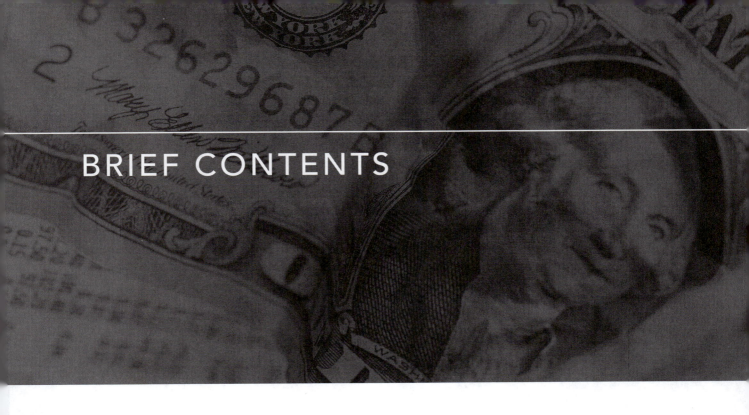

BRIEF CONTENTS

Part IV Reporting Results

DETAILED CONTENTS

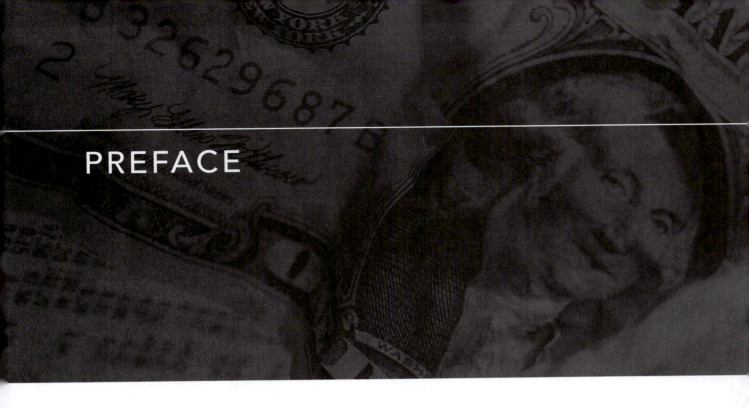

PREFACE

Some 20 years ago, after years of teaching corporate finance and writing related textbooks and casebooks, I began teaching healthcare financial management in the University of Florida's Master of Health Administration (MHA) program. The move prompted me to write my first healthcare finance textbook, *Understanding Healthcare Financial Management*. The book was designed for use in health services administration financial management courses in which students had taken prerequisite courses in both accounting and corporate finance. Often, such MHA courses are case courses, so this book served primarily as a reference tool when working healthcare finance cases.

Later on, I expanded my healthcare finance teaching to include other courses in traditional and executive MHA programs in which students do not have a formal educational background in accounting or financial management. Finance courses in these programs require a book that provides basic information on foundation topics. Furthermore, these courses often are part of programs that contain just one healthcare finance course, so the course must cover both accounting and financial management.

In reviewing the books available for use in such courses, I found some that were strong in accounting and others that were strong in financial management; however, I could not find one that gave equal emphasis to both components of healthcare finance. This situation prompted me to write *Healthcare Finance: An Introduction to Accounting and Financial Management*.

More recently, I started teaching healthcare finance outside MHA programs, in-cluding public health, health science, health education, and professional development pro-grams. I found that students in these programs were not required to have the same depth of knowledge as MHA students do. Furthermore, these students were much more interested in how healthcare finance was used by clinical as opposed to financial managers. This unique need for healthcare finance education prompted me to write this book, *Funda-mentals of Healthcare Finance*.

CONCEPT OF THE BOOK

My goal in writing *Fundamentals* was to create a text that introduces readers to those basic principles and applications of healthcare finance that are most important to entry-level op-erational managers. Thus, principles that are used primarily by financial staff members are either covered lightly or not at all. Also, background information about financial markets and securities are not included in this book.

The end result is a shorter book that contains three introductory chapters, six chap-ters that cover accounting, and four chapters devoted to financial management (corporate finance). The idea here is that entry-level managers, who typically will be working at the de-partment level or perhaps in a medical practice setting, need to understand those finance principles that they will encounter and work with on a daily basis. Other concepts can be learned later as needed. Although this book does cover some "organizational" finance issues, its focus is on topics that are most relevant to entry-level managers of clinical operations.

Another consideration in writing this book is that most readers will be seeing the material for the first time. Thus, the concepts here are explained as clearly and succinctly as possible. I have tried hard to create a book that readers will find user-friendly, enjoyable, and self-instructive. If students don't find a book interesting, understandable, and useful, they won't read it.

INTENDED MARKET AND USE

The book is not designed for any specific type of educational program. Rather, it can be used in a wide variety of settings: undergraduate and graduate, traditional and executive, on-campus and distance learning, and even independently for professional development. However, the book is ideal for undergraduate health administration programs and in un-dergraduate and graduate public health and health science programs.

The key to the book's usefulness is not the educational program but the focus of the course. If the course covers the fundamentals of healthcare finance, with a concentration on operational management, this book will be a good fit.

Practicing healthcare professionals who need to gain a better understanding of healthcare finance may greatly benefit from this book as well. Such professionals include clinicians who have management responsibilities and line managers who require additional finance skills.

ANCILLARY MATERIALS FOR INSTRUCTORS

Several teaching aids are available for instructors who adopt this book. They can be obtained through the Health Administration Press website. For access information, please e-mail hap1@ache.org.

◆ *PowerPoint slides.* The essential material in each chapter—concepts, graphs, tables, lists, and calculations—are presented in roughly 25 to 35 slides. Hard-copy versions (or the files themselves) can be provided to students as lecture notes. Instructors may use these slides as is or customize them to meet their own unique needs.

◆ *Additional online chapters.* Instructors who want to go over concepts beyond the fundamentals covered in the text may access four chapters that are posted online. (See the next section for details.)

◆ *Selected cases.* Five cases are available to instructors who want to incorporate cases into their courses. These cases are not as complex as those in *Cases in Healthcare Finance*, and they come with questions intended to both guide students and keep them on track. (See the next section for details.)

◆ *Instructor's manual.* The manual includes a sample course syllabus, solutions to the end-of-chapter questions and problems, and solutions to the online cases.

◆ *Test bank.* An online test bank is available to adopters. It consists of roughly ten multiple-choice questions per chapter.

ANCILLARY MATERIALS FOR STUDENTS

Students (and instructors) can find the following learning tools on the Health Administration Press Book Companion website at ache.org/books/FinanceFundamentals.

◆ *Additional online chapters.* These four chapters aim to expand the scope of study.

Chapter 14: Financial Markets and Securities
Chapter 15: Lease Financing and Business Valuation
Chapter 16: Distributions to Owners: Bonuses, Dividends, and Repurchases
Chapter 17: Capitation, Rate Setting, and Risk Sharing

◆ *Online appendixes*. These two appendixes (operational analysis ratios and financial analysis ratios) provide a more extensive list of ratios and their definitions than what is provided in this book.

◆ *Selected cases*. These cases are not overly complex, and they give students the opportunity to apply many of the concepts discussed in the book and in class. The cases contain a set of questions that guide students along a solution path as they work each case.

> Case 1: The Dialysis Center: Cost Allocation Concepts
> Case 2: University Hospital: Marginal Cost Pricing
> Case 3: Panhandle Medical Practice: Activity-Based Costing
> Case 4: Better Care Clinic: Breakeven Analysis
> Case 5: Twin Falls Community Hospital: Capital Investment Analysis

ACKNOWLEDGMENTS

This book reflects the efforts of many people. First and foremost, I thank the following three reviewers whose comments helped transform my rough concept into a book. Without their help, this text could not have been written.

Rod McAdams, PhD	Armstrong Atlantic State University
Kristin Reiter, PhD	University of North Carolina at Chapel Hill
Debra Tennyson, PhD	Hofstra University

Colleagues, students, and staff at the University of Florida provided inspirational support, as well as more tangible support, during the development and class testing of this book. Also, the Health Administration Press staff was instrumental in ensuring the quality and usefulness of the book.

ERRORS IN THE BOOK

In spite of the significant effort that has been expended by many individuals on this book, it is safe to say that some errors exist. In an attempt to create the most error-free and useful book possible, I strongly encourage both instructors and students to write me at the address on the next page with comments and suggestions for improving the book. I certainly welcome your input.

CONCLUSION

In the environment faced by healthcare providers today, good finance is more important than ever to the economic well-being of the enterprise. As such, clinical managers must be thoroughly grounded in finance principles and applications. But this is easier said than done.

I hope that *Fundamentals of Healthcare Finance* will help you understand the finance problems currently faced by healthcare providers and, more important, that it will provide guidance on how best to solve them.

Louis C. Gapenski, PhD
Box 100195
Health Science Center
University of Florida
Gainesville, FL 32610-0195

June 2009

HOW TO USE THIS BOOK

This section is designed to help readers get the most value from this book. It begins with a discussion of how the book is organized and then goes on to explain the learning aids designed to make its use easier and more effective.

ORGANIZATION

To paraphrase a line in Lewis Carroll's *Alice in Wonderland*: "Any road will do if you don't know where you are going." Because not just any road will take you to the main points of this book, we have carefully charted our destination: to provide you with an understanding of the fundamentals of healthcare finance. The organization of this book serves as the paved road to this destination.

Part I (Foundation Concepts) contains background material essential to the practice of healthcare finance. Chapter 1 introduces readers to healthcare finance and the healthcare environment, while Chapter 2 provides additional insights into the uniqueness of the healthcare industry and other basic business concepts. Chapter 3 deals with reimbursement, or how healthcare organizations are paid. Note that healthcare finance cannot be studied in a vacuum because it is profoundly influenced by the economic and social environment of the industry, including alternative types of ownership, taxes, and reimbursement methods.

Part II (Planning, Managing, and Control) begins by discussing costs (Chapter 4), the starting point of all planning and budgeting activities. Chapter 5 adds price to the discussion and shows how managers can use cost and revenue data to estimate profits under a wide range of assumptions. Chapter 6 focuses on planning and budgeting, or how managers plan for the future and then monitor operations to ensure that goals are met. In Chapter 7, we cover the management of financial operations, including how providers translate cash and inventories into services, then bill for those services, and ultimately collect revenues. In addition, Chapter 7 gives readers some insights into how patient service operations are monitored and controlled.

Part III (Financing and Capital Investment Decisions) addresses capital acquisition and investment. Chapter 8 examines how businesses raise money, the appropriate mix of financing, and how the cost of financing is estimated. Chapters 9 and 10 cover the vital topic of how businesses analyze new capital investment opportunities. Because major facilities projects take years to plan and execute, and because these decisions generally are not easily reversed and will affect operations for many years, their impact on the future of an organization is profound.

Part IV (Reporting Results) describes how healthcare providers create statements that compile and report financial results, and how those results are interpreted. Chapter 11 focuses on the income statement, while Chapter 12 discusses the balance sheet and statement of cash flows. Finally, Chapter 13 explains how financial statements are analyzed to assess financial condition.

All parts and chapters of the book are self-contained. For example, Part IV may be studied before Part II or Part III. By using this alternative sequencing, all of the material traditionally covered in accounting courses is bundled together. In the text, we placed Reporting Results (Part IV) at the end because readers can better understand financial statements after they learn about financing and capital investment decisions.

ONLINE CONTENT

In addition to the printed text, four chapters, two appendixes, and five cases are posted on the publisher's website at ache.org/books/FinanceFundamentals.

Chapter 14 details how businesses raise capital. Chapter 15 explains lease financing and how businesses are valued. Chapter 16 discusses how profits in investor-owned businesses are returned to owners. Chapter 17 explores capitation reimbursement and how insurers set premium rates. Appendix A contains an expanded list of ratios (metrics) for assessing operations, which complement those presented in Chapter 7. Appendix B provides an expanded list of financial condition ratios, as described in Chapter 13. The website also contains a collection of five cases, which instructors may assign, that illustrate selected healthcare finance concepts in more realistic settings.

LEARNING AIDS

The overriding goal in creating this book was to provide an easy-to-read, content-filled introductory text on healthcare finance that focuses on issues that are fundamental to the management of clinical services. The book contains several features that will assist readers in the learning process.

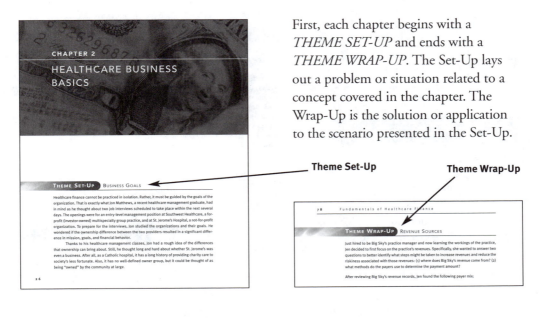

First, each chapter begins with a *THEME SET-UP* and ends with a *THEME WRAP-UP*. The Set-Up lays out a problem or situation related to a concept covered in the chapter. The Wrap-Up is the solution or application to the scenario presented in the Set-Up.

Theme Set-Up

Theme Wrap-Up

Pay particular attention to the *LEARNING OBJECTIVES* listed at the beginning of each chapter. These objectives provide a feel for the most important topics in the chapter by setting them as study goals.

Learning Objectives

Self Test Questions

As you finish reading each major section, you will find one or more *SELF-TEST QUESTIONS*. Try to provide reasonable answers to these questions. Your responses do not have to be perfect, but if you are not satisfied with your answer, reread the relevant section before proceeding. Answers to these self-test questions are not provided, but if you review the preceding section you will see that it includes all the necessary information to answer these questions.

Throughout the book, **boldface** is used to indicate important concepts, which are both explained in the text and summarized in separate sections labeled *CRITICAL CON-CEPT*. Terms that require definition, but are not critical concepts, are italicized and defined in a running glossary in the page margins.

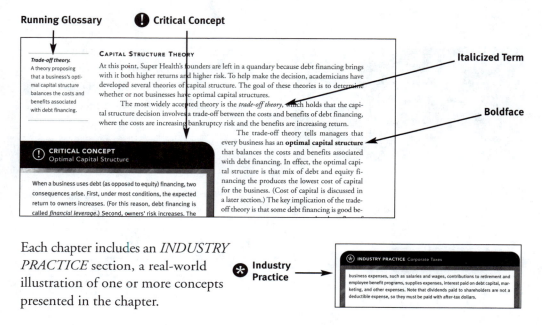

Each chapter includes an *INDUSTRY PRACTICE* section, a real-world illustration of one or more concepts presented in the chapter.

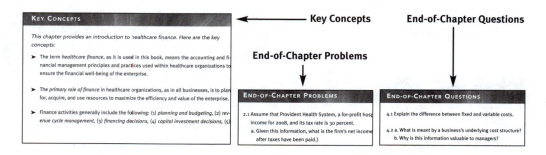

More learning aids are included at the end of each chapter. *KEY CONCEPTS* are brief summaries of the main principles and practices discussed in the chapters. *END-OF-CHAPTER QUESTIONS* are designed to assess your understanding of the *qualitative* material in the chapter. In most chapters, these questions are followed by *END-OF-CHAPTER PROBLEMS*, which are designed to assess your understanding of the *quantitative* material. Your instructor can provide answers or solutions to these questions and problems.

The structure of the book makes the learning of healthcare finance fundamentals as easy and enjoyable as possible.

PART I

FOUNDATION CONCEPTS

Two factors make healthcare services different from any other services. First, many health-care organizations, especially hospitals, are organized as not-for-profit corporations as opposed to for-profit, investor-owned businesses. For example, in Gainesville, Florida, Shands Healthcare at the University of Florida is a not-for-profit hospital, while North Florida Regional Medical Center is owned by investors. Second, payment for services rendered by healthcare providers typically is made by third-party payers, such as Blue Cross and Blue Shield, rather than by the patients who receive the services. By focusing on these differences, Part I presents the unique framework for the practice of healthcare finance.

Chapter 1 discusses the institutional setting for the delivery of healthcare services, including the organization and role of the finance staff and the types of healthcare organizations.

Chapter 2 focuses on alternative forms of business organization and ownership, and how taxes influence finance decisions. Here, the specific differences between not-for-profit and investor-owned businesses are explored. In addition, the chapter briefly describes the nature of a business and the types of finance decisions that it must make.

Chapter 3 covers the third-party payer system and alternative reimbursement methods. Healthcare managers at all levels must know who the payers are and what payment methods are used. These external factors have a profound influence on the operations of all healthcare organizations.

Some of you may already be familiar with much of the information presented in Part I, either because you have taken other courses that introduced this material or you have worked in the field. If this is your situation, a quick review cannot hurt; after all, repetition is the key to learning. For the rest of you, the material may be mostly new. In this case, Part I plays an important role in your understanding of the concepts in the remainder of the book.

CHAPTER 1

INTRODUCTION TO HEALTHCARE FINANCE

If you are using this book, you must either be working in healthcare or interested in a career in healthcare. Of course, numerous career opportunities are available in clinical fields, including medicine, dentistry, and physical therapy, and some of you are already practicing or will enter those fields upon graduation. However, most of you are considering careers in healthcare management. In addition, many clinicians find themselves balancing both clinical and administrative roles, and so healthcare management knowledge is important.

According to the Association of University Programs in Health Administration, an education in healthcare management will prepare you to enter the exciting and challenging healthcare industry, the largest in the United States, representing more than 11 million jobs. Healthcare executives have the opportunity to make a significant contribution to improving the health of citizens and to work in tens of thousands of healthcare organizations throughout the United States and the world.

An education in healthcare management can take you in many different directions. Career options for healthcare managers have never been more diverse or exciting. The kind of entry-level jobs offered to a college graduate varies in terms of the individual's interests, skills, and experience. Today, an estimated 300,000 people serve in healthcare management positions—from entry level to middle management to leadership—in organizations of all sizes—from a practice with several people to major corporations that employ thousands. After requisite experience, many healthcare management graduates are in a position to shape the future of healthcare in the United States and across the globe.

All that probably sounds good, but what types of organizations might be interested in hiring a healthcare management graduate? By the end of the chapter, you will have an idea of the settings available. See if any of them appeal to you.

LEARNING OBJECTIVES

After studying this chapter, you will be able to

➤ Define the term *healthcare finance* as it is used in this book.

➤ Discuss the structure of the finance department, the role of finance in healthcare organizations, and how this role has changed over time.

➤ Describe the major players in the healthcare industry.

➤ List the key issues currently facing healthcare managers.

1.1 INTRODUCTION

In today's healthcare environment, where financial realities play an important role in many, if not most, decisions, healthcare managers at all levels must understand the fundamentals of finance and how these concepts are used to enhance the financial well-being of the institution. In this chapter, we introduce you to the rationale that underlies this book. Furthermore, we present background information about healthcare finance and the different types of healthcare organizations. We sincerely hope that this book provides significant help in your quest to increase your professional competency in the critical area of healthcare finance.

1.2 DEFINING HEALTHCARE FINANCE

What is healthcare finance? Surprisingly, there is no single answer to that question because the definition of the term depends, for the most part, on the context in which it is used. Thus, your understanding should begin with learning the scope and meaning of the term *healthcare finance* as it is used in this book.

To start, recognize that healthcare finance is not about financing the healthcare system. *Healthcare financing* is another topic that involves how society pays for the healthcare services it consumes. This is a very complex and politically charged issue that we do not tackle directly in this book. Of course, the manner of financing healthcare affects how hospitals and physicians are reimbursed for services and hence has a significant influence on healthcare finance.

Most users of this book will become (or already are) managers at healthcare organizations, such as medical group practices, hospitals, home health agencies, or long-term-care facilities. Thus, to create a book that has the most value to its primary users, we focused on finance as it applies within *healthcare organizations*. Of course, the principles and practices of finance cannot be studied in a vacuum but must be based on the realities of the current healthcare environment, including how healthcare services are financed.

Within the health services organizations, **healthcare finance** consists of both the accounting and financial management functions. (In many settings, accounting and financial management are separate disciplines.) Accounting, as its

> **Healthcare financing**
> The system that a society uses to pay for healthcare services.

> **Healthcare organizations**
> Those that provide patient care services. Examples include hospitals, medical practices, clinics, and nursing homes. Also called providers.

CRITICAL CONCEPT
Healthcare Finance

Healthcare finance can have many different definitions, depending on the setting. For purposes here, healthcare finance encompasses the accounting and financial management functions of healthcare organizations. Accounting involves the measurement, in financial terms, of a business's operations and financial status, while financial management (corporate finance) involves the application of theory and concepts developed to help managers make better decisions. In practice, the two functions blend together, with accounting generating the data needed to make sound decisions and financial management providing the framework for those decisions.

name implies, concerns the recording, in financial terms, of economic events that reflect the operations, resources, and financing of an organization. In general, the purpose of accounting is to create and provide to interested parties, both internal (managers) and external (investors), useful information about an organization's financial status and operations.

Whereas accounting provides a rational means by which to measure a business's financial performance and to assess operations, financial management (often called corporate finance) provides the concepts and tools necessary to help managers make better decisions. Of course, the boundary between accounting and financial management is blurred; certain aspects of accounting involve decision making, and much of the application of financial management concepts requires accounting data.

(?) SELF-TEST QUESTIONS

1. What is meant by the term "healthcare finance"?

2. What is the difference between accounting and financial management?

1.3 PURPOSE OF THE BOOK

This book is designed as an introduction to the fundamentals of healthcare finance as practiced in healthcare organizations. This purpose has several important implications.

First, because the book assumes the reader has no prior knowledge of the subject matter, it is totally self-contained, with each topic explained in basic terms. Furthermore, because clarity is so important when first explaining concepts, the chapters have been written in an easy-to-read fashion. None of the topics is inherently difficult, but new concepts often take some effort to understand. This process is made easier by the writing style used and the learning aids contained in the text.

Second, because this book focuses on fundamentals, it presents a broad overview of healthcare finance rather than an in-depth treatment that might be found in accounting or financial management books.

Third, and most important, is that the book discusses tasks that are essential to the operational management of clinical services, as opposed to tasks that are exclusively financial in nature and hence are the sole province of the financial staff. This means the content is overweighted on accounting material, especially those aspects that are most relevant to entry-level managers. Of course, even managers whose primary responsibility is nonfinancial, such as those in operations, marketing, or human resources, need to know something about the finance department. Thus, the book is sprinkled with this type of information, but only in light doses.

When you finish the book, you will not be expected to fully understand every nuance of every finance principle or practice that pertains to every type of healthcare organization. Nevertheless, you will have sufficient knowledge of healthcare finance to enable you to function better as an operational manager and to judge the quality of financial analyses performed by others.

(?) SELF-TEST QUESTION

1. What is the purpose of the book?

1.4 THE ROLE OF FINANCE IN HEALTHCARE ORGANIZATIONS

The primary role of finance in healthcare organizations, as in all businesses, is to plan for, acquire, and use resources to maximize the efficiency (and value) of the enterprise. As discussed in the next major section, the two broad areas of finance—accounting and financial management—are separate functions at larger organizations, although the accounting function usually is carried out under the direction of the organization's chief financial officer (CFO) and hence falls under the overall category of finance.

FINANCE ACTIVITIES

The finance activities explored in this book include the following:

◆ **Planning and budgeting.** First and foremost, healthcare finance involves evaluating the financial effectiveness of current operations and planning for the future. Chapters 4 through 6 cover these functions.

◆ **Managing financial operations.** Healthcare organizations spend a lot of time managing cash and supplies inventories as well as collecting money owed for services rendered. Proper management of these functions is necessary to ensure operational effectiveness and to reduce costs. Typically, managers at all levels are involved, to a greater or lesser extent, in these processes, which are discussed in Chapter 7.

◆ **Financing decisions.** All organizations must raise funds to buy the assets necessary to support operations. Such decisions involve many issues, such as the choice between long-term and short-term debt and the use of lease versus conventional financing. Senior managers and the financial staff typically make the financing decisions, but these decisions have ramifications for managers at all levels. Business financing is the subject of Chapter 8.

◆ **Capital investment decisions.** One of the most critical decisions managers make is the selection of new facilities (land, buildings, and equipment). Such decisions are the primary means by which businesses implement strategic plans, and hence they play a key role in a business's financial future. These decisions, which affect everyone in the organization, are described in Chapters 9 and 10.

◆ **Financial reporting.** For a variety of reasons, businesses must record and report to outsiders the results of operations and current financial status. This task is typically accomplished with a set of financial statements, which are explained in Chapters 11 and 12.

◆ **Financial and operational analysis.** To achieve and maintain a high level of organizational performance, businesses must constantly monitor both financial and operational conditions and take actions as needed to ensure that goals are met. These topics are addressed in Chapters 7 and 13.

In addition to those finance activities that involve operational managers, the following activities are accomplished primarily by the finance staff:

◆ **Contract management.** In today's healthcare environment, healthcare institutions must negotiate, sign, and monitor contracts with managed care organizations and health insurers. The finance staff typically has primary responsibility for these tasks, although operational managers clearly are affected by external contracts and must be involved in their negotiation and management.

◆ **Financial risk management.** Many financial transactions that take place to support the operations of a business can, in themselves, increase a business's risk. Thus, an important finance staff activity is to manage financial risk.

THE FOUR Cs

The finance activities at healthcare organizations may be summarized by the **four Cs**: costs, cash, capital, and control.

The measurement and minimization of **costs** is vital to the financial success of all healthcare organizations. Rampant costs, as compared to revenues, usually spell doom for any business.

A business might be profitable but still face a crisis because of a shortage of **cash**. Cash is the lubricant that makes the wheels of a business run smoothly; without it, the business grinds to a halt. In essence, businesses must have sufficient cash on hand (or the ability to quickly raise it) to meet cash obligations as they occur. In healthcare, a critical part of managing cash is collecting money from insurers for patient services provided. In fact, this element is so important that some healthcare finance professors include **collections** as the fifth C.

Capital represents the funds (money) used to acquire land, buildings, and equipment. Without capital, healthcare businesses would not have the physical resources needed to provide patient services. Thus, capital allows healthcare organizations to meet the healthcare needs of their communities.

Finally, a business must **control** its financial and physical resources to ensure that they are being wisely employed and protected for future use. In addition to meeting current mission requirements, healthcare organizations must plan to meet society's future healthcare needs.

CRITICAL CONCEPT
The Four Cs

The finance activities within healthcare organizations can be summarized by the four Cs: (1) *cost* measurement and minimization, (2) *cash* management, (3) *capital* acquisition, and (4) *control* of resources.

IMPORTANCE OF FINANCE OVER TIME

In times of high profitability and abundant financial resources, the finance function tends to decline in significance. For example, when most healthcare organizations were reimbursed on the basis of the actual costs they incurred, the role of finance was minimal. At that time, the most critical finance function was cost accounting because it was more important to account for costs than it was to control them. In response to payer (primarily Medicare) requirements, providers (primarily hospitals) churned out a multitude of reports to comply with regulations and to maximize revenues. The complexities of cost reimbursement meant that a large amount of time had to be spent on cumbersome accounting, billing, and collection procedures. Thus, instead of focusing on value-adding activities, most finance work focused on bureaucratic functions.

In recent years, however, providers have been redesigning their finance functions to recognize the changes that have occurred in the healthcare industry. Billing and collections remain important today, but to be of maximum value to the enterprise, the finance function must support cost-containment efforts, managed care and other payer contract negotiations, joint venture decisions, and integrated delivery system participation. In essence, finance must help lead organizations into the future rather than merely record what has happened in the past.

Although in this book our emphasis is on finance, we must stress that all organizational functions are important. In addition to finance, managers must understand some elements of many different functions, such as marketing, facilities management, and human resource management. But all business decisions have financial implications, so all managers (whether in operations, marketing, personnel, or facilities) must know enough about finance to properly incorporate financial considerations into the plans and decisions within their own specialized areas.

? SELF-TEST QUESTIONS

1. What is the role of finance in today's healthcare organizations?

2. What are the four Cs?

3. How has the role of finance changed over time?

1.5 THE STRUCTURE OF THE FINANCE DEPARTMENT

Chief financial officer (CFO) The senior manager (or top finance dog) in a large organization's finance department. Also called vice president–finance.

The structure of the finance department depends on the type (e.g., hospital or medical practice) and size of the healthcare organization. The finance department in a large organization generally is structured in the following way.

The head of the finance department holds the title of *chief financial officer (CFO)*. (The title "vice president–finance" is also used.) This individual typically reports directly to the organization's chief executive officer and is responsible for all finance activities within the organization. The CFO directs two senior managers who help manage finance activities: the comptroller and treasurer.

Comptroller The finance department manager who handles accounting, budgeting, and reporting activities.

The *comptroller* (pronounced, and sometimes spelled, "controller") is responsible for accounting and reporting activities, such as routine budgeting, preparation of financial statements, and patient accounts management. For the most part, the comptroller is involved in those activities covered in Chapters 4 through 7 of this text. The *treasurer* is responsible for the acquisition and management of capital (funds). In other words, the treasurer must raise the funds needed by the organization and ensure that those funds are effectively used. Specific activities include the acquisition of capital, cash and debt management, lease financing, financial risk management, and endowment fund management (within not-for-profits). In general, the treasurer is involved in those activities discussed in Chapters 8 through 13 of this book.

Treasurer The finance department manager who handles capital acquisition, investment management, and risk management activities.

In large organizations, the comptroller and treasurer have managers under them who are responsible for specific functions, such as the patient accounts manager, who reports to the comptroller, and the cash manager, who reports to the treasurer.

In small businesses, many of the finance responsibilities are combined and assigned to one individual. For example, in a small group practice, the finance function is managed by one person, often called the *business (practice) manager*, who may be supported by one or more clerks.

**Business (practice)
manager**
The manager responsible for the finance function in a small healthcare organization, such as a medical practice with one or a few clinicians.

> ## (?) SELF-TEST QUESTIONS
>
> 1. Briefly describe the typical structure of the finance department within a large healthcare organization.
>
> 2. How does the size of the organization affect the finance department structure?

1.6 HEALTHCARE SETTINGS

Healthcare services are provided in numerous settings, including hospitals, ambulatory care offices and clinics, long-term-care facilities, and integrated delivery systems. Before the 1980s, most healthcare organizations were freestanding and not formally linked with other organizations. Those that were linked tended to be part of *horizontal systems*, which control a single type of healthcare facility, such as a group of hospitals or nursing homes. Recently, however, many healthcare organizations have created *vertical systems*, which control different types of providers such as medical practices, hospitals, and nursing homes.

Horizontal system
A single business entity that owns a group of similar providers, such as hospitals.

Vertical system
A single business entity that owns a group of related, but not identical, providers, such as a hospitals, nursing homes, and medical practices.

HOSPITALS

Hospitals provide diagnostic and therapeutic services to individuals who require more than several hours of care, although most hospitals are actively engaged in ambulatory (walk-in) services as well. To ensure a minimum standard of safety and quality, hospitals must be licensed by the state and undergo inspections for compliance with state regulations. In addition, most hospitals are accredited by the *Joint Commission* (previously called the Joint Commission on Accreditation of Healthcare Organizations, or JCAHO). Joint Commission accreditation is a voluntary process intended to promote high standards of care. Although the cost to achieve and maintain compliance with standards can be substantial, accreditation provides eligibility for participation in the Medicare and Medicaid programs, and hence most hospitals seek accreditation. (Medicare and Medicaid are discussed in Chapter 2.)

Joint Commission
The accreditation body for hospitals.

Recent environmental and operational changes have created significant challenges for hospital managers. For example, many hospitals are experiencing decreasing admission rates and shorter lengths of stay, resulting in reduced revenues and excess capacity. On the other hand, hospitals in fast-growing areas are hard pressed to keep ahead of patient demand. In addition, all hospitals are being pressured to give discounts to major insurers, limit the growth in patient charges, and assume greater risk in their contracts with payers.

Hospitals differ in function, length of patient stay, size, and ownership. These factors affect the type and quantity of assets, services offered, and management requirements and often determine the type and level of reimbursement. Hospitals are classified as either general acute care facilities or specialty facilities.

General acute care hospitals provide general medical and surgical services and selected acute specialty services. Such hospitals, which account for the majority of hospitals, have relatively short lengths of stay, typically a week or less. *Specialty hospitals*, such as psychiatric, children's, women's, rehabilitation, and cancer, limit admission of patients to specific ages, sexes, illnesses, or conditions. The number of specialty hospitals has grown significantly in the past few decades because of the belief that such hospitals can provide better patient services than can hospitals that treat all conditions. In addition, specialty hospitals often have lower costs than general hospitals because they do not require the overhead associated with providing many different types of services.

Hospitals vary in size from fewer than 25 beds to more than 1,000 beds; general acute care hospitals tend to be larger than specialty hospitals. Although economists do not all agree, the general belief is that the optimal hospital size is about 400–500 beds. Smaller hospitals do not benefit from economies of scale, while larger hospitals are too big to manage efficiently (have diseconomies of scale). Small hospitals, those with fewer than 100 beds, tend to be located in rural areas. Many rural hospitals have experienced financial difficulties in recent years because they have less ability than large hospitals to lower costs in response to ever-tighter reimbursement rates. Most of the largest hospitals are academic health centers or teaching hospitals. These large hospitals offer a wide range of services, including tertiary care, which consists of specialized services for patients with unusually severe, complex, or uncommon problems.

Hospitals are classified by ownership as governmental, private not-for-profit, or investor owned. *Governmental hospitals*, which make up about 25 percent of all hospitals, are broken down into federal and public (nonfederal) entities. Federal hospitals, such as those operated by the military services or the U.S. Department of Veterans Affairs, serve special purposes. Public hospitals are funded wholly or in part by a city, county, tax district, or state. In general, federal and public hospitals provide substantial services to indigent patients. In recent years, many public hospitals have converted to other ownership categories (primarily, private not-for-profit) because local governments have found it increasingly difficult to fund healthcare services and at the same time provide other necessary public services.

Private not-for-profit hospitals are nongovernmental entities organized for the sole purpose of providing inpatient healthcare services. Because of the charitable origins of U.S. hospitals and a tradition of community service, roughly 80 percent of all private hospitals (60 percent of all hospitals) are not-for-profit entities. In return for serving a charitable purpose, these hospitals receive numerous benefits, including exemption from federal and state income taxes, exemption from property and sales taxes, eligibility to receive tax-deductible charitable contributions, favorable postal rates, favorable tax-exempt financing, and tax-favored annuities for employees.

The remaining 20 percent of private hospitals (15 percent of all hospitals) are *investor-owned hospitals*, whose owners (typically shareholders) benefit directly from the profits generated by the business. Historically, most investor-owned hospitals were owned by physicians, but now most are owned by large corporations, such as HCA (Hospital Corporation of America), which owns about 190 hospitals in the United States and England; Tenet Healthcare, which owns about 65 hospitals; and Hospital Management Associates (HMA), which owns about 60 hospitals. Unlike not-for-profit hospitals, investor-owned hospitals pay taxes and forgo the other benefits of not-for-profit status.

Despite the expressed differences in mission between investor-owned and not-for-profit hospitals, not-for-profit hospitals are being forced to place greater emphasis on the financial implications of operating decisions than in the past. This trend has raised concerns in some quarters that many not-for-profit hospitals are failing to meet their charitable mission. As this perception grows, some people argue that these hospitals should lose some, if not all, of the benefits associated with their not-for-profit status. (The differences between investor-owned and not-for-profit hospitals are discussed in detail in Chapter 2.)

Hospitals are labor intensive because they need to provide continuous nursing supervision to patients, in addition to the services given by other clinical, professional, and semiprofessional staffs. Physicians petition for privileges to practice in hospitals. While they admit and provide care to hospitalized patients, physicians, for the most part, are not hospital employees and hence are not directly accountable to hospital management. However, physicians retain a major responsibility for determining which hospital services will be provided to patients and how long patients are hospitalized. Thus, physicians play a critical role in determining a hospital's costs and revenues and hence its financial condition.

AMBULATORY (OUTPATIENT) CARE

Ambulatory (outpatient) care encompasses services provided to patients who are not admitted to a hospital or nursing home. Traditional outpatient settings include clinics, medical practices, hospital outpatient departments, and emergency departments. In addition, there has been substantial growth in nontraditional settings, such as home health care, ambulatory surgery centers, urgent care centers, diagnostic imaging centers, rehabilitation/sports medicine centers, and clinical laboratories. The latest innovation in ambulatory care is the retail clinic, a small clinic operated in a retail store (such as Wal-Mart) and staffed by a physician assistant or nurse practitioner. Compared to hospital-based services, these innovative settings offer patients more amenities and convenience and, in many situations, lower prices. For example, urgent care and ambulatory surgery centers are typically less expensive than their hospital counterparts because hospitals have higher overhead costs. (The same lower-cost logic applies to urgent care centers and retail clinics as compared to medical practices).

Many factors have contributed to the expansion of ambulatory services, but technology has been a leading factor. Often, patients who once required hospitalization because

Investor-owned hospital
A hospital that is owned by investors who benefit financially from its operation. Also called for-profit hospital.

Ambulatory (outpatient) care
Care that is provided to patients that are not hospitalized or in nursing homes.

of the complexity, intensity, invasiveness, or risk associated with certain procedures can now be treated in outpatient settings. In addition, health insurers have encouraged providers to expand their outpatient services by requiring authorization for inpatient services and payment mechanisms that provide incentives to perform services on an outpatient basis.

Finally, it is easier to start a business providing outpatient care than to start a new hospital. Ordinarily, ambulatory facilities are less costly, are less frequently subject to licensure and certificate-of-need regulations (exceptions are hospital outpatient units and ambulatory surgery centers), and generally are not accredited. (Licensure and certificate-of-need regulation are discussed in detail in the next major section of this chapter.)

As outpatient care consumes an increasing portion of the healthcare dollar, and efforts to control outpatient spending are enhanced, the traditional role of the ambulatory care manager is changing. Historically, ambulatory care managers have handled routine management tasks such as billing, collections, staffing, scheduling, and patient relations, while the owners, often physicians, have tended to the important business decisions. However, a more complex healthcare environment, coupled with growing competition, is forcing managers of ambulatory care facilities to become more sophisticated in making business decisions, including finance decisions.

Long-Term Care

Long-term care consists of healthcare (and some personal care) services provided to individuals who lack all or some functional ability, specifically in the activities of daily living such as eating, bathing, and locomotion. This type of care usually covers an extended period and may be given as an inpatient or an outpatient service. Although the most common users of long-term care are the elderly, the services are available to individuals of all ages.

Individuals become candidates for long-term care when they become too mentally or physically incapacitated to perform daily living tasks and when their family members are unable to provide the help needed. Long-term care is a hybrid of healthcare and social services. Nursing homes are a major provider of such care.

Three levels of nursing home care exist: (1) skilled nursing facilities, (2) intermediate care facilities, and (3) residential care facilities. Skilled nursing facilities (SNFs) provide the level of care closest to hospital care. Services must be under the supervision of a physician and must include 24-hour daily nursing care. Intermediate care facilities (ICFs) are intended for individuals who do not require hospital or SNF care but whose mental or physical conditions require daily continuity of one or more medical services. Residential care facilities are sheltered environments that do not provide professional healthcare services. Thus, most health insurance programs do not provide coverage for residential care.

Nursing homes are more abundant than hospitals. They are also smaller, with an average of about 100 beds, compared with about 170 beds for hospitals. Large for-profit nursing home companies exist (such as Manor Care, which operates 275 homes in 30 states), but many nursing homes are "mom-and-pop" facilities. Nursing homes are licensed and inspected by states, which also license nursing home administrators. Although the Joint Commission accredits nursing homes, only a small percentage of these facilities obtain accreditation because accreditation is not required for reimbursement, and the standards to achieve accreditation are much higher than licensure requirements.

The long-term-care industry has experienced tremendous growth in recent decades. In 1960, long-term care accounted for only 1 percent of U.S. healthcare expenditures, but by 2007 it accounted for more than 6 percent. Demand increases are anticipated, as the percentage of the U.S. population aged 65 or older is expected to grow from less than 17 percent in 2007 to 20 percent in 2030. The elderly are disproportionately high users of healthcare services in general and are major users of long-term care in particular.

Although long-term care is often perceived as nursing home care, many new services have been developed that are less institutional, such as adult day care, life care centers, and hospice programs. These services tend to offer a higher quality of life, although they are not necessarily less expensive than institutional care. Home health care, provided for an extended time period, is an alternative to nursing home care but is not as readily available in many rural areas. Furthermore, third-party payers, especially Medicare, have sent mixed signals about adequately paying for home health care. In fact, many home health care businesses have been forced to close in recent years as a result of a new, and less generous, Medicare payment system.

Finally, a lot of Americans suffer from a long-lasting or chronic illness (from the Greek word "chronos," meaning time). Some chronic diseases, such as cancer or AIDS, are life threatening. Other chronic illnesses, such as asthma and diabetes, are also incurable but allow patients to live for many years. Symptoms of chronic diseases can be managed and treated, even though the basic cause cannot.

Traditionally, the treatment of chronic illnesses was fragmented, with primary care physicians, specialists, hospitals, and other providers separately contributing their services without much planning or coordination with the other parties. Today, there is finally recognition that the most effective way to provide chronic care is using a long-term integrated approach, wherein a single case manager is responsible for the patient's care, regardless of the setting.

INTEGRATED DELIVERY SYSTEMS

Many healthcare experts have extolled the benefits of providing hospital care, ambulatory care, long-term care, and business support services through a single **integrated delivery system**. The potential benefits of such a system include the following:

◆ Patients are kept in the corporate network of services (*patient capture*).

◆ Providers have access to managerial and functional specialists, such as reimbursement and marketing professionals.

Patient capture
The concept that once a patient enters the system at one point (e.g., a doctor's office), all services needed by that patient will be provided by the system.

◆ Information systems that track all aspects of patient care, as well as insurance and other data, can be developed more easily, and the costs to develop them can be shared.

◆ Larger, multipurpose organizations have better access to capital.

◆ The ability to recruit and retain management and professional staff is enhanced.

◆ Healthcare insurers can be offered a complete package of services ("one-stop shopping").

◆ A full range of healthcare services, including chronic disease management and health status improvement programs, can be better planned and delivered to meet the needs of a defined population. Many of these population-based efforts typically are not offered by stand-alone providers.

◆ Incentives that encourage all providers in the system to work together for the common good of the system can be created, which has the potential to improve quality and control costs.

Although integrated delivery systems can be structured in many ways, the defining characteristic of such systems is that the organization has the ability to assume full clinical responsibility for the healthcare needs of a defined population. Because of state laws, which typically mandate that the insurance function can be assumed only by licensed insurers, integrated delivery systems typically contract with insurers rather than directly with employers. Sometimes the insurer, often a managed care plan, is owned by the integrated delivery system itself, but generally it is separately owned. In contracts with some insurers, the integrated delivery system receives a fixed payment per plan-covered life and hence assumes both the financial and clinical risks associated with providing healthcare services.

To be an effective competitor, integrated delivery systems must minimize the provision of unnecessary services because additional services create added costs but do not necessarily result in additional revenues. Thus, the objective of integrated delivery systems is to provide all needed services to its member population in the lowest cost setting. To achieve this goal, integrated delivery systems invest heavily in primary care services, especially prevention, early intervention, and wellness programs. While hospitals con-

CRITICAL CONCEPT
Integrated Delivery System

An integrated delivery system consists of a number of different types of healthcare organizations, such as hospitals, clinics, and nursing homes, owned and operated as a single provider. Although integrated delivery systems offer the opportunity to coordinate all aspects of patient care under a single "umbrella," their complexity makes the overall management process much more difficult than in smaller organizations that focus on one type of service.

tinue to be centers of technology, integrated delivery systems have the incentive to shift patients toward lower cost settings. Thus, clinical integration among the various providers and components of care is essential to achieving quality, cost efficiency, and patient satisfaction.

In spite of the benefits of integration, health system executives have found that managing large, diverse enterprises is difficult. In many cases, the financial and patient care gains predicted were not realized, and some of the integrated delivery systems formed in the 1990s have broken up. Today, it is not clear whether large integrated health systems are better suited for success than are smaller, more-focused organizations. Only time will tell.

(?) SELF-TEST QUESTIONS

1. What are some different types of hospitals, and what trends are occurring in the hospital industry?

2. What trends are occurring in outpatient and long-term care?

3. What is an integrated delivery system?

4. Do you think that integrated delivery systems will be more or less prevalent in the future? Explain your answer.

(*) INDUSTRY PRACTICE What We Spend on Healthcare

Most people think that healthcare spending in the United States is out of control. For example, in 2007, about 16 percent of the nation's total value of goods and services (gross domestic product [GDP]) was spent on healthcare. The proportion of GDP devoted to healthcare is expected to rise to 20 percent by 2017, an amount that is expected to be higher than the expenditure for housing and food combined. In effect, rapidly rising healthcare costs are "squeezing out" the spending on other goods and services. By comparison, most other industrialized nations, such as Germany, England, and Canada, currently spend about 8 percent to 10 percent of their GDP on healthcare.

Where does all this money go? 2007 data indicate that Americans spend healthcare dollars this way:

(Continued)

(*) INDUSTRY PRACTICE What We Spend on Healthcare

Hospital care	29.7%
Physician and other ambulatory care	23.2
Retail health products	12.6
Prescription drugs	9.7
Administration costs	9.7
Nursing home care	5.9
Dental care	4.2
Miscellaneous medical products	2.7
Home health care	2.3
Total	100.0%

According to this table, the largest area of healthcare expenditure is hospital care, while the second largest is physician and other outpatient services, such as diagnostics and surgeries, physical therapy, and chiropractic care. Combined, hospitals and ambulatory care providers consume more than half of each healthcare dollar.

The next biggest healthcare expense, at 12.6 percent, is for retail health products, such as over-the–counter drugs and medical supplies. Prescription drugs follow closely, at 9.7 percent. However, the proportion spent on prescription drugs is expected to increase over time as more and more individuals gain access to insurance programs that cover prescription drugs.

Interestingly, almost 10 percent of each healthcare dollar is spent on administrative costs. In 2007, over $2.2 trillion was spent on healthcare, and about $200 billion of that money paid for administrative costs. Administrative costs can be defined and measured in numerous ways, but regardless of how they are measured, these costs eat up a great deal of money. One persuasive argument for establishing a universal or national healthcare system is that it can dramatically reduce administrative costs and hence make more money available for patient services. In fact, some people have argued that the savings in administrative costs alone would be sufficient to insure the currently uninsured.

Will we ever get healthcare spending under control? Who knows! What we know is that it cannot continue to grow at the current rate without causing financial damage to other parts of the economy. Thus, sooner or later, we will need to do something.

Source: This industry practice is based on data from "By the Numbers," *Modern Healthcare*, December 24, 2007.

1.7 REGULATORY AND LEGAL ISSUES

Healthcare services are subject to many regulations. For example, pharmacy services are regulated by state and federal laws, and radiology services are highly regulated because of the handling and disposal of radioactive materials. Entry into the healthcare industry is also heavily regulated. Examples of such regulation include licensure, certificate of need, rate setting, and review programs.

States require *licensure* of certain healthcare providers in an effort to protect the health, safety, and welfare of the public. Licensure regulations establish minimum standards that must be met to provide a service. Many types of providers are licensed, including entire facilities (such as hospitals and nursing homes) and individuals (such as physicians, dentists, nurses, and even some managers).

Licensed facilities must submit to periodic inspections and review activities. Such reviews focus more on physical features and safety than on patient care and outcomes, although progress is being made to change this practice. Thus, licensure has not necessarily ensured that the public will receive quality services.

Critics of licensure contend that it is designed to protect providers, not consumers. For example, licensed paramedical professionals (say, physician assistants or dental hygienists) usually are required to work under the supervision of a physician or a dentist, making it impossible for paramedical professionals to compete with physicians or dentists. Despite the limitations of licensure, it is undoubtedly here to stay.

Certificate of need (CON) regulation was enacted by Congress in 1974 in an effort to control growing healthcare costs. CON legislation required providers to obtain state approval on the basis of community need for construction and renovation projects that either relate to specific services or exceed a defined cost threshold. This attempt to control capital expenditures by controlling expansion and preventing duplication of services lasted less than a decade before the Reagan administration began to downplay CON regulation and promote cost controls through competition. However, CON regulation, in one form or another, still exists in roughly 35 states.

Critics of CON regulation argue that it does not provide as much control over capital expenditures as originally envisioned and that it increases costs by requiring additional administrative costs when new facilities are needed. Perhaps the biggest criticism of CON is that it creates a territorial franchise for services that it covers; that is, it makes it difficult for new entities to enter markets, even though the new businesses may be more cost efficient and offer better patient care than the existing ones.

> ⓘ **CRITICAL CONCEPT**
> Certificate of Need
>
> A certificate of need (CON) is the approval required by many states before a new healthcare facility can be constructed. CON proponents claim the system helps control costs by preventing excess capacity. Critics, however, contend that CON regulation impedes competition and the spread of new technologies while protecting established providers even when inefficient.

Cost-containment programs
State programs that require providers (primarily hospitals) to submit budgets each year for approval.

Professional liability
The responsibility of organizations and individuals who provide professional services, such as hospitals and physicians, for losses that result from malpractice.

In addition to CON, *cost-containment programs* were enacted in many states at the time when most healthcare reimbursement was based on costs. By the late 1970s, nine states had mandatory cost-containment programs, and many other states had voluntary programs (those that did not mandate compliance). The primary tool for cost-containment programs is the rate review system.

Three types of rate review systems have been used: (1) detailed budget reviews with approval or setting of rates; (2) formula methods, which use inflation formulas to set target rates; and (3) negotiated rates, which involve joint decision making between the provider and the rate setter. Some states that use rate review systems have reduced the rate of cost increase to below the national average, while others have failed to do so. However, rate review, as a sole means of cost containment, has been criticized because it does not address the issue of demand for healthcare services.

Outside of regulation, healthcare providers have many other legal concerns. For most providers, the primary legal concern is *professional liability*. Malpractice suits are the oldest forms of quality assurance in the U.S. healthcare system, and today such suits are used to an extreme extent. Many people believe that the United States is facing a malpractice insurance crisis. Total malpractice premiums, which have doubled in the last ten years, have been passed on to healthcare purchasers. Some specialist physicians pay malpractice premiums of more than $100,000 per year, and each month U.S. courts manage approximately 20,000 new malpractice suits, with awards averaging $300,000 for cases that go to trial.

Although providers in some states have been successful in achieving tort reforms, malpractice litigation continues to be perceived as inefficient because it diverts resources to lawyers and courts and creates disincentives for physicians to practice high-risk specialties and for hospitals to offer high-risk services. In addition, such litigation encourages the practice of defensive medicine, in which physicians overuse diagnostic services in an effort to protect themselves.

Professional liability is the most visible legal concern in healthcare, but the industry is subject to many other legal issues, including the typical general liability and antitrust claims. Finally, healthcare providers are confronted with unique ethical issues, such as the right to die or the right to prolong life, that are often resolved through the legal system.

? SELF-TEST QUESTIONS

1. What are some forms of regulation in the healthcare industry?

2. What is the most pressing legal issue facing healthcare providers today?

1.8 CURRENT CHALLENGES

For the past several years, the American College of Healthcare Executives (ACHE) has surveyed hospital chief executive officers (CEOs) regarding their major concerns. In their most recent survey (2007), the top-ranked issue was financial challenges, by almost a two to one margin over the next highest concern (personnel shortages). In fact, financial worries have headed the list of challenges on every survey. Tom Dolan, ACHE president and CEO, said: "These survey results are a continuation of previous concerns. First and foremost is finance." When asked to rank their specific financial concerns, CEOs put revenues (reimbursement) at the forefront, with concerns over Medicaid, Medicare, and bad debt losses topping the list. (Reimbursement is discussed in Chapter 3.) Clearly, the ability of government payers to adequately reimburse providers leads this list.

Another survey, which appeared in the January 2006 issue of *Healthcare Financial Management*, focused on the concerns of CFOs. The most pressing issue cited here was balancing clinical and financial needs. In essence, how can financial performance be improved without having a negative impact on clinical performance? Other issues revealed included improving the revenue cycle (billing and collecting on a timely basis) and developing different ways to access (raise) capital.

Taken together, these surveys confirm the fact that finance is of primary importance to today's healthcare managers. The remainder of this book is dedicated to helping you confront and solve these issues.

(?) SELF-TEST QUESTION

1. What are some important issues facing healthcare managers today?

THEME WRAP-UP   CAREERS IN HEALTHCARE MANAGEMENT

What are some settings that require healthcare management graduates? The largest employers of healthcare managers are hospitals. In the United States, about 5,000 community hospitals, as well as Veterans Affairs (VA), military, and public health facilities, are in operation. Within hospitals, healthcare managers are needed in a multitude of functional areas, such as operations, marketing, human resources (personnel), facilities, information technology, and finance. About 40 percent of all healthcare management graduates initially take positions at hospitals. Most start their careers in operations, but some find that they are better suited for one of the other functional areas and move to specialized staff positions.

Another career opportunity is in medical practice management. Almost one million physicians practice in the United States in settings that range from one physician (a solo practice) to large group practices (such as the Mayo Clinic, which has more than 2,000 physicians). Physicians practice within specialties, the largest of which is internal medicine. Other specialties include cardiology (heart), dermatology (skin), pediatrics (children), and surgery. Some group practices consist of only one specialty, while other practices include physicians from several specialties (multispecialty practices). Obviously, the larger the group practice, the greater the need for management expertise.

The structure of the management staff at large group practices is similar to that at hospitals, while small practices may have only a practice manager and a few clerks. In addition to physician practices, other healthcare professionals, such as physical therapists and psychologists, can have stand-alone medical practices that require managerial skills beyond those possessed by clinicians. The bottom line here is that healthcare organizations need managers, and the larger the organization, the greater the need.

As the population ages, and as life expectancy increases, the requirement for nursing homes will continue to grow at a rapid rate. Currently, about 20,000 nursing homes operate in the United States. As do other institutional providers, these nursing homes require significant managerial expertise to prosper in an era of financial constraints.

A multitude of career opportunities is also available in insurance, health services research, consulting, public health, and even homeland security.

Regardless of your specific healthcare management goals, knowledge of the fundamentals of healthcare finance is a critical skill. This book will help you obtain this professional competency.

KEY CONCEPTS

This chapter provides an introduction to healthcare finance. Here are the key concepts:

➤ The term *healthcare finance*, as it is used in this book, means the accounting and financial management principles and practices used within healthcare organizations to ensure the financial well-being of the enterprise.

➤ The *primary role of finance* in healthcare organizations, as in all businesses, is to plan for, acquire, and use resources to maximize the efficiency and value of the enterprise.

➤ Finance activities generally include the following: (1) *planning and budgeting,* (2) *financial operations management,* (3) *financing decisions,* (4) *capital investment decisions,*

(5) *financial reporting,* (6) *financial and operational analysis,* (7) *contract management,* and (8) *financial risk management.*

➤ Finance activities can be summarized by the "four Cs": costs, cash, capital, and control.

➤ The size and structure of the finance department within healthcare organizations depend on the type and size of the provider.

➤ The finance department in large provider organizations generally consists of a *chief financial officer (CFO)*, who typically reports directly to the chief executive officer (CEO) and is responsible for all finance activities within the organization. Under the CFO are the *comptroller*, who is responsible for accounting and reporting activities, and the *treasurer*, who is responsible for the acquisition and management of capital (funds).

➤ In large organizations, the comptroller and treasurer direct managers with responsibility for specific functions, such as the *patient accounts manager*, who reports to the comptroller, and the *cash manager*, who reports to the treasurer.

➤ In small healthcare businesses, the finance responsibilities are combined and assigned to one individual, often called the *business (practice) manager.*

➤ All business decisions have *financial implications*, so all managers (whether in operations, marketing, personnel, or facilities) must know enough about finance to incorporate its implications into their own specialized decision processes.

➤ Healthcare services are provided in numerous settings, including hospitals, ambulatory care facilities, long-term-care facilities, and even the home.

➤ *Hospitals* differ in function (*general acute care* versus *specialty*), patient length of stay, size, and ownership (*governmental* versus *private,* or *for-profit* versus *not-for-profit*).

➤ *Ambulatory care*, also known as *outpatient care*, encompasses services provided to non-institutionalized patients. Outpatient settings include medical practices, hospital outpatient departments, ambulatory surgery centers, urgent care centers, diagnostic imaging centers, rehabilitation/sports medicine centers, and clinical laboratories.

➤ *Home health care* brings many of the same services provided in ambulatory care settings into the patient's home.

➤ *Long-term care* entails healthcare services provided for an extended period, including inpatient, outpatient, and home health care, often with a focus on mental health, rehabilitation, or nursing home care.

➤ The defining characteristic of an *integrated delivery system* is that it has the capability of providing all healthcare services needed by a defined population.

➤ Entry into the healthcare industry has been heavily regulated. Examples of regulations include *licensure*, *certificate of need (CON)*, and *rate setting and review* programs.

➤ Legal issues, such as *malpractice*, are prominent in discussions about controlling healthcare costs.

➤ Two recent surveys of healthcare executives confirm the fact that healthcare managers view financial concerns as the most important current issue.

In Chapter 2, we continue our discussion of foundation concepts and move on to finance-related topics, such as business basics, forms of organization, and taxes.

END-OF-CHAPTER QUESTIONS

1.1 a. What is meant by the term *healthcare finance* as it is used in this book?
   b. What are the two broad areas of healthcare finance?
   c. Why is it necessary to have a book on healthcare finance as opposed to a generic finance book?

1.2 a. Briefly discuss the role of finance in the healthcare industry.
   b. Has this role increased or decreased in importance in recent years?

1.3 a. Briefly describe the following healthcare settings:
- Hospitals
- Ambulatory care
- Home health care
- Long-term care
- Integrated delivery systems

   b. What are the benefits attributed to integrated delivery systems?

1.4 What role does regulation play in the healthcare industry?

1.5 What is the structure of the finance function within healthcare organizations?

1.6 What is the primary legal issue facing providers today?

CHAPTER 2

HEALTHCARE BUSINESS BASICS

Healthcare finance cannot be practiced in isolation. Rather, it must be guided by the goals of the organization. That is exactly what Jon Matthews, a recent healthcare management graduate, had in mind as he thought about two job interviews scheduled to take place within the next several days. The openings were for an entry-level management position at Southwest Healthcare, a for-profit (investor-owned) multispecialty group practice, and at St. Jerome's Hospital, a not-for-profit organization. To prepare for the interviews, Jon studied the organizations and their goals. He wondered if the ownership difference between the two providers resulted in a significant difference in mission, goals, and financial behavior.

Thanks to his healthcare management classes, Jon had a rough idea of the differences that ownership can bring about. Still, he thought long and hard about whether St. Jerome's was even a business. After all, as a Catholic hospital, it has a long history of providing charity care to society's less fortunate. Also, it has no well-defined owner group, but it could be thought of as being "owned" by the community at large.

On the other hand, Southwest is owned by its physicians and does not have the same tradition of serving the poor. Does the motivation to make money cause Southwest's mission and goals to be different from St. Jerome's? If so, does this mean its approach to financial decision making differs? Jon wanted to answer these questions before his interviews.

By the end of this chapter, you will know more about the various types of provider organizations, their goals, and how these goals influence the finance function. See if your take on the situation will be the same as Jon's.

LEARNING OBJECTIVES

After studying this chapter, you will be able to

➤ Define the concept of a business in financial terms.

➤ Describe the alternative legal forms of business.

➤ Articulate the key differences between for-profit and not-for-profit businesses.

➤ Explain how business goals are influenced by the form of organization and ownership.

➤ Briefly discuss the implications of tax laws for individuals, for-profit businesses, and not-for-profit corporations.

2.1 INTRODUCTION

Fortunately, most of the basic concepts of healthcare finance are the same regardless of the specific industry (for example, hospital versus long-term care versus medical practice) and organizational setting. However, some aspects of healthcare finance are influenced by the unique nature of healthcare organizations. In this chapter, we present the context in which finance is practiced in healthcare organizations.

First, we consider the nature of businesses. Is the provision of healthcare services a business, and if so, how are businesses formed and what are the implications of being a business as opposed to a pure charity? Then, we explore the consequences of the fact that many healthcare businesses are organized as not-for-profit corporations. Does not-for-profit status influence an organization's goals and objectives and, if so, does that affect the practice of finance?

These, along with a brief look at the impact of taxes, are some of the issues we explore in this chapter.

2.2 CONCEPT OF A BUSINESS

What is a **business**? If this question were asked of a group of accountants, the answer probably would involve financial statements, such as the income statement and balance sheet, which we cover in Chapters 11 and 12. However, if the question were posed to a group of lawyers, the answer likely would include legal forms of business, which we describe in the next section.

However, from a financial (economic) perspective, a business can be thought of as an entity (its legal form does not matter) that (1) obtains financing (capital) from the marketplace; (2) uses those funds to buy land, buildings, and equipment; (3) operates those assets to create goods or services; and then (4) sells those goods or services to create revenue. To be financially viable, a business has to have sufficient revenue to pay all of the costs associated with creating and selling its goods or services.

Although this description of a business is surprisingly simple, it tells a great deal about the basic decisions that business managers must make. One of the first decisions is what legal form the business will take. The next decision is how the business will raise the capital it needs to get started. Should it borrow the money (use debt financing), raise the money from owners (or from the community if not-for-profit), or use some combination of the two sources? Next, once the start-up capital is raised, what physical assets (facilities and equipment) should be acquired to create the services (in the case of healthcare providers) that will be offered to patients?

Note that businesses are profoundly different from **pure charities**. A business, such as a hospital or medical practice, sustains itself financially by selling goods or services. Thus, it is in competition with other businesses for the consumer dollar. A pure charity, such as the American Heart Association, on the other hand, does not sell goods or services. Rather, it obtains funds by soliciting contributions and then uses those funds to supply charitable (free) services. In essence, a pure charity is a budgetary organization in that the amount of contributions fixes its budget for the year. Similarly, a governmental agency has a budget that is fixed by appropriations.

Pure charities and governmental agencies must operate in a businesslike manner, but they do not operate like businesses because they do not obtain their operating funds by selling goods or services. Of course, some healthcare providers do solicit contributions, and many provide some charitable care, but healthcare organizations primarily sustain themselves by selling services.

> **(!) CRITICAL CONCEPT**
> Business Versus Pure Charity
>
> A business is an entity that raises capital in the marketplace; invests those funds in land, buildings, and equipment; and uses the assets to create goods or services, which it sells. Businesses differ from pure charities in the sense that businesses sustain themselves by revenue obtained from sales, while pure charities are sustained primarily by contributions. In a sense, pure charities, as well as governmental agencies, are *budgetary organizations* in that their funding is constrained by external forces (contributions or appropriations), and each year they must "live within the budget." Businesses, however, are not so constrained; they can influence their "funding" by selling more products or services.

> **(?) SELF-TEST QUESTIONS**
>
> 1. Briefly describe a business from a financial perspective.
>
> 2. What is the difference between a business and a pure charity?

2.3 LEGAL FORMS OF BUSINESSES

Because the focus of this book is on the practice of finance within healthcare businesses, a good starting point is to understand the different **legal forms of businesses**. Many healthcare managers work for corporations, including not-for-profit corporations, because these businesses often are large and require extensive management structures. However, some medical practices are organized as proprietorships or partnerships, and hybrid forms (which have features of both partnerships and corporations) are becoming common in medical practices. Healthcare managers need to be familiar with all legal forms of businesses, regardless of the form of their own organization. To illustrate this point, hospital managers, whether at for-profit or not-for-profit hospitals, work closely with the physician staff, so knowledge of how physicians organize their practices is useful.

CRITICAL CONCEPT
Legal Forms of Businesses

Business entities can be one of three basic legal forms: (1) proprietorship or partnership, (2) corporation, or (3) hybrid (a combination of the first two types). Each legal form has its advantages and disadvantages, but most large businesses, including all not-for-profits, are organized as corporations. Proprietorships and partnerships are easy to form, but sale of an ownership interest is difficult and owners have unlimited liability. For-profit corporations are more complex to set up, but they offer easier ownership transfer and limited liability. However, for-profit corporations are often subject to double taxation—once at the corporate level and then again at the stockholder (owner) level. Hybrid forms tend to offer some advantages of each of the other ownership types without the disadvantages.

Proprietorship
A simple form of business owned by one person. Also called sole proprietorship.

Partnership
An unincorporated business that is created and owned by two or more people.

PROPRIETORSHIPS AND PARTNERSHIPS

A *proprietorship* (or sole proprietorship) is a business owned by one person. Going into business as a proprietor is easy—the owner merely begins business operations. However, most cities require even the smallest businesses to be licensed, and state licensure is required for most healthcare professionals.

The proprietorship form of organization is easily and inexpensively formed, subject to few governmental regulations, and pays no corporate (business) income taxes. All earnings of the business, whether reinvested in the business or withdrawn by the owner, are taxed as personal income to the proprietor. In general, a sole proprietorship will pay lower total taxes than a comparable, taxable corporation because corporate profits are taxed twice—once at the corporate level and again by stockholders (owners) at the personal level when profits are distributed as dividends or when the stock is sold.

A *partnership* is similar to a proprietorship, but it is owned by two or more individuals. Partnerships may operate under different degrees of formality, ranging from informal oral agreements between the partners to formal agreements filed with the state in which the partnership does business. Like a proprietorship, the major advantage of the partnership form of organization is its low cost and ease of formation. In addition, the tax treatment of a partnership is similar to that of a proprietorship: the partnership's earnings are allocated to the partners and taxed as personal income, regardless of whether the earnings are actually paid out to the partners or retained in the business.

Proprietorships and partnerships have several disadvantages, including the following:

◆ Selling an ownership interest in the business is difficult. There is no well-established market for selling a proprietorship or partnership position.

◆ Proprietors and partners have unlimited personal liability for the debts of the business, which can result in losses greater than the amount invested in the business. In a proprietorship, unlimited liability means that the owner is personally responsible for the debts of the business. In a partnership, it means that if any partner is unable to meet his or her pro rata obligation in the event of bankruptcy, the remaining partners are responsible for the unsatisfied claims and must draw on their personal assets if necessary.

◆ The life of the business is limited to the life of the owners.

For these reasons, proprietorships and most partnerships are restricted to small businesses.

The three disadvantages of proprietorships and partnerships lead to the fourth, and perhaps most important, disadvantage from a finance perspective: the difficulty that proprietorships and partnerships have in attracting large amounts of capital. This is no particular problem for a small business or when the proprietor or partners are wealthy, but in most situations the difficulty of attracting capital becomes a handicap if the business needs to grow substantially to take advantage of market opportunities. Thus, many for-profit businesses start out as sole proprietorships or partnerships but then ultimately convert to corporations.

FOR-PROFIT CORPORATIONS

A for-profit (investor-owned) business may be organized as a corporation, but a not-for-profit business *must* be organized as a corporation. In this section, we focus on the advantages and disadvantages of for-profit corporations. Not-for-profit corporations, along with more facets of for-profit corporations, are discussed in the next major section.

A *for-profit corporation* is a legal entity that is separate and distinct from its owners and managers. The creation of a separate business entity provides these primary advantages:

For-profit corporation
A legal business entity that is separate and distinct from its owners and managers.

◆ A for-profit corporation has unlimited life and can continue in existence after its original owners and managers have died or left the company.

◆ Transferring ownership in a for-profit corporation is easy because ownership is divided into shares of stock that can be easily sold (assuming the business is large and its stock is frequently traded).

◆ Owners of a for-profit corporation have limited liability. To illustrate, suppose Kate Anderson made an investment of $10,000 in a partnership that subsequently went bankrupt, owing $100,000. Because the partners are liable for the debts of the partnership, Kate could be assessed for a share of the partnership's debt in addition to the loss of her initial $10,000 contribution. In fact, if the other partners were unable to pay their shares of the indebtedness, Kate could be held liable for the entire $100,000. However, if the $10,000 had been invested in a corporation that went bankrupt, Kate's potential loss would be limited to her initial $10,000 investment. (Note that in the case of small, financially weak corporations, the limited liability feature of ownership is often fictitious because bankers and other lenders require personal guarantees from the stockholders.)

With these three major advantages—unlimited life, ease of ownership transfer, and limited liability—for-profit corporations can more easily raise money in the financial markets than sole proprietorships or partnerships can.

For-profit corporations have two primary disadvantages. First, corporate earnings typically are subject to double taxation—once at the corporate level and then again at the personal level, when dividends are paid or the stock is sold. Second, setting up a corporation, and then filing the required periodic state and federal reports, is more costly and time consuming than what is required to establish a proprietorship or partnership.

Although a proprietorship or partnership can begin operations without much legal paperwork, setting up a corporation requires that the founders, or their attorney, prepare a charter and a set of bylaws. Today, attorneys have standard forms for charters and bylaws on their computers, so they can set up a "no frills" corporation with modest effort. Indeed, there are websites that allow most of the setup work to be done by the founders. Still, setting up a corporation remains relatively difficult when compared to a proprietorship or partnership, and it is even more difficult if the corporation has nonstandard features.

The value of any for-profit business, other than a small one, generally will be maximized if it is organized as a corporation for the following reasons:

◆ Limited liability reduces the risks borne by the owners (stockholders). With all else the same, the lower the risk, the higher the value of the ownership investment.

◆ A business's value is dependent on growth opportunities, which in turn are dependent on the business's ability to attract capital. Because corporations can obtain capital more easily than other forms of business can, they are better able to take advantage of growth opportunities.

◆ The value of any investment depends on its *liquidity*, which means the ease at which it can be sold for a fair price. Because an ownership interest in a for-profit corporation is much more liquid than a similar interest in a proprietorship or partnership, the corporate form of organization creates more value for its owners.

HYBRID FORMS

In addition to the two basic forms of organization—proprietorship/partnership and corporation—several *hybrid forms* of business are used by healthcare businesses.

Liquidity
The ability to quickly sell an investment at a "fair" price.

Hybrid form
A legal business entity that has features associated with both partnerships and for-profit corporations.

To begin, several specialized types of partnerships have characteristics different from those of a standard partnership. First, limiting some of the partners' liabilities is possible by establishing a limited partnership, wherein certain partners are designated general partners and others are limited partners. The limited partners, like the owners of a corporation, are liable only for the amount of their initial investment in the partnership, while the general partners have unlimited liability. However, the limited partners typically have restricted or no control; control rests solely with the general partners. Limited partnerships are quite common in some industries (think real estate). They are not as prevalent in the healthcare industry because finding one partner who is willing to accept all of the business's risk and another partner who is willing to relinquish control is difficult.

A *limited liability partnership (LLP)* is a type of partnership available in many states. Here, the partners have joint liability for all actions of the partnership, including personal injuries and indebtedness. However, all partners enjoy limited liability regarding professional malpractice because partners are only liable for their own individual malpractice actions, not those of the other partners.

A *limited liability company (LLC)* has some characteristics of both a partnership and a corporation. The owners of an LLC are called members, and they are taxed as if they are partners in a partnership. However, a member's liability is like that of a stockholder of a corporation because liability is limited to the member's initial contribution in the business. Personal assets are only at risk if the member assumes specific liability, such as signing a personal loan guarantee.

A *professional corporation (PC)*, called a professional association (PA) in some states, is a corporate form of organization common among physicians and other individual and group practice healthcare professionals. All 50 states have statutes that prescribe the requirements for such businesses, providing the usual benefits of incorporation, but not relieving the participants of professional liability. Indeed, the primary motivation behind a professional corporation, which is a relatively old business form compared to the LLP and LLC, was to provide a way for professionals to incorporate yet still be held personally liable for professional malpractice.

For tax purposes, standard for-profit corporations are called *C corporations*. However, if certain requirements are met, one or a few individuals can form a for-profit corporation but elect to pay taxes as if the business were a proprietorship or partnership, and hence avoid double taxation. Such corporations, which differ only in how the owners are taxed, are called *S corporations*. (The name comes from subchapter S of the tax code.) Although S corporations are similar to LLPs and LLCs in terms of taxes, LLPs and LLCs provide more flexibility and benefits to owners. Many businesses, especially group practices, are therefore converting to the newer forms.

Limited liability partnership (LLP)

A partnership that limits the professional (malpractice) liability of its members.

Limited liability company (LLC)

A corporation that combines some features of a partnership with others of a corporation.

Professional corporation (PC)

A type of corporate business organization in which the owner/managers retain professional (medical) liability. Called a professional association in some states.

C corporation

A traditional for-profit corporation.

S corporation

A for-profit corporation with a limited number of stockholders that, after filing an application with the Internal Revenue Service, is taxed as a proprietorship or partnership.

? SELF-TEST QUESTIONS

1. What are the three forms of business organization, and how do they differ?

2. What are the different types of partnerships?

3. What is the difference between a C corporation and an S corporation?

2.4 ALTERNATIVE FORMS OF OWNERSHIP

Unlike other industries, not-for-profit corporations play a major role in the healthcare industry. As we discussed in Chapter 1, about 60 percent of the hospitals in the United States are private not-for-profit hospitals. Only 15 percent of all hospitals are for-profit (investor owned); the remaining 25 percent are governmental. Furthermore, not-for-profit ownership is common in nursing home, home health care, and health insurance businesses. Before we go into not-for-profit corporations in detail, we offer some additional information about for-profit corporations.

! CRITICAL CONCEPT
Investor-Owned (For-Profit) Corporation

Investor-owned corporations are for-profit businesses whose ownership (stock) is either publicly traded (owned by a large number of investors) or privately held (owned by a small number of investors). The stockholders of for-profit corporations exercise control of the business by voting for the board of directors. Stockholders have a claim on the residual earnings of the business, which is the amount of revenue that remains after all expenses have been paid. All or a portion of the residual earnings may be paid out to stockholders as dividends or may be used to repurchase shares currently owned by stockholders. For-profit corporations must pay taxes, including both property and income taxes.

ADDITIONAL INFORMATION ON FOR-PROFIT CORPORATIONS

When you think of a corporation, you probably think in terms of an **investor-owned (for-profit) corporation**. Large businesses, such as Microsoft, IBM, and General Electric, are investor-owned corporations. In healthcare, HCA and Tenet Healthcare are for-profit hospital corporations, as are Apria Healthcare, which offers home health services, and Brookdale Senior Living, which provides long-term care.

Investors become owners of such businesses by buying shares of common stock in the company. When stock is sold by the company, the funds raised from the sale go to the corporation. However, stock owners (stockholders) can sell their shares to other individuals. These sales typically take place on exchanges, such as the New York Stock Exchange (NYSE) or in the over-the-counter (OTC) market, which is composed of a large number of stockbrokers connected by a sophisticated electronic trading system. When shares are bought and sold by individuals through exchanges, the corporations whose stocks are traded receive no funds from the trades. Corporations receive funds only when the shares are first sold to investors.

Investor-owned corporations may be publicly held or privately held. The shares of *publicly held companies* are owned by a large number of investors and are widely traded. For example, Health Management Associates (HMA), which owns and operates roughly 60 hospitals, has about 240 million shares outstanding owned by some 30,000 individual and institutional stockholders. Another example is Kindred Healthcare, which owns and operates about 240 nursing homes and 80 long-term acute care hospitals and has about 38 million shares outstanding owned by some 8,000 stockholders. Drug companies, such as Merck and Pfizer, and medical equipment manufacturers, such as St. Jude Medical (which makes heart valves), are all publicly held corporations.

Conversely, the shares of *privately (closely) held companies* are owned by just a handful of investors and are not publicly traded. In general, the managers of privately held companies are major stockholders. For example, HCA, the nation's largest for-profit hospital chain with about 170 hospitals, was a publicly held company until November 2006. At that time, the outstanding stock of the company was purchased by a small group of investors, taking the company private. In reality, privately held companies are more similar to partnerships than to publicly held companies. Often, the privately held corporation is a transitional form of organization that exists for a short time between a proprietorship or partnership and a publicly owned corporation. This organization may be motivated to "go public" either by the need for additional capital or by the desire of the owners to "cash out." In the case of HCA, the expectation is that the new owners will sell off poorly performing hospitals, improve the operations of the remaining hospitals, and then in several years go public again to recover their investment and, hopefully, earn a profit.

Stockholders (shareholders) are the owners of investor-owned corporations. As owners, they have these basic rights:

◆ *The right of control.* Common stockholders have the right to vote for the corporation's board of directors, which oversees the management of the company. Each year, a company's stockholders receive a ballot called a proxy, which they use to vote for directors and to vote on other issues proposed by management or stockholders. In this way, stockholders exercise control. In the voting process, stockholders cast one vote for each common share held.

◆ *A claim on the residual earnings of the firm.* A for-profit corporation sells goods or services and realizes revenue from the sales. To produce this revenue, the corporation must incur expenses for materials, labor, insurance, debt capital, and so on. Any excess of revenue over expenses—the residual earnings—belongs to the shareholders of the business. Often, a portion of these earnings is paid out in the form of dividends, which are cash payments to stockholders, or stock repurchases, in which the company buys back shares held by stockholders. However, management typically elects to rein-

Publicly held company

A for-profit corporation whose shares are held by the general public (a large number of shareholders) and traded on the New York Stock Exchange or in the over-the-counter market.

Privately (closely) held company

A for-profit corporation whose stock is owned by a small number of individuals—usually the business's managers—and is not publicly traded.

Stockholders (shareholders)

The owners of a for-profit corporation by virtue of holding one or more shares of the company's stock.

Residual earnings
The earnings that remain after all expenses have been paid. In other words, a corporation's profit.

vest some (or all) of the *residual earnings* in the business, which presumably will produce even higher earnings in the future. (If you are interested in more information about how corporate earnings are distributed to stockholders, see Chapter 16, which is available online at ache.org/books/FinanceFundamentals.)

◆ *A claim on liquidation proceeds.* In the event of bankruptcy and liquidation, shareholders are entitled to any proceeds that remain after all other obligations of the business have been satisfied. In most liquidations, however, there is little or nothing left for stockholders.

In summary, for-profit corporations have three key traits. First, the owners (the stockholders) of the business are well defined and exercise control of the firm by voting for directors. Second, the residual earnings of the business belong to the owners, so management is responsible only to the stockholders for the profitability of the firm. Third, investor-owned corporations are subject to taxation at the local, state, and federal levels.

CRITICAL CONCEPT
Not-for-Profit (Tax-Exempt) Corporation

Not-for-profit healthcare businesses must be incorporated under the provisions of 501(c)(3) of the IRS Tax Code. Because such corporations have no owners, none of their profits can be paid out as dividends. In essence, not-for-profit businesses are "owned" by the community at large and are controlled by a board of trustees, which generally includes community representation. In general, not-for-profit corporations are exempt from local, state, and federal income and property taxes.

NOT-FOR-PROFIT CORPORATIONS

If an organization meets a set of stringent requirements, it can qualify for incorporation as a **not-for-profit (tax-exempt) corporation**. Such corporations are sometimes called nonprofit corporations. Because nonprofit businesses (as opposed to pure charities, such as the American Red Cross) need profits to sustain operations, and because it is hard to explain why nonprofit corporations should earn profits, the term not-for-profit is more descriptive of such healthcare corporations.

Tax-exempt status is granted to healthcare businesses that meet the tax definition of a charitable corporation as defined by Internal Revenue Service (IRS) Tax Code Section 501(c)(3). Hence, such corporations are also known as 501(c)(3) corporations. The IRS Tax Code defines a charitable organization as "any corporation, community chest, fund, or foundation that is organized and operated exclusively for religious, charitable, scientific, public safety, literary, or educational purposes." Because the promotion of health is commonly considered a charitable activity, a corporation that provides healthcare services can qualify for tax-exempt status, provided that it meets the other requirements.

In addition to the charitable purpose, a not-for-profit corporation must be organized and operated so that it operates exclusively for the public, rather than private, interest. Thus, no profits can be used for private gain and no direct political activity can be conducted. Also, if the corporation is liquidated or sold to an investor-owned business, the proceeds from the liquidation or sale must be used for a charitable purpose. Because individuals cannot benefit from the profits of not-for-profit corporations, such organizations cannot pay dividends. However, prohibition of private gain from profits does not prevent parties, such as managers or physicians, from benefiting through salaries, perquisites, contracts, and so on.

Not-for-profit corporations differ significantly from investor-owned corporations. Because not-for-profit corporations have no shareholders, no single body of individuals has ownership rights to the firm's residual earnings or exercises control of the firm. Rather, control is exercised by a board of trustees that, for all practical purposes, is not constrained by external parties (such as shareholders). However, unlike for-profit corporations, the boards of not-for-profit corporations are made up mostly of community leaders, who presumably are motivated to ensure that the organization meets community needs.

Not-for-profit corporations are generally exempt from taxation, including both property and income taxes, and have the right to issue tax-exempt debt. (The ability to issue tax-exempt debt means that not-for-profit corporations pay relatively low interest rates on their debt financing.) Finally, individual contributions to not-for-profit organizations can be deducted from taxable income by the donor, so not-for-profit firms have access to tax-subsidized contribution capital. (The tax benefits enjoyed by not-for-profit corporations, including the benefits associated with tax-exempt debt, are discussed in more detail later in the section on tax laws.)

The financial problems facing federal, state, and local governments have caused politicians to take a closer look at the tax subsidies provided to not-for-profit hospitals. Several bills that require hospitals to meet minimum levels of care to the indigent to retain tax-exempt status have been introduced in the U.S. Congress. Such efforts by Congress have prompted the American Hospital Association to issue guidelines for charity care that include (1) giving discounts to uninsured patients of "limited means"; (2) establishing a common definition for *community benefits*, which encompasses the full range of services provided to the population served such as health education and community outreach; and (3) improving *transparency*, or the ability of outsiders to understand a business's governance structure and policies, including executive compensation.

In addition to congressional action, legislators in more than 20 states have proposed bills that mandate the amount of charity care provided by not-for-profit hospitals and the billing and collections procedures applied to the uninsured. For example, Texas has established minimum requirements for charity care that, in effect, hold not-for-profit hospitals accountable to the public for the tax exemptions they receive. The Texas law specifies four tests, and each hospital must meet at least one of them. The test that most hospitals use to comply with the law requires that at least 4 percent of patient revenue be spent on charity

Community benefits
Initiatives taken by providers, such as education programs, that enhance the health and well-being of the community.

Transparency
The ability of outsiders to know what is happening within a business.

care. Under a proposed Illinois law, not-for-profit hospitals would be required to devote at least 8 percent of their operating costs on charity care and to establish discounts to the uninsured on the basis of income level.

Finally, money-starved municipalities in several states have attacked the property tax exemption of not-for-profit hospitals that have "neglected" their charitable missions. For example, tax assessors in several states have forced selected hospitals to pay property taxes, arguing that the hospitals had strayed too far from their charitable purpose. According to one estimate, if all not-for-profit hospitals had to pay taxes comparable to their investor-owned counterparts, local, state, and federal governments would garner an additional $4 billion in tax revenues.

(?) SELF-TEST QUESTIONS

1. What are the major differences between investor-owned and not-for-profit corporations?

2. What pressures recently have been placed on not-for-profit hospitals to ensure that they meet their charitable mission?

2.5 ORGANIZATIONAL GOALS

Healthcare finance is practiced with some objective in mind. Finance goals must be consistent with, as well as support, the overall goals of the organization. Thus, we discuss goals to establish a framework for financial decision making within healthcare organizations.

SMALL FOR-PROFIT BUSINESSES

In a proprietorship or partnership, small privately owned corporation, or in any other form of for-profit small business, the owners generally are also the managers. In theory, the business can be operated for the exclusive benefit of the owners. If the owners want to work hard every day to maximize income and wealth, they can. On the other hand, if they want to devote every Wednesday to playing golf, they can do that instead. (Of course, the business still has to satisfy the needs of its customers or else it will not survive.)

Typically, in small businesses, goals of income (wealth) and other benefits (such as leisure time) are blended in such a way as to satisfy the owners' wishes. It is in large, publicly held corporations, in which owners and managers are separate parties, that organizational goals become important guideposts for managers.

LARGE FOR-PROFIT BUSINESSES

From a finance perspective, the primary goal of large publicly held corporations is generally assumed to be **shareholder (ownership) wealth maximization**, which translates to stock price maximization. Investor-owned corporations do, of course, have other goals. Managers, who make the actual decisions, are interested in their own personal welfare, in their employees' welfare, and in the good of the community and society at large. Still, the goal of stock price maximization is a reasonable operating objective on which to build financial decision rules.

The primary obstacle to shareholder wealth maximization in large investor-owned corporations is the *agency problem.* An agency problem exists when one or more individuals hire another individual or group of individuals (agents) to perform a service on their behalf, thereby delegating decision-making authority to those agents. Such a problem occurs between stockholders and managers of large investor-owned corporations because the managers typically hold only a small proportion of the firm's stock, and hence they benefit relatively little from stock price increases. On the other hand, managers benefit substantially from such actions as increasing the size of the firm to justify greater salaries, bonuses, and fringe benefits; awarding themselves generous retirement plans; and spending too much on office space, personal staff, and travel—actions often detrimental to shareholders' wealth. Many situations arise in which managers are motivated to take actions that are in their, rather than the stockholders', best interests.

Shareholders recognize the agency problem and counter it by creating compensation incentives, such as stock options and performance-based bonus plans, that encourage managers to act in shareholders' interests. Additionally, other factors, such as the threat of takeover or removal, keep managers focused on shareholder wealth maximization.

Of course, managers of investor-owned corporations can have motivations that are inconsistent with shareholder wealth maximization. Still, sufficient incentives and sanctions exist to motivate managers to view shareholder wealth maximization as an important goal. Thus, shareholder wealth maximization is a reasonable goal for financial decision making within investor-owned corporations in spite of the agency problem.

NOT-FOR-PROFIT CORPORATIONS

Not-for-profit corporations consist of a number of *stakeholders*, which include all parties that have an interest, usually of a financial nature, in the organization. For example, a not-

! CRITICAL CONCEPT
Shareholder (Ownership) Wealth Maximization

The primary goal of large, investor-owned businesses is shareholder wealth maximization or maximization of owners' wealth. For corporations, this goal translates to stock price maximization. Of course, many other managerial goals exist, such as the fair treatment of all parties to the business. Still, when alternative courses of action are being considered, the impact on shareholder wealth should play a dominant role in the decision process.

Agency problem
The problem that arises when the managers of a corporation are separate from the owners. In this situation, managers are motivated to act in their own interests as opposed to the interests of stockholders.

Stakeholder
A party that has an interest—typically financial—in an organization. For example, owners (in for-profit businesses), managers, patients, and suppliers are some of the stakeholders of healthcare businesses.

for-profit hospital's stakeholders include the board of trustees; managers; employees; physicians; creditors; suppliers; patients; and even potential patients, which may include the entire community. An investor-owned hospital has the same set of stakeholders plus owners (stockholders in corporations), who dictate the goal of ownership wealth maximization. While managers of investor-owned companies have to please primarily one class of stakeholders (the owners) to keep their jobs, managers of not-for-profit firms face a different situation. They have to please all of the organization's stakeholders because no single well-defined group exercises control.

Some people argue that managers of not-for-profit corporations do not have to please anyone at all because they tend to dominate the board of trustees, who are supposed to exercise oversight. Others argue that managers of not-for-profit firms have to please all of the firm's stakeholders to a greater or lesser extent because all are necessary to the successful performance of the business. Of course, even managers of investor-owned firms should not attempt to enhance shareholder wealth by treating other stakeholders unfairly because such actions ultimately will be detrimental to shareholders.

Typically, the goal of not-for-profit corporations is stated in terms of a mission statement. For example, here is the current mission statement of New River Memorial Hospital, a 250-bed, not-for-profit acute care hospital:

New River Memorial Hospital, along with its medical staff, is a recognized, innovative healthcare leader dedicated to meeting the needs of the community. We strive to be the best comprehensive healthcare provider through our commitment to excellence.

Although this mission statement provides New River's managers and employees with a framework for developing specific goals and objectives, it does not provide much insight into the goal of the hospital's finance function. For the hospital to accomplish its mission, its managers have identified the following five financial goals:

1. The hospital must maintain its financial viability.

2. The hospital must generate sufficient profits to continue to provide the current range of healthcare services to the community. This means that current buildings and equipment must be replaced as they become obsolete.

3. The hospital must generate sufficient profits to invest in new medical technologies and services as they are developed and needed.

4. Although the hospital has an aggressive philanthropy program in place, it does not want to rely on this program or government grants to fund its operations.

5. The hospital will strive to provide services to the community as inexpensively as possible, given the above financial requirements.

In effect, New River's managers are saying that to achieve the hospital's commitment to excellence as stated in its mission statement, the hospital must remain financially strong and profitable. Financially weak organizations cannot accomplish their stated missions over the long run. What is interesting is that New River's five financial goals are probably not much different from the finance goals of Jackson Regional Medical Center (JRMC), a for-profit competitor.

Clearly, JRMC has to worry about providing a return to its shareholders, and it receives only a small amount of contributions and grants. However, to maximize shareholder wealth, JRMC also must maintain its financial viability and have the financial resources necessary to offer new services and technologies. Furthermore, competition in the market for hospital services will not permit JRMC to charge appreciably more for services than its not-for-profit competitors.

(?) SELF-TEST QUESTIONS

1. What is the difference in goals between investor-owned and not-for-profit businesses?

2. What is the agency problem, and how does it apply to investor-owned firms?

3. What factors tend to reduce the agency problem?

2.6 TAX LAWS

The value of any investment—whether the investment is a security, such as a stock for an individual's retirement account, or a business's investment in new diagnostic equipment—depends on the *usable* cash flows that the investment is expected to provide. Because taxes affect usable cash flows, both individuals and managers of for-profit healthcare businesses must be concerned about taxes.

U.S. tax laws are complicated and are constantly changing. Indeed, some tax law provisions automatically expire over time if not renewed by congressional action. Consequently, covering even the most basic features of tax laws in an introductory healthcare finance book is nearly impossible. Still, healthcare managers must understand those features of the tax system that directly affect financial decision making.

Personal (individual) taxes

Taxes paid by individuals to federal and state (in most states) authorities on wages, interest, dividends, capital gains, and proprietorship and partnership income.

PERSONAL (INDIVIDUAL) TAXES

Individuals must pay *personal (individual) taxes* to federal and state (in most states) authorities that can approach 50 percent of income. Thus, income from proprietorships and partnerships, as well as interest, dividends, and *capital gains* on securities investments, will be reduced when personal taxes are taken into account.

To illustrate the **impact of personal taxes**, assume that Dr. Cynthia Morgan's tax rate is 35 percent and she receives $200,000 in partnership income from her medical practice. Using the letter T to represent tax rate, she must pay T × $200,000 = 0.35 × $200,000 = $70,000 in taxes on that income, which leaves her with only $200,000 – $70,000 = $130,000 in usable (after-tax) income. This tax analysis leads to the following useful equation:

$$AT = BT - (T \times BT)$$
$$= BT \times (1 - T),$$

where AT = after tax and BT = before tax. Thus, Dr. Morgan's after-tax income can be calculated as follows:

$$AT = BT \times (1 - T)$$
$$= \$200,000 \times (1 - 0.35)$$
$$= \$200,000 \times 0.65$$
$$= \$130,000.$$

Capital gains

The profit that arises when securities (or other investments) are sold for more than their purchase price.

Note that this equation can be applied to interest rates as well as dollar amounts. (See Problem 2.3 at the end of the chapter as an example.) Clearly, taxes will influence personal investment decisions, so any tax implications on investment alternatives must be considered in the decision process. This is especially important when two investments under consideration have differential tax implications.

CORPORATE TAXES

Corporate taxes affect both for-profit and not-for-profit companies.

For-Profit Corporations

In addition to personal taxes paid by individuals, investor-owned (for-profit) corporations must pay

CRITICAL EQUATION
Impact of Taxes

The impact of taxes on income can be calculated with a simple equation:

$$AT = BT \times (1 - T),$$

where AT = after taxes, BT = before taxes, and T = tax rate. For example, if your taxable income is $75,000 and your federal and state tax rate is a combined 25 percent, then BT = $75,000, T = 25% = 0.25, and your after-tax income is $56,250:

$$AT = BT \times (1 - T)$$
$$= \$75,000 \times (1 - 0.25)$$
$$= \$75,000 \times 0.75$$
$$= \$56,250.$$

both federal and state *corporate taxes*, which can exceed 40 percent of taxable income. For-profit corporations pay taxes on earnings before dividends are distributed, so corporate income is subject to double taxation. (Income is taxed once when corporations pay their income taxes and again when stockholders pay their income taxes on dividends and capital gains.) Small corporations can avoid double taxation by filing with the IRS as an S corporation, which, for tax purposes only, prorates the corporate income among the owners to be taxed as personal income. Also, hybrid forms of business avoid double taxation. (See the Industry Practice box on page 44 for more information on corporate taxes.)

(See the Industry Practice box on page 44 for more information on corporate taxes.)

Corporate taxes
Income taxes paid by for-profit (taxable) corporations to federal and state authorities.

Not-for-Profit Corporations

Not-for-profit corporations, for the most part, are not subject to income, property, or sales taxes. The exemption from taxes is, by far, the biggest benefit granted to not-for-profit providers. In addition, such organizations enjoy two other tax benefits.

First, not-for-profit organizations are able to borrow funds (use debt financing) that have interest payments exempt from the lender's personal taxes. Thus, if Jake Jaworski buys a $5,000 bond issued by New River Memorial Hospital, a not-for-profit corporation, the interest paid by the hospital to Jake is not subject to personal taxes.

To illustrate the advantage of being able to issue tax-exempt debt, first assume that Jake owns some bonds issued by Jackson Regional Medical Center (JRMC), a for-profit hospital. These bonds have an interest rate of 10 percent, so Jake receives $0.10 \times \$100 = \$10$ in annual interest for every $100 worth of bonds that he owns. If Jake pays 40 percent in federal and state income taxes, each $10 of interest provides him with $AT = BT \times (1 - T) = \$10 \times (1 - 0.40) = \$10 \times 0.6 = \$6$ of usable (after-tax) interest.

However, if the bonds had been issued by New River, Jake would not have to pay taxes on the interest and hence would keep the entire $10. If investors truly require a $6 after-tax (usable) return, New River can issue debt with an interest rate of only 6 percent and, with all else the same, investors (such as Jake) in the 40 percent tax bracket would be as willing to buy these bonds as they are the JRMC 10 percent bonds.

Thus, the interest rate that New River must set on its debt issues is lower than the rate that JRMC must set because of the tax exemption on debt issued by not-for-profit corporations. This appears to give not-for-profit healthcare businesses a big advantage over for-profit businesses, but we have not told the full story. For-profit providers can deduct their interest payments on debt financing from taxable income and hence gain a tax benefit that, over time, reduces the effective interest rate on for-profit hospital debt to about the same amount as paid by similar not-for-profit (tax-exempt) providers.

In addition to the tax-exempt debt benefit, the contributions made by individuals to not-for-profit corporations are tax deductible to the donor. If Miguel Corales, who is in the 40 percent personal income tax bracket (including both federal and state taxes), donates $1,000 to New River, his taxable income would be reduced by $1,000. A reduction in taxable income of this amount would save Miguel T × $1,000 = 0.40 × $1,000 = $400 in taxes. Thus, the effective cost of his contribution would only be $600, because he saved $400 in taxes by making the contribution. In effect, the government will pay Miguel 40 cents for every dollar he contributes. Thus, not-for-profit providers have access to a source of financing (contributions) that, for all practical purposes, is not available to investor-owned providers.

Because of the impact that taxes have on usable earnings of investor-owned businesses and because not-for-profit ownership has important tax consequences, we highlight and explain, as needed, these tax implications throughout the book. For now, recognize that taxes play a critical role in many finance decisions.

(?) SELF-TEST QUESTIONS

1. Why does a finance book have to consider taxes?

2. What is the primary tax advantage of not-for-profit corporations?

3. Why is the ability to issue tax-exempt debt an advantage for not-for-profit corporations?

4. What advantage accrues to businesses that qualify for tax-exempt contributions?

(*) INDUSTRY PRACTICE Corporate Taxes

For-profit, as well as not-for-profit, corporations are organized (chartered) under state laws. More than 60 percent of large for-profit corporations are chartered in Delaware, which over the years has provided a favorable legal environment for corporations. (A business does not have to locate its headquarters, or even operate, in the state of incorporation.)

The taxable income of a corporation is composed of revenues less allowable deductions. Revenues may be derived from any source, including the sale of products or services, rents, royalties, interest and dividends on securities investments, and gains from the sale of assets. Allowable deductions include ordinary

INDUSTRY PRACTICE Corporate Taxes

business expenses, such as salaries and wages, contributions to retirement and employee benefit programs, supplies expenses, interest paid on debt capital, marketing, and other expenses. Note that dividends paid to shareholders are not a deductible expense, so they must be paid with after-tax dollars.

The amount of federal income taxes paid (for tax year 2008) is based on the following table:

Taxable Income	Tax Rate %
$0–$50,000	15
$50,001–$75,000	25
$75,001–$100,000	34
$100,001–$335,000	39
$335,001–$10,000,000	34
$10,000,001–$15,000,000	35
$15,000,001–$18,333,333	38
Over $18,333,333	35

For example, suppose Southwest Healthcare, a for-profit multispecialty group practice, had $250,000 in taxable income. Its tax liability would be $80,750:

$$Tax = 0.15(\$50,000) + 0.25(\$25,000) + 0.34(\$25,000)$$
$$+ 0.39(\$250,000 - \$100,000)$$
$$= \$7,500 + \$6,250 + \$8,500 + \$58,500$$
$$= \$80,750.$$

Although the incremental tax rates in the table bounce around (go up to 39 then down to 34 then up to 35 percent, and so on), there is a rational pattern to the rates. In effect, the rate table produces a flat tax rate of 34 percent for taxable incomes

(Continued)

✳ INDUSTRY PRACTICE Corporate Taxes

between $335,001 and $10 million, and then a flat rate of 35 percent for all income above $18,333,333. (A flat rate is a single rate applied to all income.)

Note that Southwest's *marginal* tax rate (the rate on the next dollar of income) is 39 percent. Thus, in any analyses that involve additional taxable income, the appropriate rate is 39 percent (at least up to $335,000 in taxable income). But, Southwest's average tax rate is only 32.3 percent: $80,750 in taxes paid on $250,000 of taxable income, or $80,750 / $250,000 = 32.3%. The federal corporate income tax system is progressive, which means that higher incomes lead to higher tax rates. However, the system is only mildly so, and, as we pointed out earlier, the rate structure flattens out at higher levels of income. Corporations must also pay state income taxes, which generally are flat (a single rate) and range roughly from 5 to 10 percent.

To avoid taxation at both the corporate and individual levels, small corporations that are owner-managed can file as an S corporation. Alternatively, small corporate businesses, such as a five-physician primary care practice, can create zero taxable corporate income by distributing any income earned by the business to the owner-physicians in the form of salaries or bonuses. By doing so, the corporation pays no income taxes, but, of course, the physicians have to pay personal taxes on the added income. Still, a situation of double taxation is converted into single taxation. Note, however, that the IRS is wary of small corporations that pay its owners/managers salaries and bonuses far in excess of prevailing wage standards and can impose corporate taxes on the amount deemed excessive.

THEME WRAP-UP BUSINESS GOALS

After doing more research on forms of business organization and goals, here's what Jon concluded. For starters, the not-for-profit St. Jerome's is indeed a business. It must accomplish all of the actions associated with businesses: (1) raise capital; (2) invest the funds raised in land, buildings, and equipment; (3) provide patient services; and (3) earn enough profit to sustain and grow the organization. Even though it offers a significant amount of charity care, which is mostly funded from profits earned on services provided to those who do pay, the hospital must be operated as a business, not as pure charity.

Now, what about the difference in goals between Southwest Healthcare and St. Jerome's? Southwest's mission is to "provide timely, high-quality, and efficient healthcare to its service area in a competent and compassionate manner by offering a wide variety of services from primary care to specialized procedures." St. Jerome's mission is to "extend the Catholic healthcare ministry by continually improving the health and quality of life of the people in the communities we serve."

These mission statements sound great, but do they translate into different financial goals? Probably not. Southwest does not address the issue of owner's wealth in its mission statement, but the doctor-owners are concerned with earning a return on the capital they invested in the business. To succeed, the practice must offer the services needed by the communities served at a price and quality that make its services competitive in the marketplace. St. Jerome's must do the same thing. To accomplish its mission, the hospital needs to offer state-of-the-art technology and services at competitive prices.

Thus, both organizations have to maintain the financial wherewithal to expand the number and types of services they provide to meet the changing needs of the populations they serve. In addition, each organization must be able to invest in new technologies to provide the best patient care and to remain competitive. As one prominent Catholic healthcare administrator put it: "no margin, no mission." This simply means you have to be profitable to accomplish your mission.

In the end, Jon figured that the finance function at for-profit and not-for-profit healthcare providers must be run in just about the same way. All businesses must maintain financial viability to be competitive in the marketplace.

Based on the information given in the chapter, did you arrive at the same conclusion?

KEY CONCEPTS

This chapter presents background material on business organizations and goals. Here are the key concepts:

➤ A *business* maintains its financial viability by selling goods or services, while a *pure charity* relies solely on contributions.

➤ The three legal forms of business are *proprietorship* and *partnership*, *corporation*, and *hybrid*. Although each form of organization has its own unique advantages and disadvantages, most large businesses, and all not-for-profit entities, are organized as *corporations*.

➤ *Investor-owned corporations* have *stockholders* who are the owners of the corporation. Stockholders exercise control through the *proxy* process in which they elect the corporation's *board of directors* and vote on matters of major consequence to the firm. As owners, stockholders have a claim on the *residual earnings* of the corporation. Investor-owned corporations are fully taxable.

➤ Healthcare organizations that meet certain criteria can be organized as *not-for-profit corporations*, which are governed by a *board of trustees*. Rather than having a well-defined set of owners, such organizations have a large number of *stakeholders* who have an interest in the organization. In effect, not-for-profit corporations are owned by the communities they serve, although technically they have no owners.

➤ From a financial management perspective, the primary goal of investor-owned corporations is *shareholder wealth maximization*, which translates to stock price maximization. For not-for-profit corporations, a reasonable goal for financial management is to ensure that the organization can fulfill its mission, which translates to *maintaining financial viability*. Both goals lead to roughly the same managerial behavior.

➤ An *agency problem* is the conflict of interest that arises between the owners and managers (agents) of large, for-profit corporations. The problem is mitigated by creating incentives for managers to act in the best interest of owners.

➤ The value of any income stream depends on the amount of *usable*, or *after-tax*, *income*. Thus, tax laws play an important role in financial management decisions.

➤ Before-tax (BT) income can be converted to after-tax (AT) income using this equation:
$$AT = BT \times (1 - T),$$
where T is the tax rate.

➤ Individuals pay *personal (individual) taxes* to federal and state (in most states) authorities on proprietorship, partnership, interest, dividend, and capital gains income.

➤ For-profit corporations pay *corporate income taxes* to federal and state authorities. Because corporations pay taxes, and then individuals pay taxes on dividend and capital gains income, corporate income typically is subject to double taxation.

➤ Small corporations can file with the IRS for S corporation status, which means they are taxed as proprietorships or partnerships and hence avoid double taxation.

➤ Not-for-profit corporations generally are exempt from all levels of property, income, and sales taxes. Furthermore, not-for-profits can use *tax-exempt debt* financing, which means that lenders do not have to pay taxes on the interest earned. *Contributions* to not-for-profit corporations can be deducted from the donor's taxable income, which encourages such contributions.

Because managers of healthcare organizations must make financial decisions within the constraints imposed by the economic environment, we draw on the concepts described here throughout the remainder of the book.

END-OF-CHAPTER QUESTIONS

2.1 a. From a financial perspective, briefly describe the concept of a business.
   b. What is the difference between a business and a pure charity?

2.2 What are the three legal forms of business organization? What are their advantages and disadvantages?

2.3 What are the primary organizational differences between investor-owned and not-for-profit corporations?

2.4 a. What is the primary goal of investor-owned corporations?
   b. What is the primary goal of most not-for-profit healthcare corporations?
   c. Are there substantial differences between the finance goals of investor-owned and not-for-profit corporations? Explain your answer.
   d. What is an agency problem?

2.5 a. Why are tax laws important to healthcare finance?

b. What three major advantages do tax laws give to not-for-profit corporations?

END-OF-CHAPTER PROBLEMS

2.1 Assume that Provident Health System, a for-profit hospital, has $1 million in taxable income for 2008, and its tax rate is 30 percent.

a. Given this information, what is the firm's net income? (Net income is what remains after taxes have been paid.)

b. Suppose the hospital pays out $300,000 in dividends. A stockholder, Carl Johnson, receives $10,000. If Carl's tax rate on dividends is 15 percent, what is his after-tax dividend?

2.2 A firm that owns the stock of another corporation does not have to pay taxes on the entire amount of dividends received. In general, only 30 percent of the dividends received by one corporation from another are taxable. The reason for this tax law feature is to mitigate the effect of triple taxation, which occurs when earnings are first taxed at the first firm, then its dividends paid to the second firm are taxed again, and then the dividends paid to stockholders by the second firm are taxed yet again. Assume that a firm with a 35 percent tax rate receives $100,000 in dividends from another corporation. What taxes must be paid on this dividend, and what is the after-tax amount of the dividend?

2.3 Kim Davis is in the 40 percent personal tax bracket. She is considering investing in HCA (taxable) bonds that carry a 12 percent interest rate.

a. What is her after-tax yield (interest rate) on the bonds?

b. Suppose Twin Cities Memorial Hospital has issued tax-exempt bonds that have an interest rate of 6 percent. With all else the same, should Kim buy the HCA or the Twin Cities bonds?

c. With all else the same, what interest rate on the tax-exempt Twin Cities bonds would make Kim indifferent between these bonds and the HCA bonds?

2.4 Jane Smith currently holds tax-exempt bonds of Good Samaritan Healthcare that pay 7 percent interest. She is in the 40 percent tax bracket. Her broker wants her to buy some

Beverly Enterprises taxable bonds that will be issued next week. With all else the same, what rate must be set on the Beverly bonds to make Jane interested in making a switch?

2.5 George and Margaret Wealthy are in the 48 percent tax bracket, considering both federal and state personal taxes. Norman Briggs, the CEO of Community General Hospital, has been aggressively pursuing the couple to contribute $500,000 to the hospital's soon-to-be-built Cancer Care Center. Without the contribution, the Wealthy's taxable income for 2008 would be $2 million. What impact would the contribution have on the Wealthy's 2008 tax bill?

CHAPTER 3

PAYING FOR HEALTH SERVICES

Big Sky Dermatology Specialists is a small group practice in Jackson, Wyoming. The city is located in the scenic Jackson Hole valley and is a major gateway to the Grand Teton and Yellowstone National Parks. In addition, it is home to the world's largest ball of barbed wire. (It's amazing what you learn when studying healthcare finance!)

Jen Latimer, a recent graduate of Idaho State University's healthcare administration program, was just hired to be Big Sky's practice manager. One of her first tasks was to review the group's payer mix. After all, revenues are the first step (of many) needed to ensure the financial success of any business. (Payer mix is a listing of the individuals and organizations that pay for a provider's services, along with each payer's percentage of revenues.)

To better understand Big Sky's revenues, Jen focused on two questions. First, who are the payers? In other words, where does Big Sky's revenue come from? Second, what methods do the payers use to determine the payment amount? By gaining an appreciation of the group's revenues, Jen believed she could better judge the financial riskiness of the practice. Furthermore, she would then be able to identify the steps that might be taken to increase the practice's revenues and reduce the riskiness associated with those revenues.

By the end of the chapter, you will have a better understanding of healthcare provider revenue sources and how the specific payment method influences provider behavior. Specifically, you, like Jen, will know more about how these issues affect Big Sky.

LEARNING OBJECTIVES

After studying this chapter, you will be able to

➤ List the key features of insurance.

➤ Describe the major types of third-party payers.

➤ Discuss, in general terms, the reimbursement methods used by third-party payers, and the incentives and risks that they create for providers.

➤ Explain how coding affects reimbursement.

➤ Define the specific reimbursement methods used by Medicare.

3.1 INTRODUCTION

In most industries, the consumer of the product or service (1) has a choice among many suppliers, (2) can distinguish the quality of competing goods or services, (3) makes a (presumably) rational decision regarding the purchase on the basis of quality and price, and (4) pays for the full cost of the purchase.

However, the provision of healthcare services typically takes place in unique circumstances. First, often there are only a few providers of a particular service. Second, judging the quality of competing providers is difficult, if not impossible. Third, the decision (or at least recommendation) on which provider to use typically is not made by the consumer but rather by a physician or some other clinician. Fourth, the bulk of the payment to the provider is not normally made by the user (the patient) but by an insurer. Finally, for most individuals, the purchase of health insurance is paid for (or heavily subsidized) by employers or government agencies, so patients are insulated from the true cost of healthcare services.

This highly unusual marketplace has a profound effect on the supply of, and demand for, healthcare services. To get a better understanding of the unique payment mechanisms involved, we must examine the healthcare reimbursement system.

3.2 BASIC INSURANCE CONCEPTS

Because insurance is the cornerstone of healthcare reimbursement, an appreciation of basic insurance concepts will help you better understand the marketplace for healthcare services.

A SIMPLE ILLUSTRATION

Assume that no health insurance exists, and that you face only two medical outcomes in the coming year:

Outcome	Probability	Cost
Stay healthy	0.99	$ 0
Get sick	0.01	50,000
	1.00	

What is your expected healthcare cost (in the statistical sense) for the coming year? To find the answer—$500—multiply the cost of each outcome by its probability of occurrence and then sum the products:

$$
\begin{aligned}
\text{Expected cost} &= (\text{Probability of outcome 1} \times \text{Cost of outcome 1}) \\
&+ (\text{Probability of outcome 2} \times \text{Cost of outcome 2}) \\
&= (0.99 \times \$0) + (0.01 \times \$50,000) \\
&= \$0 + \$500 = \$500.
\end{aligned}
$$

Now, assume that everyone else faces the same medical outcomes and hence "sees" the same odds and costs associated with healthcare. Furthermore, assume that you, and everyone else, make $60,000 a year. With this salary, you can easily afford the $500 expected healthcare cost. The problem is, however, that no one's actual cost will be $500. If you stay healthy, your cost will be zero. But if you get sick, your cost will be $50,000, and this amount could force you, and most people who get sick, into personal bankruptcy, which is a ruinous event. (Don't forget, you have to pay all of your living expenses out of your $60,000 annual income in addition to any healthcare costs.)

Now, suppose an insurance policy that pays all of your healthcare costs for the coming year is available for $600. Would you take the policy, even though it costs $100 more than your "expected" healthcare costs?

> ## ⊙ CRITICAL CONCEPT
> ### Risk Aversion
>
> Risk aversion is the tendency of individuals and businesses to dislike financial risk. In other words, "risk" is a four-letter word. Risk-averse individuals and businesses are motivated to use insurance and other techniques to protect against risk. For example, a favorite tool to control risk is diversification, which in the context of revenues means lowering risk by having different sources of income. By not depending on one source—say, Medicare patients—a provider can reduce the uncertainty (riskiness) of its revenue stream. Insurance is another way to limit risk. Individuals buy insurance on the houses they own to limit the consequences of calamitous events, such as fires or hurricanes.

Most people would. Because individuals are **risk averse**, they would be willing to pay a $100 premium over their expected benefit to eliminate the risk of financial ruin. In effect, policyholders are passing the costs associated with the risk of getting sick to the insurer who, as you will see, is spreading those costs over a large number of subscribers.

Would an insurer be willing to offer the policy for $600? If the insurer could sell enough policies, it would know its revenues and costs with some precision. For example, if the insurer sold 1 million policies, it would collect 1,000,000 × $600 = $600 million in health insurance premiums, pay out roughly 1,000,000 × $500 = $500 million in claims, and hence have about $100 million to cover administrative costs, provide a reserve in case claims are greater than predicted, and make a profit. By writing a large number of policies, the financial risk inherent in medical costs can be spread over a large number of people and hence reduce the risk for the insurance company (and for each individual).

Basic Characteristics of Insurance

The simple example we gave illustrates why individuals would seek health insurance and why insurance companies would be formed to provide such insurance. Let's dig a little deeper into insurance basics.

Insurance typically has four distinct characteristics:

Pooling
The spreading of
losses over a large
group of individuals (or
organizations).

1. *Pooling of losses.* The *pooling* (sharing) of losses is the heart of insurance. Pooling means that losses are spread over a large group of individuals so that each individual realizes the average loss of the pool rather than the actual loss incurred. In addition, pooling involves the grouping of a large number of homogeneous exposure units (people or things having the same risk characteristics) so that the law of large numbers can apply. Thus, pooling implies (1) the sharing of losses by the entire group, and (2) the prediction of future losses with some accuracy based on the law of large numbers. (The law of large numbers implies that predicting losses is easier when many individuals are involved. For example, if a coin is flipped only once, you do not know whether the results will be a head or a tail. But if the coin is flipped 1,000 times, the result will be very close to 500 heads and 500 tails. Thus, you cannot predict the results of a single toss with any confidence, but you can predict the aggregate results if you have a large pool of tosses.)

Random loss
An unpredictable loss,
such as one that results
from a fire or hurricane.

2. *Payment only for random losses.* A *random loss* is unforeseen, is unexpected, and occurs as a result of chance. Insurance is based on the premise that payments are made only for losses that are random. We discuss the moral hazard problem, in which losses are not random, in a later section.

Risk transfer
The passing of risk
from one individual or
business to another
(usually an insurer).

3. *Risk transfer.* An insurance plan almost always involves *risk transfer.* The sole exception to the element of risk transfer is self-insurance, which occurs when an individual or business does not buy insurance. (Self-insurance is discussed in a later section.) Risk transfer means that the risk is transferred from the insured to the insurer, which typically is in a better financial position to pay the loss than the insured because of the premiums collected. Also, because of the law of large numbers, the insurance company is better able to predict its losses.

Indemnification
The agreement to pay
for losses incurred by
another party.

4. *Indemnification. Indemnification* is the reimbursement of the insured if a loss occurs. Within the context of health insurance, indemnification occurs when the insurer pays, in whole or in part, the insured or the provider for the expenses related to an insured illness or injury.

In summary, we applied these four characteristics to our insurance example: (1) The losses are pooled over 1 million individuals, (2) the losses on each individual are random (unpredictable), (3) the risk of loss is passed to the insurance company, and (4) the insurance company pays for any losses.

REAL-WORLD PROBLEMS

Insurance works fine when the four basic characteristics are present. However, if any of these characteristics is violated, problems arise. Here are the two most common problems.

Adverse Selection

One of the major problems for insurers is **adverse selection**. Adverse selection occurs because those individuals and businesses likely to have losses are more inclined to purchase insurance than those less likely to incur losses. For example, an otherwise healthy individual without insurance who needs a costly surgical procedure is more apt to get health insurance if he or she can afford it, whereas an identical individual without the threat of surgery is less likely to purchase insurance. Similarly, consider the health insurance purchase likelihood of a 20-year-old versus that of a 65-year-old. All

CRITICAL CONCEPT
Adverse Selection

Adverse selection, in its simplest form, means that individuals most likely to need healthcare services are most likely to buy health insurance. This creates a problem for insurers, because it drives the costs of healthcare for a defined population to higher-than-anticipated levels.

else the same, the older individual, with much greater health risk because of age, will probably buy insurance. (Individuals aged 65 or older consume more than three times as many healthcare services as younger individuals do.)

If the tendency toward adverse selection goes unchecked, a disproportionate number of sick people, or those most likely to become sick, will seek health insurance, causing the insurer to experience higher-than-expected claims. This increase in claims will trigger a premium increase, which worsens the problem, because healthier members of the plan will either pursue cheaper rates from another company (if available) or totally forgo insurance.

One way health insurers attempt to control the adverse selection problem is by *underwriting* provisions. Thus, smokers may be charged a higher premium than nonsmokers. Another way is by including preexisting condition clauses in contracts. (A preexisting condition is a physical or mental condition of the insured individual that existed before the issuance of the policy.) A typical clause states that preexisting conditions are not covered until the policy has been in force for some period of time—say, one or two years. Preexisting conditions present a true problem for the health insurance industry because an important characteristic of insurance is randomness. If an individual has a preexisting condition, the insurer no longer bears random risk but rather assumes the role of payer for the treatment of a known condition.

Underwriting
The selection and classification of candidates for insurance.

Because of the tendency of insurers to shy away from large predictable claims, Congress passed the Health Insurance Portability and Accountability Act (HIPAA) in 1996. Among other things, HIPAA sets national standards, which can be modified within limits by the states, regarding what provisions can be included in health insurance policies. For example, under a group health policy—say, one that covers employees of a furniture manufacturer—coverage to individuals cannot be denied or limited, nor can employees be required to pay more if they suffer from poor health.

Although preexisting condition clauses are not banned, there are limits on what counts as a preexisting condition and how long it takes for coverage to begin. Also, time credit for preexisting conditions under one plan can be credited toward a second plan should the employee change jobs, provided there is no break in coverage.

Finally, health insurance cannot be canceled if the policyholder becomes sick, and if a policyholder leaves the company, he or she has the right to purchase insurance (for a limited time) from the insurer that provided the company's group policy. All in all, the provisions of HIPAA give individuals protection against arbitrary actions by insurers when their health status changes for the worse or when they leave the employer.

Moral Hazard

The fact that insurance is based on the premise that payments are made only for random (unforeseen) losses creates the problem of moral hazard. The most common illustration of **moral hazard** is the owner who deliberately sets a failing business on fire to collect the insurance.

Moral hazard is also present in health insurance, but its form typically is not so dramatic—not too many people are willing to voluntarily sustain injury or illness for the purpose of collecting health insurance benefits. However, undoubtedly some people do purposely use healthcare services that are not medically required. For example, some people who live alone might visit a physician or a walk-in clinic for the social value of human companionship rather than to address a medical necessity.

More importantly, when the full cost or most of the cost of healthcare services is covered by insurance, individuals are more inclined to agree to a $1,000 MRI (magnetic resonance imaging) scan or other high-cost procedure even when its need is questionable. If the same test required total out-of-pocket payment, an individual would probably think carefully before agreeing to such an expensive procedure, unless it is a true medical necessity. The fact that somebody else is paying leads to a greater consumption of healthcare services than would occur if patients bore the full costs.

An even more insidious aspect of moral hazard is the impact of insurance on individual behavior. Individuals are less likely to take preventive actions when the costs of not taking those actions will be borne by insurers. Why worry about getting a flu shot if the monetary costs associated with the treatment are borne by the insurer, or why stop smoking if others will pay for the likely adverse health consequences? The fact that insurance exists causes individuals to forgo preventive actions

CRITICAL CONCEPT
Moral Hazard

Moral hazard is the risk to an insurer that excess healthcare services are being consumed because individuals do not bear the full cost of the services provided. For example, a patient may be quick to agree to an expensive test, even though that test is not medically necessary, because most of the cost is covered by insurance. Another illustration is the increased willingness of individuals to take health risks, such as forgoing vaccinations, because they know that the financial cost of getting sick is borne mostly by others.

and embrace unhealthy behaviors, both of which might be approached differently in the absence of insurance.

Insurers attempt to protect themselves from moral hazard claims by paying less than the full amount of healthcare costs. Making insured individuals bear some of the cost lessens their tendency to consume unneeded services or engage in unhealthy behaviors. One way to do this is to require a *deductible*. Medical policies usually stipulate a dollar amount that must be satisfied before benefits are paid.

Although deductibles have some positive effect on the moral hazard problem, their primary purpose is to eliminate the payment of a small claim, if that is the only healthcare expense for the year. In such cases, the administrative cost of processing the claim may be larger than the claim itself. To illustrate, a policy may state that the first $500 (or more) of medical expenses incurred each year will be paid by the individual. Once the deductible is met, the insurer will pay all eligible medical expenses (less any copayments and coinsurance) for the remainder of the year.

The primary weapons that insurers have against the moral hazard problem are copays and coinsurance. *Copayment* (or copay) is a fixed amount paid by the patient each time a service is rendered, such as $20 per office visit or $75 for each emergency department visit. *Coinsurance* is the sharing of costs between the patient and insurer, typically on a percentage basis. For example, the patient bears 20 percent of the costs of a hospital stay.

Copays and coinsurance serve two primary purposes. First, these payments discourage overutilization of healthcare services and hence reduce insurance benefits. Additionally, by being forced to pay some of the costs, insured individuals will presumably seek fewer and more cost-effective treatments and embrace a healthier lifestyle. Second, because insured individuals pay part of the cost, premiums can be reduced. Health insurance premiums (costs) have almost doubled since 2000 and now exceed $12,000 annually for family coverage. Employers, on average, pay about 75 percent of the premium costs. Because of the alarming trend in health premiums, employers are seeking ways to reduce these costs, and one way is to pass more of the costs on to employees through copays and coinsurance.

Some health insurance policies contain out-of-pocket maximums, whereby the insurer pays all covered costs, including coinsurance, after the insured individual pays a certain amount of costs—say, $2,000. Finally, most insurance policies have policy limits; for example, $1 million in total lifetime coverage, $1,500 per year for mental health benefits, or $100 for eyeglasses. These limits are designed to control excessive use of certain services and protect the insurer against catastrophic losses. Of course, a lifetime coverage limit means that patients must bear the risk of catastrophic losses.

Before we move on, we should briefly mention a new type of health insurance that is gaining popularity: *high-deductible health plans (HDHPs)*. An HDHP has a higher annual deductible (more than $2,000 for family coverage) than traditional plans do. But it allows individuals to set up savings accounts for the sole purpose of paying healthcare costs. Furthermore, contributions to such accounts are tax deductible (up to a set limit) and can roll over from year to year. HDHPs are becoming popular with executives and other highly

Deductible
The dollar amount that must be spent on healthcare services before any benefits are paid by the insurer. For example, $500 per year.

Copayment
A fixed cost to the patient each time a service is rendered. For example, $20 per outpatient visit.

Coinsurance
A sharing of costs between the patient and the insurer. For example, the patient pays 20 percent of the costs of hospitalization.

High-deductible health plan (HDHP)
A type of health insurance that requires high deductibles but allows insured individuals to set up tax-advantaged savings accounts to pay those deductibles.

paid workers because of the tax shelter benefit, but they have not been as widely accepted by blue-collar workers because of the high deductible amount.

? SELF-TEST QUESTIONS

1. Briefly explain the concept of health insurance.

2. What is adverse selection, and how do insurers deal with the problem?

3. What is moral hazard, and how do insurers handle it?

3.3 THIRD-PARTY PAYERS

As mentioned earlier, a large proportion of provider revenues does not come directly from patients (the users of healthcare services) but from insurers known collectively as **third-party payers**. Because a healthcare organization's revenues are key to its financial viability, we first discuss the sources of most revenues in the healthcare industry. In the next section, we examine the types of reimbursement methods employed by these payers.

Health insurance originated in Europe in the early 1800s when mutual benefit societies were formed to reduce the financial burden associated with illness or injury. Today, health insurers fall into two broad categories: private insurers and public programs.

! CRITICAL CONCEPT
Third-Party Payers

Third-party payers are the insurers that reimburse healthcare organizations and hence are the major source of revenues for most providers. Third-party payers include private insurers, such as Blue Cross and Blue Shield, and public (government) insurers, such as Medicare and Medicaid. Third-party payers use several methods to pay providers, depending on the specific payer (for example, Blue Cross versus Medicare) and the type of service rendered (for example, inpatient versus outpatient).

PRIVATE INSURERS

In the United States, the concept of public, or government, health insurance is relatively new, while private health insurance has been in existence since the early twentieth century. In this section, we discuss the major private insurers.

Blue Cross and Blue Shield

Blue Cross and Blue Shield organizations trace their roots to the Great Depression, when both hospitals and physicians were concerned about their patients' abilities to pay healthcare bills.

Blue Cross originated as a number of separate insurance programs offered by individual hospitals. At that time, many patients were unable to pay their hospital bills, but most people, except the poorest, could afford to pay small monthly premiums to purchase some type of hospitalization insurance. Thus, the programs were initially designed to benefit both patients and hospitals.

The programs were all similar in structure: Hospitals agreed to provide a certain number of services to program members who made periodic payments to the hospitals whether services were used or not. In a short time, these programs were expanded from single-hospital programs to community-wide, multihospital plans that were called hospital service plans. The American Hospital Association (AHA) recognized the benefits of such plans to hospitals, so a close relationship was formed between the AHA and the organizations that offered hospital service plans.

In the early years, several states ruled that the sale of hospital services by prepayment did not constitute insurance, so the plans were exempt from regulations governing insurance companies. However, the legal status of hospital service plans clearly would be subject to future scrutiny unless their status was formalized. Thus, the states, one by one, passed legislation that provided for the founding of not-for-profit hospital service corporations that were exempt both from taxes and from the capital requirements (reserves) mandated for other insurers. However, state insurance departments had (and continue to have) oversight over most aspects of the plans' operations. The Blue Cross name was officially adopted by most of these plans in 1939.

Blue Shield plans developed in a manner similar to that of the Blue Cross plans, except that the providers were physicians instead of hospitals and the professional organization was the American Medical Association (AMA) instead of the AHA. Today, 39 Blue Cross/Blue Shield (the Blues) organizations exist, some of which offer only one of the two plans, but most offer both plans. The Blues are organized as independent corporations, but all belong to a single national association that sets the required standards for using the Blue Cross/Blue Shield name. Collectively, the Blues provide healthcare coverage for more than 100 million people in all 50 states, the District of Columbia, and Puerto Rico.

Historically, the Blues have been not-for-profit corporations that enjoyed the full benefits accorded to that status, including freedom from taxes. But in 1986, Congress eliminated the Blues' tax exemption on the grounds that they engaged in commercial-type insurance activities. However, the plans were given special deductions, which resulted in taxes that are generally less than those paid by commercial insurers.

In spite of the 1986 change in tax status, the national association continued to require all Blues to operate entirely as not-for-profit corporations, although they could establish for-profit subsidiaries. In 1994, the national association lifted its traditional ban on member plans becoming investor-owned companies, and several Blues have since converted to for-profit status.

Commercial Insurers

Commercial health insurance traditionally was issued by life insurance and casualty insurance (home and auto) companies. Today, however, most health insurance is provided by companies that exclusively write health insurance. Examples of commercial insurers include

Aetna, Humana, and UnitedHealth Group. Most commercial insurance companies are stockholder-owned, and all are taxable entities.

Commercial insurers moved strongly into health insurance following World War II. At that time, the United Auto Workers (UAW) negotiated the first contract with employers in which fringe benefits were a major part of the contract. Like the Blues, the majority of individuals with commercial health insurance are covered under *group policies* with employee groups, professional and other associations, and labor unions.

Self-Insurers

An argument can be made that all individuals who do not have some form of health insurance are self-insurers, but this is not correct. Self-insurers make a conscious decision to bear the risks associated with healthcare costs and then set aside (or have available) funds to pay for costs they may incur in the future. Individuals, except the very wealthy, are not good candidates for self-insurance because, as discussed earlier, individuals who do not pool risks face much uncertainty in future healthcare costs.

On the other hand, large organizations, especially employers, are good candidates for self-insurance. In fact, most large companies, and many midsized companies, are self-insured. The advantages of self-insurance include the potential to reduce costs (cut out the middleman) and the opportunity to offer plans tailored to meet the unique characteristics of the organization's employees. Organizations that self-insure typically pay an insurance company to administer the plan. For example, employees of the state of Florida are covered by health insurance whose costs are paid directly by the state, but the plan is administered by Blue Cross/Blue Shield of Florida.

PUBLIC INSURERS

Government is a major insurer and a direct provider of healthcare services. For example, the government provides healthcare services directly to qualifying individuals through the Department of Veterans Affairs (VA), Department of Defense (DOD), and Public Health Service (PHS) medical facilities. In addition, the government either provides or mandates a variety of insurance programs, such as Worker's Compensation and TRICARE (health insurance for military members and families, formerly CHAMPUS). In this section, however, our focus is on the two major government insurance programs: Medicare and Medicaid, which fund roughly one-third of all healthcare services provided in the United States.

Medicare

Medicare was established by Congress in 1965 primarily to provide medical benefits to individuals aged 65 or older. About 50 million people have Medicare coverage, which pays for about 17 percent of all U.S. healthcare services.

Over the decades, Medicare has evolved to include four major coverages: (1) Part A, which provides hospital and some skilled nursing home coverage; (2) Part B, which covers physician services, ambulatory surgical services, outpatient services, and certain other miscellaneous services; (3) Part C, which is managed care coverage that can be selected in lieu of Parts A and B; and (4) Part D, which covers prescription drugs. In addition, Medicare covers healthcare costs associated with selected disabilities and illnesses (such as kidney failure), regardless of age.

Part A coverage is free to all individuals eligible for Social Security benefits. Elderly individuals who are not eligible for Social Security benefits can obtain Part A medical benefits by paying premiums of $423 per month (for 2008). Part B is optional to all individuals who have Part A coverage, and it requires a monthly premium for most enrollees of between $96.40 and $238.40 (for 2008), depending on income. About 97 percent of Part A participants purchase Part B coverage. Because of deductibles, copays, coinsurance, and coverage limits, Medicare Parts A and B coverage can still require beneficiaries to bear significant out-of-pocket costs. Thus, many Medicare participants purchase additional coverage from private insurers to help cover the "gaps" in Medicare coverage. Such coverage is called *Medigap insurance.*

Part C coverage is an alternative to coverage under Parts A and B that is offered by private insurance companies but paid for by Medicare. These plans, called *Medicare Advantage plans*, generally provide Parts A and B coverage along with many of the same benefits that a Medigap policy would include, so additional insurance is not required. (Also, some plans include prescription drug [Part D] coverage.) However, because the plans are essentially managed care plans (which we discuss shortly), they typically have more restrictions on access than in standard coverage under Parts A and B. Also, some Medicare Advantage plans charge members a small premium above the amount paid by Medicare.

Part D, which began in 2006, offers prescription drug coverage through plans offered by more than 70 private companies. Each plan may offer somewhat different coverage, so the benefits and costs of Part D coverage vary widely, depending on the plan chosen.

The Medicare program falls under the U.S. Department of Health and Human Services (HHS), which creates the specific rules of the program on the basis of federal legislation. Medicare is administered by an agency in HHS called the *Centers for Medicare and Medicaid Services (CMS).*

> **! CRITICAL CONCEPT**
> **Medicare**
>
> Medicare is a federal health insurance program that primarily covers elderly individuals (those aged 65 or older). It consists of four major parts: Part A covers inpatient services, Part B covers outpatient services, Part C is managed care coverage that replaces Parts A and B, and Part D covers prescription drugs. Medicare is administered by the Centers for Medicare and Medicaid Services, which falls under the U.S. Department of Health and Human Services.

Medigap insurance
Insurance taken out by Medicare beneficiaries that pays many of the costs not covered by Parts A and B. (It fills in the "gaps.")

Medicare Advantage plan
Managed care plan coverage offered to Medicare beneficiaries that replaces Parts A and B coverage.

Centers for Medicare and Medicaid Services (CMS)
The federal agency, within the U.S. Department of Health and Human Services, that administers the Medicare and Medicaid programs.

CMS has ten regional offices that oversee the Medicare program and ensure that regulations are followed. Medicare payments to providers are not made directly by CMS but by contractors at the state or local level called intermediaries for Part A payments and carriers for Part B payments.

Medicaid

Medicaid began in 1965 as a modest program jointly funded and operated by the individual states and the federal government. The idea was to provide a medical safety net for low-income mothers and children and for elderly, blind, and disabled individuals.

Congress mandated that state programs, at a minimum, cover hospital and physician care but encouraged states to provide additional benefits either by increasing the range of benefits or extending the program to cover more people. States with large tax bases were quick to expand coverage to many groups, while states with limited revenues were forced to establish more restrictive programs. In addition to state expansions, a mandatory nursing home benefit was added in 1972. As a consequence, Medicaid is now the largest payer of long-term-care benefits and the largest single budget item in many states. In total, Medicaid covers roughly 15 million individuals and pays for about 16 percent of healthcare services in the United States.

Over the years, Medicare and Medicaid have provided access to healthcare services for many low-income individuals who otherwise would have no health insurance coverage. Furthermore, these programs have become an important source of revenue for healthcare providers, especially for nursing homes and other providers that treat large numbers of low-income patients. However, both Medicare and Medicaid expenditures have been growing at an alarming rate, which has forced both federal and state policymakers to search for more cost-effective ways to provide healthcare services.

> **! CRITICAL CONCEPT**
> Medicaid
>
> Medicaid is a joint federal–state health insurance program that primarily covers low-income individuals and families. The federal government funds about half of the costs of the program, while the states fund the remainder. Although general guidelines are established by CMS, the program is administered by the individual states. Thus, each state, as long as it follows basic federal guidelines, can set its own rules regarding eligibility, benefits, and provider payments.

> **? SELF-TEST QUESTIONS**
>
> 1. What are the different types of private insurers?
>
> 2. Briefly, what are the origins and purpose of Medicare?
>
> 3. What is Medicaid, and how is it administered?

3.4 MANAGED CARE ORGANIZATIONS

Managed care organizations (MCOs) strive to combine the provision of healthcare services and the insurance function into a single entity. Typically, MCOs are created by insurers who either directly own a provider network or create one through contractual arrangements with independent providers. Occasionally, however, MCOs are created by integrated delivery systems that establish their own insurance companies.

There are several types of MCOs. Historically, the most common type was the **health maintenance organization (HMO).** HMOs are based on the premise that the traditional insurer–provider relationship creates perverse incentives that reward providers for treating patients' illnesses but offers little incentive for providing prevention and rehabilitation services. By combining the financing and delivery of healthcare services into a single system, HMOs theoretically have as strong an incentive to prevent as to treat illnesses. However, because of their different types of organizational structures, ownership, and financial incentives, HMOs can vary widely in cost and quality.

HMOs use a variety of methods to control costs. These include limiting patients to particular providers, called the *provider panel*, and using *gatekeeper* physicians who must authorize all specialized and referral services. In general, services are not covered if beneficiaries bypass their gatekeeper physician or use providers that are not part of the HMO panel.

The federal Health Maintenance Act of 1973 encouraged the development of HMOs by providing federal funds for HMO-operating grants and loans. In addition, the act required larger employers that offer healthcare benefits to their employees to include an HMO as one alternative, if one was available, in addition to traditional insurance plans.

Although the number and sizes of HMOs grew rapidly during the 1980s and 1990s, since then they have lost some of their luster because healthcare consumers have been unwilling to accept access limitations, even though such limitations might reduce costs. To address consumer concerns and falling enrollments, another type of MCO—the **preferred provider organization (PPO)**—was developed. These organizations, which are not as "tightly" managed as HMOs, combine some of the cost-savings strategies of HMOs with features of traditional health insurance plans.

PPOs do not mandate that beneficiaries use specific providers, although financial incentives are created that encourage members to use providers that are part of the panel, which typically has discounted price contracts with the PPO. Furthermore,

Provider panel

The group of providers—say, doctors and hospitals—that is an integral part of a managed care plan. Services provided outside of the panel may be only partially covered by the plan or not covered at all.

Gatekeeper

A primary care physician who controls specialist and ancillary service referrals. Some managed care plans will only pay for those services approved by the gatekeeper.

(!) CRITICAL CONCEPT
Managed Care Organizations: HMOs and PPOs

Managed care organizations (MCOs) combine insurer and provider functions into a single administrative organization. The idea here is not only to pay for care but also to manage the care provided. MCOs come in different types, and their primary difference is in how "tightly" the care is managed. Health maintenance organizations (HMOs) tend to exercise most control over the types and amount of care provided, while preferred provider organizations (PPOs) tend to be less controlling. In all managed care plans, the goal is to provide only services that are medically required in the lowest cost setting.

PPOs do not require plan members to use preselected gatekeeper physicians. Finally, PPOs are less likely than HMOs to provide preventive services, and they do not assume any responsibility for quality assurance because enrollees are not constrained to use only the PPO panel of providers.

In an effort to achieve the potential cost savings of MCOs, health insurers are now applying managed care strategies, such as preadmission certification, utilization review, and second surgical opinions, to their conventional plans. Thus, the term managed care now describes a continuum of plans, which can vary significantly in their approaches to providing combined insurance and healthcare services. The common feature in MCOs is that the insurer has a mechanism to control, or at least influence, patients' utilization of healthcare services. Today, most employer-sponsored health coverage is provided by some type of MCO.

(?) SELF-TEST QUESTIONS

1. What is meant by the term "managed care organization (MCO)"?

2. What are two different types of MCOs?

3.5 ALTERNATIVE REIMBURSEMENT METHODS

Regardless of the payer for a particular healthcare service, only a limited number of payment methods are used to reimburse providers. Payment methods fall into two broad classifications: fee-for-service and capitation. In this section, we discuss the most used reimbursement methods.

FEE-FOR-SERVICE

In fee-for-service payment methods, of which many variations exist, the more services provided, the higher the reimbursement. The three primary **fee-for-service** methods of reimbursement are cost based, charge based, and prospective payment.

Cost-Based

Under cost-based reimbursement, the payer agrees to reimburse the provider for the costs incurred in providing services to the insured population. Cost-based reimbursement is retrospective in the sense that reimbursement is based on what has happened in the past. Cost-based reimbursement is limited to allowable costs, usually defined as costs directly related to the provision of healthcare services. For all practical purposes, cost-based reimbursement guarantees that a provider's costs will be covered by revenues.

Charge-Based

When payers pay billed charges, they pay according to a rate schedule, called a *chargemaster*, established by the provider. To a certain extent, this reimbursement system places payers at the mercy of providers, especially in markets where competition is limited. In the very early days of health insurance, all payers reimbursed providers on the basis of charges. Now, the trend is toward other, less-generous reimbursement methods, and the only payers that are expected to pay the full amount of charges are self-pay (private-pay) patients. Even then, low-income uninsured patients often are given discounts from charges.

Most insurers that still base reimbursement on charges now pay negotiated, or discounted, charges. Insurers with managed care plans, as well as conventional insurers, often have bargaining power because of the large number of patients they bring to a provider, so they can negotiate discounts that generally range from 20 percent to 50 percent (or more) of charges. The effect of these discounts is to create a system similar to hotel or airline pricing, where few people pay the listed rates (rack rates or full fares). Many people argue that chargemaster prices have become meaningless, and hence the entire concept should be abandoned. But old habits die hard, and chargemaster prices still play a role in some reimbursement methods, so we expect that they will be around for some time.

Prospective Payment

In a *prospective payment* system, the rates paid by payers are determined by the payer before the services are provided. Furthermore, payments are not directly related to either costs or charges. Here are the common units of payment used in prospective payment systems:

- ◆ *Per procedure.* Under per procedure reimbursement, a separate payment is made for each procedure performed on a patient. Because of the high administrative costs associated with this method when applied to complex diagnoses, per procedure reimbursement is primarily used in outpatient settings.

> **① CRITICAL CONCEPT**
> Fee-for-Service Reimbursement
>
> Under fee-for-service reimbursement, healthcare organizations are paid on the basis of the amount of services provided. A "service" can be defined several ways. For example, a physician may be paid for each procedure performed, such as an office visit or the reading of CT scan. A hospital may be reimbursed for costs incurred, for each admission, or perhaps for each patient day. A clinical laboratory may be paid for each test performed. Regardless of the specific definition of a service, in fee-for-service reimbursement the greater the amount of services provided, the greater the revenues. Thus, the risk of utilization uncertainty is borne by the insurer rather than by the provider.

Chargemaster
A provider's official list of charges (prices) for supplies and services rendered.

Prospective payment
A reimbursement system meant to cover expected costs as opposed to historical (retrospective) costs.

◆ *Per diagnosis.* In the per diagnosis reimbursement method, the provider is paid a rate that depends on the patient's diagnosis. Diagnoses that require higher resource utilization, and hence are more costly to treat, have higher reimbursement rates. Medicare pioneered this basis of payment in its diagnosis-related group system, which it first used for hospital inpatient reimbursement in 1983. (See the Industry Practice box for examples of per procedure and per diagnosis reimbursement.)

◆ *Per day (per diem).* Some insurers reimburse institutional providers, such as hospitals and nursing homes, on a per day (per diem) basis. Here, the provider is paid a fixed amount for each day that service is provided. Often, per diem rates are stratified, which means that different rates are applied to different services. For example, a hospital may be paid one rate for a medical/surgical day, a higher rate for a critical care unit day, and yet a different rate for an obstetric day. Stratified per diems recognize that providers incur widely varied daily costs for providing different types of inpatient care.

◆ *Global reimbursement.* Under global reimbursement, payers pay a single prospective payment that covers all services delivered in a single episode, whether the services are rendered by a single or by multiple providers. For example, a global fee may be set for all obstetric services associated with a pregnancy provided by a single physician, including all prenatal and postnatal visits, as well as the delivery. For another example, a global price may be paid for all physician and hospital services associated with a cardiac bypass operation.

CRITICAL CONCEPT
Capitation

With capitation, providers are paid a set amount on the basis of the number of members (patients) assigned to that provider. Thus, the reimbursement amount is fixed on the basis of the population served, regardless of the amount of services provided to that population. In effect, the provider, rather than the insurer, now faces utilization risk, because higher per member utilization means higher provider costs with no additional revenues. Critics of capitation contend that it creates the incentive to withhold needed services, while proponents argue that it discourages unneeded services and hence reduces costs.

CAPITATION

As compared to fee-for-service, **capitation** is an entirely different approach to reimbursement. Under capitated reimbursement, the provider is paid a fixed amount per covered life per period (usually a month), regardless of the amount of services provided. For example, a primary care physician might be paid $15 per member per month for handling 100 members of a managed care plan.

Capitation payment, which is used mostly by managed care organizations to reimburse primary care physicians, dramatically changes the financial environment of healthcare providers. Its implications are addressed in the next section and as needed in the remainder of this book. (For additional information about capitation, see Chapter 17, which is available online at ache.org/books/Finance-Fundamentals.)

PAY FOR PERFORMANCE

Before closing our discussion of reimbursement, we should note that many insurers are now creating reimbursement systems that explicitly reward providers for doing certain things. These reimbursement systems, which are really modified fee-for-service or capitation systems, are called *pay-for-performance (P4P)* systems.

In most P4P reimbursement, insurers pay providers an "extra" amount if certain standards, usually related to quality of care, are met. For example, a primary care practice may receive additional reimbursement if it meets goals, such as 85 percent of female patients older than 50 receiving mammograms or 90 percent of diabetic patients being on medication and having quarterly blood tests. A hospital may also receive additional reimbursement if it falls in the lower 10 percent of hospitals experiencing medical errors and hospital-acquired infections.

The idea here is to create incentives for better quality care, which may cost insurers in the short run but will lead to lower medical costs in the long run. In some pay-for-performance plans, insurers make providers bear the cost of the plan by reducing payments to poor performers and using the savings to make enhanced payments to good performers.

Pay for performance
A reimbursement system that rewards providers for meeting specific goals—for example, patient satisfaction.

? SELF-TEST QUESTIONS

1. What is the major difference between fee-for-service reimbursement and capitation?

2. Briefly explain the following fee-for-service payment methods:
   - Cost-based
   - Charge-based and discounted charges
   - Per procedure
   - Per diagnosis
   - Per diem
   - Global

3. What is pay-for-performance reimbursement?

✳ INDUSTRY PRACTICE How Medicare Pays Providers

Medicare uses different reimbursement methods to pay for hospital services and physician services. In this section, we briefly describe the two methods. Understanding the basics of Medicare reimbursement is critical because many other third-party payers have adopted these or similar systems.

Hospitals

From its inception in 1965 until 1983, Medicare hospital payments for inpatients were based on a retrospective system that reimbursed hospitals for all reasonable costs. However, in an attempt to curb Medicare spending, Congress established a new reimbursement system for hospitals in 1983 called the inpatient prospective payment system (inpatient PPS or IPPS). Under the IPPS, a single payment for each inpatient stay covers the cost of routine inpatient care, special care, and ancillary services. The amount of the prospective payment is based on the patient's diagnosis-related group (DRG) assigned at discharge.

The starting point in determining the amount of reimbursement is the DRG itself. Potential patient diagnoses have been divided into 334 base DRGs (base diagnoses). Then, these base diagnoses are split into subgroups on the basis of complications or comorbidities. (A comorbidity is the presence of one or more diseases or disorders in addition to the primary diagnosis.) In all, there are 745 total MS-DRGs, where MS stands for Medicare Severity.

To illustrate, consider the MS-DRGs for heart failure. DRG 293 is the base DRG (no complications or comorbidities [CC]), while DRG 292 is with CC and DRG 291 is with major CC. Each MS-DRG is assigned a relative weight that represents the average resources consumed in treating that particular diagnosis relative to resources consumed in treating an average diagnosis, and the greater the weight, the greater the reimbursement amount. The weights and sample payment amounts for the three heart failure DRGs are as follows:

MS-DRG	Weight	Payment
293	0.8765	$4,351
292	1.0134	5,030
291	1.2585	6,247

(*) INDUSTRY PRACTICE How Medicare Pays Providers

As can be seen from the data, the DRG with no CC (293) has a lower weight than the one with CC (292), which has a lower weight than the one with major CC (291). In fact, the amount of hospital resources consumed to treat a patient with DRG 293 (basic heart failure) is less than that required to treat an average inpatient because the weight is less than 1.0. An inpatient diagnosed with heart failure with CC (DRG 292) is about average in resource consumption, while a heart failure patient with major CC (DRG 291) uses roughly 25 percent more resources than the average inpatient.

The translation from DRG weight to payment amount (the actual reimbursement) depends on several factors, such as hospital location and teaching status, and hence is somewhat complex. In essence, the DRG weight is multiplied by an adjusted base rate (dollar amount) that incorporates several factors unique to the hospital and its geographic location. In the table above, we show representative payment amounts calculated using an adjusted base rate of $4,964. For example, the reimbursement for a typical hospital for DRG 292 would be 1.0134 x $4,964 = $5,030. The bottom line is that the greater the amount of resources needed to treat the diagnosis, the greater the DRG weight and reimbursement amount.

Note that the single DRG payment reimburses the hospital for all inpatient costs. To provide some cushion for the high costs associated with severely ill patients within each diagnosis, Medicare includes a provision for outlier payments. Outliers are classified into two categories: (1) length of stay (LOS) outliers and (2) cost outliers. Medicare will make additional payments when a patient's LOS or cost exceeds established cutoff points. Such payments are designed to compensate hospitals for treating patients that consume resources that fall outside of normal bounds.

Also, note that hospital outpatient visits are reimbursed on a prospective payment system that is similar in concept, but different in structure, to the inpatient MS-DRG system. The outpatient prospective payment system (OPPS) categorizes outpatient visits into groups called Ambulatory Payment Classifications (APCs), which are similar clinically and in the amount of resources consumed. Like MS-DRGs, each APC has a weight that is multiplied by a hospital-specific payment rate to obtain the reimbursement amount.

(Continued)

INDUSTRY PRACTICE How Medicare Pays Providers

Physicians

Through 1991, Medicare reimbursement for physicians was based on the concept of reasonable charges. In essence, Medicare defined a reasonable charge as the lowest of (1) the actual charge for the service performed, (2) the physician's customary charge, or (3) the prevailing charge for that service in the community.

However, Medicare changed its physician payment system in 1992 to a resource-based relative value scale (RBRVS) system. Under RBRVS, reimbursement is based on three resource components: (1) physician work, (2) practice (overhead) expense, and (3) malpractice insurance expense. Each of roughly 8,000 procedure codes have relative value units (RVUs) assigned for the three resource components, which, after adjustment for geographic cost differentials, are summed to get the total number of RVUs per procedure performed. The total RVUs are then multiplied by a conversion factor that equals the dollar value of one unit to get the dollar reimbursement amount.

For example, consider code 99213, which is one category of office visit. The physician work RVU is 0.92, the practice expense RVU is 0.72, and the malpractice insurance RVU is 0.03. For a physician practicing in Marco Island, Florida, the adjusted RVU values are 0.92, 0.67, and 0.04, respectively. (The overhead costs associated with a practice in Marco Island are slightly less than the national average, but malpractice insurance is slightly more.) The 2008 Medicare conversion factor is $38.09, so the Medicare reimbursement amount would be (0.92 + 0.67 + 0.04) x $38.09 = 1.63 x $38.09 = $62.09.

Like Medicare's MS-DRG system for inpatients, the more complicated the patient treatment, the greater the reimbursement amount. However, because the codes used for physician reimbursement are specific to the services rendered, no provisions for outlier payments are given to physicians. Later in this chapter, we explain medical coding, which is the starting point for most reimbursement methods.

3.6 THE IMPACT OF REIMBURSEMENT ON FINANCIAL INCENTIVES AND RISKS

Different methods of reimbursement create different incentives and risks for providers. In this section, we briefly discuss these issues.

PROVIDER INCENTIVES

Providers, like individuals or other businesses, react to the incentives created by the financial environment. For example, individuals can deduct mortgage interest from income for tax purposes, but they cannot deduct interest payments on personal loans. Loan companies have responded by offering home equity loans that are a type of second mortgage. The intent is not that such loans would be used to finance home ownership, as the tax laws assumed, but that the funds would be used for other purposes, including paying for vacations and purchasing cars or appliances. In this situation, tax laws created incentives for consumers to have mortgage debt rather than personal debt, and the mortgage loan industry responded accordingly.

In the same vein, alternative reimbursement methods have an impact on provider behavior. Under cost-based reimbursement, providers are issued a "blank check" to acquire facilities and equipment and incur operating costs. If payers reimburse providers for all service-related costs, the incentive is to incur such costs. Facilities will be lavish and conveniently located, and staff will be available to ensure that patients are given red-carpet treatment. Furthermore, services that are not required will be provided because more services lead to higher costs, which lead to higher revenues.

Under charge-based reimbursement, providers have the incentive to set high prices and offer more services. However, in competitive markets, there will be a constraint on prices. Still, to the extent that insurers, rather than patients, are footing the bill, considerable leeway exists. Also, because reimbursement based on charges is a fee-for-service type of reimbursement, a strong incentive exists to provide the highest possible amount of services. In essence, providers can increase utilization, and hence revenues, by creating more visits, ordering more tests, extending inpatient stays, and so on. Although charge-based reimbursement does encourage providers to contain costs, the incentive is weak because charges can be more easily increased than costs can be decreased. In recent years, the ability of providers to increase revenues by raising charges has been greatly offset by insurers through negotiated discounts, which place additional pressure on profitability and hence sweeten the incentive for providers to reduce costs.

Under prospective payment reimbursement, provider incentives are altered. First, under per procedure reimbursement, the profitability of individual procedures will vary depending on the relationship between the actual costs incurred and the payment for that procedure. In other words, because of inconsistencies in reimbursement, some procedures are more profitable than others. Providers, typically physicians, have the incentive to perform procedures that have the highest profit potential. Furthermore, the more procedures performed the better because each procedure typically generates additional profit.

The incentives under per diagnosis reimbursement are similar. Providers, usually hospitals, will seek patients with diagnoses that have the greatest profit potential and discourage (or even discontinue) services that have the least potential. (Why, in recent years, have so many hospitals created cardiac care centers?)

Bundling
The payment of a single amount for several procedures. When reimbursement is unbundled, separate amounts are paid for each procedure.

In all prospective payment methods, providers have the incentive to reduce costs because the amount of reimbursement is fixed and independent of the costs actually incurred. For example, when hospitals are paid under per diagnosis reimbursement, they have the incentive to reduce length of stay and hence costs. Note, however, when per diem reimbursement is used, hospitals have an incentive to increase length of stay. Because the early days of a hospitalization typically are more costly than the later days, the later days are more profitable. However, as mentioned previously, hospitals have the incentive to reduce costs during each day of a patient stay.

Under global reimbursement, providers do not have the opportunity to be reimbursed for a series of separate services. For example, a physician's treatment of a fracture could be *bundled*, and hence billed as one episode, or it could be unbundled with separate bills submitted for making the diagnosis, taking the x-rays, setting the fracture, removing the cast, and so on. The rationale for unbundling is usually to provide more detailed records of treatments rendered, but often the result is higher total charges for the parts than would be charged for the entire package under global payment.

Also, global reimbursement, when applied to multiple providers for a single episode of care, forces involved providers (physicians and hospitals) to jointly offer the most cost-effective treatment. Such a joint view of cost containment may be more effective than each provider separately attempting to minimize its treatment costs because the actions of one provider to lower costs could increase the costs of the other provider.

Finally, capitation reimbursement totally changes the playing field by completely reversing the actions that providers must take to ensure financial success. Under all fee-for-service methods, the key to provider success is to work harder, increase the amount of services provided (utilization) and hence maximize profits. Under capitation, the key to profitability is to work smarter and decrease utilization.

As with prospective payment, capitated providers have the incentive to lower the cost of the services provided, but now they also have the incentive to reduce the amount of services provided. Thus, only those procedures that are truly medically necessary should be performed, and treatment should take place in the lowest cost setting that can provide the appropriate quality of care. Furthermore, providers have the incentive to promote health, rather than just treat illness and injury, because a healthier population consumes fewer healthcare services.

PROVIDER RISKS

One key issue providers contend with is the impact of various reimbursement methods on financial risk. We can think of financial risk in terms of the effect that the reimbursement methods have on profit uncertainty—the greater the uncertainty in profitability (and hence the greater the chance of losing money), the higher the risk.

Cost- and charge-based reimbursements are the least risky for providers because payers more or less ensure that provider costs are covered, and hence profits will be earned.

In cost-based systems, costs are automatically covered. In charge-based systems, providers typically can set charges high enough to ensure that costs are covered, although discounts introduce some uncertainty into the reimbursement process.

In all reimbursement methods, except cost-based, providers bear the cost-of-service risk in the sense that costs can exceed revenues. However, a primary difference among the reimbursement types is the ability of the provider to influence the revenue–cost relationship. If providers set charge rates for each type of service provided, they can most easily ensure that revenues exceed costs. Furthermore, if providers have the power to set rates above those that would exist in a truly competitive market, charge-based reimbursement could result in higher profits than cost-based reimbursement can realize.

Prospective payment creates additional risk for providers. In essence, payers are setting reimbursement rates on the basis of what they believe to be sufficient. If the payments are set too low, providers cannot make money on their services without sacrificing quality. Today, many hospitals and physicians believe that Medicare and Medicaid reimbursement rates are too low. Thus, the only way to survive is to recoup these losses from privately insured patients or stop treating government-insured patients, which for many providers would take away more than half of their revenues. Whether or not government reimbursement is too low is open to debate. Still, prospective payment can place significant risk on providers.

Under capitation, providers assume **utilization risk** along with the risks assumed under the other reimbursement methods. The assumption of utilization risk has traditionally been an insurance, rather than a provider, function. In the traditional fee-for-service system, the financial risk of providing healthcare services is shared between providers and insurers: If costs are too high, providers suffer; if too many services are consumed, insurers suffer. Capitation, however, places both cost and utilization risk on providers.

When provider risk under different reimbursement methods is discussed in this descriptive fashion, an easy conclusion to make is that capitation is by far the riskiest to providers, while cost- and charge-based reimbursement are by far the least risky. Although this conclusion is not a bad starting point for analysis, financial risk is a complex subject, and we have just scratched its surface. For now, keep in mind that different payers use

CRITICAL CONCEPT
Utilization Risk

Utilization risk is the risk that patients, often members of a managed care plan, will use more healthcare services than initially assumed. For example, each employee of General Electric may be expected to make three visits per year to a primary care physician. However, the utilization risk is that each employee will actually make four visits. If the primary care physicians who treat the employees are paid on a fee-for-service basis, utilization risk is borne by the insurer (General Electric, because it is self-insured). The physicians will be paid for the actual number of visits and, if more than expected, the insurer must bear the added costs. However, if the physicians are capitated, they will be paid a fixed amount per employee based on the assumption of three visits. When employees make four visits, the primary care physicians bear the extra cost and hence the utilization risk.

differing reimbursement methods. Thus, providers can face conflicting incentives and differing risk, depending on the predominant method of reimbursement.

In closing, note that all prospective payment methods create financial risk for providers. This assumption of risk does not mean that providers should avoid such reimbursement methods; indeed, refusing to accept contracts with prospective payment provisions would be organizational suicide for most providers. However, providers must understand the risks involved in prospective payment arrangements, especially the effect on profitability, and make every effort to negotiate a level of payment that is consistent with the risk incurred.

? SELF-TEST QUESTIONS

1. What provider incentives are created under (a) cost-based reimbursement, (b) prospective payment, and (c) capitation?

2. Which of the three payment methods listed in Question 1 carries the least risk for providers? The most risk? Explain your answer.

3.7 CODING: THE FOUNDATION OF FEE-FOR-SERVICE REIMBURSEMENT

In practice, the basis for most fee-for-service reimbursement is the patient's diagnosis (in the case of hospitals) or the procedures performed on the patient (in the case of physicians). Clinicians indicate diagnoses and procedures by codes, so a brief background on clinical coding will help your understanding of reimbursement. (See the Industry Practice box for a description of Medicare reimbursement methods for hospitals and physicians.)

DIAGNOSIS CODES

ICD codes
International Classification of Diseases (ICD) codes are used by hospitals and other organizations to specify patient diagnoses.

The International Classification of Diseases (most commonly known by the abbreviation ICD) has become the standard for designating diseases and a wide variety of signs, symptoms, and external causes of injury. Published by the World Health Organization, *ICD codes* are used internationally to record many types of health events, including hospital inpatient stays and death certificates. (The first use of ICD codes, in 1893, was to report death statistics.)

The codes are periodically revised, with the most recent version being ICD-10. However, U.S. hospitals are still using a modified version of the 9th revision, called ICD-9-CM, where CM stands for Clinical Modification. (It is expected that conversion to ICD-10 codes will occur in 2013.) The ICD-9 codes consist of 3, 4, or 5 digits, with the first 3 digits being the disease category and the 4th and 5th digits providing additional information. For example, code 410 describes an acute myocardial infarction (heart attack), while code 410.1 is an attack involving the anterior wall of the heart.

In practice, the application of ICD codes to diagnoses is complicated and technical. Hospital coders have to understand both the coding system and the medical terminology and abbreviations used by clinicians. Because of its complexity, and the fact that proper coding can mean higher reimbursement from third-party payers, ICD coders require a great deal of training and experience to be most effective.

PROCEDURE CODES

While ICD codes are used to specify diseases, Current Procedural Terminology (CPT) codes are used to specify medical procedures (treatments). *CPT codes* were developed and are copyrighted by the American Medical Association. The purpose of CPT is to create a uniform language (set of descriptive terms and codes) that accurately describes medical, surgical, and diagnostic procedures. CPT terminology and codes are revised periodically to reflect current trends in clinical treatments. The Health Insurance Portability and Accountability Act (HIPAA) of 1996, in an attempt to increase standardization and the use of electronic medical records, requires that CPT be used for the coding and transfer of healthcare information by physicians and other clinical providers, including laboratory and diagnostic services. (HIPAA also requires that ICD-9-CM codes be used for hospital inpatient services.)

CPT codes
Current procedural terminology (CPT) codes are used by clinicians to specify procedures performed on patients.

To illustrate CPT codes, there are ten codes for physician office visits. Five of the codes apply to new patients, and the other five apply to established patients (repeat visits). The differences among the five codes in each category are based on the level of complexity of the visit as indicated by three components: (1) extent of patient history review, (2) extent of examination, and (3) difficulty of medical decision making. For repeat patients, the least complex (typically shortest) office visit has the code 99211, while the most complex (typically longest) has the code 99215.

Although not as complex as the ICD codes, CPT codes still require coders to have a high level of training and experience to do the job correctly. As in ICD coding, correct CPT coding ensures correct reimbursement. Coding is so important that many businesses offer services, such as books, software, education, and consulting, to hospitals and medical practices to improve coding efficiency.

⁇ SELF-TEST QUESTIONS

1. Briefly describe the coding system used at hospitals (ICD codes) and medical practices (CPT codes).

2. What is the link between coding and reimbursement?

THEME WRAP-UP   REVENUE SOURCES

Just hired to be Big Sky's practice manager and now learning the workings of the practice, Jen decided to first focus on the practice's revenues. Specifically, she wanted to answer two questions to better identify what steps might be taken to increase revenues and reduce the riskiness associated with those revenues: (1) where does Big Sky's revenue come from? (2) what methods do the payers use to determine the payment amount?

After reviewing Big Sky's revenue records, Jen found the following payer mix:

Commercial:		
Fee-for-service	37%	
Managed care	15	
Total	52%	
Government:		
Medicare	29%	
Medicaid	8	
Total	37%	
Miscellaneous:		
Self-pay	6%	
Other	5	
Total	11%	
Total	100%	

The largest category of payer for the practice is commercial insurance, with a total of 52 percent of revenues. (Note that commercial revenues include Blue Shield.) Of the commercial patients, 37 percent are enrolled in fee-for-service plans, while 15 percent are enrolled in managed care plans. Next largest is government programs (Medicare and Medicaid) with 37 percent, followed by self-pay with 6 percent and other sources at 5 percent. (Other sources consist of Workers' Compensation and other government programs, a small amount of charity care, and about 2 percent bad debt losses. Bad debt losses arise when patients who have the ability to pay fail to do so.) Although not shown in the table, 5 percent of Big Sky's revenues come from capitated contracts, while the remaining 95 percent are on a fee-for-service basis.

This payer mix should present few problems for Big Sky. In general, commercial insurers are considered to be more generous than government programs, so the revenue stream should be adequate and not overly dependent on payments influenced by political decisions. Also, bad debt losses appear not to be a major concern for the practice.

Because Big Sky's revenue stream is mostly fee-for-service, the physicians have an overall incentive to increase production—that is, to perform more procedures and hence increase revenues. However, the incentive for capitated patients (which make up 5 percent of revenues) is to provide only the services that are absolutely needed. Do the physicians know which patients are fee-for-service and which are capitated? You bet! Although capitated revenues provide a steady stream of monthly payments to the practice, they bring with them utilization risk. However, with only a small percentage of capitated revenues, this risk is minimal.

All in all, Big Sky's revenue stream appears sound, with no significant negatives. That's the good news for Jen. The bad news is that now she must tackle an issue that is potentially more difficult to deal with: examining Big Sky's costs and balancing them against the revenue stream.

KEY CONCEPTS

This chapter explores the insurance function, the third-party-payer system, and reimbursement methods. Here are the key concepts:

➤ Health insurance is widely used in the United States because individuals are *risk averse* and insurers can spread the financial risk over a large population.

➤ *Adverse selection* occurs when individuals most likely to have claims purchase insurance, while those least likely to have claims do not.

➤ *Moral hazard* occurs when an insured individual purposely sustains a loss, as opposed to a random loss. In a health insurance setting, moral hazard is more subtle, producing such behaviors as seeking more services than needed and engaging in unhealthy behavior because the potential costs are borne by someone else.

➤ Insurers are classified as either private or public (governmental). The major private insurers are *Blue Cross and Blue Shield*, *commercial insurers*, and *self-insurers*.

➤ The government is a major insurer and direct provider of healthcare services. The two major forms of government health insurance are *Medicare* and *Medicaid*.

➤ When payers pay *billed charges*, they pay according to the schedule of charge rates established by the provider in its *chargemaster*.

➤ *Negotiated charges*, which are *discounted* from billed (chargemaster) charges, are often used by insurers in conjunction with managed care plans.

➤ Under a *retrospective cost* system, the payer agrees to pay the provider certain allowable costs that are incurred in providing services to the payer's enrollees.

➤ In a *prospective payment system*, the rates are determined in advance and are not tied directly to either reimbursable costs or billed charges. Typically, prospective payments are made on the basis of the following service definitions: (1) *per procedure*, (2) *per diagnosis*, (3) *per diem* (per day), or (4) *global reimbursement*.

➤ In 1983, the federal government adopted the *inpatient prospective payment system (IPPS)* for Medicare hospital inpatient reimbursement. Under this system, the amount of payment is fixed by the patient's diagnosis, as indicated by the *diagnosis-related group (DRG)*.

➤ Physicians are reimbursed by Medicare using the *resource-based relative value scale (RBRVS)* system. Under RBRVS, reimbursement is based on three resource components: (1) *physician work*, (2) *practice (overhead) expenses*, and (3) *malpractice insurance*.

➤ *International Classification of Diseases* (most commonly known by the abbreviation *ICD*) codes are used for designating diseases plus a wide variety of signs, symptoms, and external causes of injury.

➤ *Current Procedural Terminology (CPT)* codes are used to specify medical procedures (treatments).

The information in this chapter plays a vital role in financial decision making in heathcare organizations. Thus, we will use it over and over in future chapters.

END-OF-CHAPTER QUESTIONS

3.1 Briefly describe the major third-party payers.

3.2 a. What are the primary characteristics of managed care organizations (MCOs)?
     b. Describe two different types of MCOs.

3.3 What is the difference between fee-for-service reimbursement and capitation?

3.4 What is pay for performance?

3.5 Describe provider incentives and risks under each of the following reimbursement
     methods:
     a. Cost-based
     b. Charge-based, including discounted charges
     c. Prospective payment
     d. Capitation

3.6 Briefly describe the coding systems for diseases (diagnoses) and procedures.

3.7 How does Medicare reimburse hospitals for inpatient stays?

3.8 How does Medicare reimburse physician services?

PLANNING, MANAGING, AND CONTROL

In Part II, we begin our discussion of the actual practice of healthcare finance. Here, the major topics are planning, managing, and control, which span four chapters.

Chapter 4 addresses cost estimation, the foundation of managerial accounting. If an organization does not know its costs, its business decisions are doomed to failure.

Chapter 5 adds pricing and revenues to the cost picture. After both revenues and costs are estimated, managers can estimate profits and, more importantly, the effect of changing assumptions about volume, costs, and prices on profits.

Chapter 6 covers the important subject of planning and budgeting. If healthcare businesses did not plan for the future, they would be operating at the whims of the economic environment. During planning and budgeting, specific operational goals are set along with a plan for meeting these goals.

Chapter 7 contains several topics related to operational and financial management, with emphasis on how managers monitor operations to ensure that the goals set in the planning and budgeting process are met.

CHAPTER 4

ESTIMATING COSTS

THEME SET-UP   COST STRUCTURE

As you know from Chapter 3, Big Sky Dermatology Specialists is a small group practice located in Jackson, Wyoming. Jen Latimer, a recent health administration graduate and newly hired manager for the group, completed her review of Big Sky's revenue sources. Now she wants to take a closer look at Big Sky's cost structure.

Jen remembers from her healthcare finance courses that a business's costs can be classified in several ways, with the two major ones being (1) the relationship of the cost to the amount of services offered (does the cost increase as volume increases?) and (2) the relationship of the cost to the subunit being analyzed (does the cost go away if the subunit is abolished?).

As she thought about these classifications, she breathed a sigh of relief. Big Sky was not formally divided into departments (subunits), so a system would not have to be developed to allocate overhead costs, such as billing expenses, to separate departments within the practice. Still, she had to identify costs that are not tied to volume (fixed costs) and costs that are tied to volume (variable costs). By identifying these two types of costs, Jen would be able to forecast Big

Sky's profit potential under different volume (number of visits) assumptions.

By the end of this chapter, you will have a better appreciation for the costs inherent in healthcare businesses and how those costs are classified. Then you, like Jen, will be able to apply this knowledge to estimate the cost structure of Big Sky Dermatology Specialists.

LEARNING OBJECTIVES

After studying this chapter, you will be able to

➤ Discuss the nature and purpose of managerial accounting.

➤ Explain how costs are classified according to their relationship with volume.

➤ Describe how costs are classified according to their relationship with the unit being analyzed.

➤ Answer why proper cost allocation is important to healthcare organizations.

➤ Define the terms cost pool and cost driver, and describe the characteristics of a good cost driver.

➤ List the three primary methods used to allocate overhead costs among revenue-producing (patient services) departments.

➤ Articulate the differences between traditional costing and activity-based costing.

4.1 INTRODUCTION

Healthcare managers have many responsibilities. The more important ones include planning for the future, establishing policies that control the operations of the organization, and overseeing the day-to-day activities of line employees.

For example, the practice manager of a primary care practice must estimate future demand (volume) and see to it that the practice has the facilities, staff, and supplies necessary to meet this demand. This is accomplished primarily with budgets that use forecasted future volume to estimate the resources needed to meet expected patient needs. As the future unfolds, the practice manager must monitor operations to see if the volume estimates were correct. If not, supplies and staffing requirements must be adjusted to reflect variations from forecasts. Finally, the practice manager must constantly review the resources used to ensure that they are being acquired at the lowest possible costs.

All of these activities require information, a great deal of it. Furthermore, this information has to be presented in a format that facilitates analysis, interpretation, and decision making. Without timely and relevant information, healthcare managers would be making decisions in the dark. Of course, accurate information does not ensure good decision making, but without it the chances of making good decisions are almost nil.

The foundation of a good information system is the ability to estimate costs with confidence. This is not an easy task. You may be able to precisely estimate the cost of your college education—just add up the costs of tuition, books and supplies, room and board, and so on. However, what about the costs of healthcare organizations? Their overall (total) costs can be measured with some precision, such as the total costs of running a hospital or a medical practice. But what about the costs of running the emergency department, or the costs associated with Medicare patients, or the costs of treating patients who have had heart attacks? Estimating these costs with confidence is essential to sound management, yet estimating costs associated with departments, payers, and patients is not easy.

Although cost estimation has a multitude of problems, it is far too important to the financial well-being of healthcare providers to do in a sloppy way. Thus, organizations put a lot of time and effort into doing the best possible job at it.

4.2 THE BASICS OF MANAGERIAL ACCOUNTING

Accounting is split into two primary areas: managerial accounting and financial accounting. Whereas financial accounting (which is discussed in Chapters 11 and 12) focuses on the reporting of operational and financial results to outsiders, **managerial accounting** focuses on the development of information used internally for managerial decision making.

Managerial accounting information is used for routine budgeting processes, allocation of managerial bonuses, and pricing and service decisions, all of which deal with subunits of an organization. In addition, managerial accounting data can be compiled for special purposes, such as assessing alternative modes of delivery or projecting the profitability of a particular reimbursement contract.

CRITICAL CONCEPT
Managerial Accounting

The accounting function within businesses is broken down into two major areas: managerial accounting and financial accounting. Financial accounting, which is covered later in the book, involves the creation of statements that report what has occurred at the organization. Managerial accounting concerns the creation and use of data to manage current operations. Thus, managerial accounting produces reports that focus on future activities at various levels within an organization, such as departments or contracts or specific services.

Cost

A resource use associated with providing, or supporting, a specific service.

Because managers are more concerned with what will happen in the future than with what has happened in the past, managerial accounting is for the most part forward-looking. Because most of the future is unknown, managerial accounting information requires many assumptions about future events. For example, as managers create budgets, they often must make assumptions regarding utilization (volume), reimbursement, and costs.

A critical part of managerial accounting is the measurement of costs. Unfortunately, there is no single definition of the term *cost*. Rather, different costs exist for different purposes. As a general rule for healthcare providers, a cost involves a resource use associated with providing, or supporting, a specific service. However, the cost-per-service identified for pricing purposes can differ from the cost-per-service used for management control purposes. Also, the cost-per-service used for long-range planning purposes may differ from the cost-per-service defined for short-term purposes. Thus, when dealing with costs, managers have to understand the context so that the correct cost is identified. To further complicate matters, costs do not necessarily reflect actual cash outflows.

Costs are classified in two primary ways: by their relationship to the volume (amount) of services provided and by their relationship to the unit (i.e., department) being analyzed. This chapter focuses on these two cost classifications. Then, in Chapter 5, we add revenues to the mix and show how to convert cost estimates into profit estimates.

(?) SELF-TEST QUESTIONS

1. What is the primary purpose of managerial accounting information?

2. What is meant by cost?

3. What are the two primary ways that costs can be classified?

4.3 COST CLASSIFICATION I: FIXED VERSUS VARIABLE COSTS

One way to define (classify) costs is on the basis of their relationship to the amount of services provided, often referred to as volume or utilization. Future volume—the number of patient days, visits, enrollees, laboratory tests, and so on—is almost always uncertain.

Volume may be forecast in a number of ways. One way is to review historical trends, say, over the past five to ten years. In many situations, the past is a good predictor of the future. If this is thought to be the case, then statistical analysis (linear regression) can be applied to the historical data to predict future volumes. If past data are not available or if significant changes in the operating environment are taking place, then volume forecasting becomes more difficult. In that case, it is necessary to evaluate population and disease trends in the service area, actions of competitors, pricing strategies, the impact of new contracts with insurers, and a whole host of additional factors that influence future volume.

If a provider's volume forecast is off, the consequences can be severe. First, if the market for any particular service expands more than expected and planned for, then the provider will not be able to meet its patients' needs. Potential patients will end up going elsewhere, and the business will lose market share and perhaps miss a major opportunity. On the other hand, if projections are overly optimistic, the provider could end up with excess equipment, supplies, and staff, and hence costs that are higher than necessary.

In spite of the difficulties in forecasting volume, managers typically have some idea of the potential range. For example, the manager of Northside Clinic, a small walk-in clinic, might estimate that the total number of patient visits for next year could range from 12,000 to 14,000 or from about 34 to 40 per day. If utilization is not likely to fall outside of these bounds, then the range of 12,000 to 14,000 annual visits defines the clinic's *relevant range*. Note that the relevant range pertains to a particular time period—in this case, next year. For other time periods, the relevant range might differ from this estimate.

Volume
The amount of services provided; for example, number of visits or inpatient days. Also called utilization.

Relevant range
The likely range of volume (utilization) over some time period. It defines the volume limits over which the organization's cost structure holds.

FIXED COSTS

Some costs, called **fixed costs**, are more or less known with certainty, regardless of the level of volume within the relevant range. For example, Northside Clinic has a labor force that would be increased or decreased only under unusual circumstances. Thus, as long as volume falls within the relevant range of 12,000 to 14,000 patient visits, labor costs at the clinic are fixed for the coming year. The actual number of visits might turn out to be 12,352 or 13,877, but labor costs will remain at their forecasted level as long as volume falls within the relevant range. Other examples of the clinic's fixed costs include expenditures on facilities (e.g., rent, property

> ### ⚠ CRITICAL CONCEPT
> Fixed Versus Variable Costs
>
> One way of classifying costs is by their relationship to volume. Fixed costs are known and predictable regardless of volume (within some relevant range). Conversely, variable costs depend on the volume of services supplied. Consider a clinical laboratory. The costs of the building, equipment, and personnel to run the lab are known with some certainty for the coming year. Furthermore, these costs are independent of the number of tests actually conducted. Such costs are fixed. But the annual costs of reagents and other test supplies depend on the number (and type) of tests conducted—the greater the number of tests, the greater these costs. Thus, these costs are classified as variable costs.

taxes, and utilities), diagnostic equipment, and information systems. After an organization has acquired these assets, it typically is locked into them for some period of time regardless of volume fluctuations, so these costs are known beforehand.

Of course, no costs are fixed over the long run and over large volume changes. At some point of increasing volume, healthcare businesses must incur additional fixed costs for new property and equipment, additional staffing, and so on. Likewise, if volume decreases by a substantial amount, an organization likely would reduce fixed costs by shedding part of its fixed assets and labor base.

VARIABLE COSTS

Whereas some costs are fixed regardless of volume (within the relevant range), other resources are more or less consumed as volume dictates. Costs that are related to (depend on) volume are called **variable costs**. For example, the costs of the clinical supplies (e.g., rubber gloves, tongue depressors, and hypodermics) used by Northside would be classified as variable costs. Also, some of the clinic's diagnostic equipment is leased on a per use basis (a fixed payment each time the equipment is used), which converts the cost of the equipment from a fixed cost to a variable cost. Finally, some healthcare organizations pay their employees on the basis of the amount of work performed, which would convert labor costs from fixed to variable. The bottom line here is that fixed costs are independent of the volume of services delivered (within the relevant range), while variable costs depend on volume.

UNDERLYING COST STRUCTURE (COST BEHAVIOR)

Healthcare managers are vitally interested in how costs are affected by changes in the amount of services supplied (volume). The relationship between costs and volume, called underlying cost structure, is used by managers in planning, control, and decision making. The primary reason for defining an organization's **underlying cost structure** is to provide managers with a tool for forecasting costs (and ultimately profits) at different volume levels.

(!) CRITICAL CONCEPT
Underlying Cost Structure

The underlying cost structure of a business defines the relationship between volume and costs. To illustrate, assume you plan to sell customized pens to your classmates to make some extra money. To get started, you paid someone $50 to design the logo for the pens. Then, each pen costs you $1.75. The cost structure of your pen business consists of $50 in fixed costs and a variable cost rate of $1.75. Thus, the cost structure of the business can be written as:

Total costs = $50 + ($1.75 x Volume).

If you sell 100 pens, your total costs are $225:

Total costs = $50 + ($1.75 x Volume)
$\qquad$ = $50 + ($1.75 x 100)
$\qquad$ = $50 + $175
$\qquad$ = $225.

To illustrate the concept of cost behavior, consider the hypothetical cost data presented in Table 4.1 for a hospital's clinical laboratory. The underlying cost structure consists of both fixed and variable costs—that is, some of the costs are expected to be volume sensitive and some are not. This structure of both fixed and variable costs is typical in healthcare organizations as well as most other businesses. For illustrative purposes, let's assume the relevant range is from zero to 20,000 tests. (Of course, the actual relevant range might be from 15,000 to 20,000 tests.)

As noted in Table 4.1, the laboratory has $150,000 in fixed costs that consist primarily of labor, facilities, and equipment costs. These costs will occur even if the laboratory does not perform one test, assuming it is kept open. In addition to the fixed costs, each test, on average, requires $10 in laboratory supplies, such as glass slides and reagents.

The per unit (per test, in this example) variable cost of $10 is defined as the *variable cost rate*. If laboratory volume doubles—for example, from 500 to 1,000 tests—total variable costs will double from $5,000 to $10,000. However, the variable cost rate of $10 per test remains the same whether the test is the first, the hundredth, or the thousandth. *Total variable costs*, therefore, increase or decrease proportionately as volume changes, but the variable cost rate remains constant.

Fixed costs, in contrast to total variable costs, remain unchanged as the volume varies. When volume doubles from 500 to 1,000 tests, fixed costs remain at $150,000. Because all costs in this example are either fixed or variable, *total costs* are merely the sum of the two. For example, at 5,000 tests, total costs are Fixed costs + Total variable costs = $150,000 + (5,000 × $10) = $150,000 + $50,000 = $200,000. Because variable costs are tied to volume, total variable costs, and hence total costs, increase as the volume increases, even though fixed costs remain constant.

The rightmost column in Table 4.1 contains *average cost* per unit of volume, which in this example is average cost per test. It is calculated by dividing total costs by volume. For example, at 5,000 tests, with total costs of $200,000, the average cost per test is $200,000 / 5,000 = $40. Because fixed costs are spread over more tests as volume increases, the average cost per test declines as volume increases. For example, when volume doubles from 5,000 to 10,000 tests, fixed costs remain at $150,000, but fixed cost per test declines from $150,000 / 5,000 = $30 to $150,000 / 10,000 = $15.

With fixed cost per test declining from $30 to $15, the average cost per test goes down from $30 + $10 = $40 to $15 + $10 = $25. The fact that higher volume reduces average fixed cost and average cost per unit of volume has important implications on the effect of volume changes on profitability. This point will be made clear in a later section. (In economics, the situation of declining average cost as volume increases is called *economies of scale*.)

The cost behavior presented in Table 4.1 in tabular format is presented in graphical format in Figure 4.1. Here, costs are shown on the vertical (Y) axis, and volume (number of tests)

Variable cost rate
The added cost for each additional unit of service. For example, the variable cost rate at a walk-in clinic might be $5 per patient visit.

Total variable costs
The variable cost rate multiplied by volume. For example, if a walk-in clinic has a variable cost rate of $5 per visit and 10,000 visits annually, total variable costs for the year equal $50,000.

Total cost
For purposes here, the sum of fixed costs and total variable costs.

Average cost
Total costs divided by volume. For example, if laboratory costs total $300,000 to conduct 15,000 tests, the average cost (per test) is $20.

Economies of scale
The situation in which higher volume leads to lower per unit cost.

TABLE 4.1

Cost Behavior
Illustration: Fixed
and Variable Costs

Variable Cost per Test		Fixed Costs per Year	
Laboratory supplies	$10	Labor	$100,000
		Other fixed costs	50,000
			$150,000

Volume	Fixed Costs	Total Variable Costs	Total Costs	Average Cost per Test
0	$150,000	$ 0	$150,000	—
1	150,000	10	150,010	$150,010.00
50	150,000	500	150,500	3,010.00
100	150,000	1,000	151,000	1,510.00
500	150,000	5,000	155,000	310.00
1,000	150,000	10,000	160,000	160.00
5,000	150,000	50,000	200,000	40.00
10,000	150,000	100,000	250,000	25.00
15,000	150,000	150,000	300,000	20.00
20,000	150,000	200,000	350,000	17.50

FIGURE 4.1

Cost Behavior
Graph

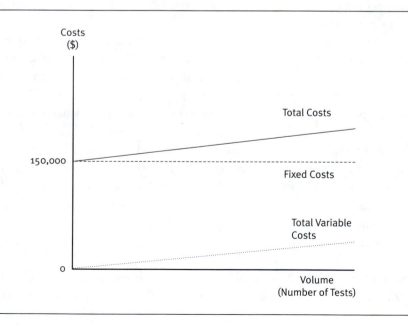

is shown on the horizontal (X) axis. Because fixed costs are independent of volume, they are shown as a horizontal dashed line at $150,000. Total variable costs appear as an upward-sloping dotted line that starts at the origin (0 tests, $0 costs) and rises at a rate of $10 for each additional test. When fixed and total variable costs are combined to obtain total costs, the result is the upward-sloping solid line parallel to the total variable costs line but beginning at the Y axis at a value of $150,000 (the fixed costs amount). In effect, the total costs line is nothing more than the total variable costs line shifted upward by the amount of fixed costs.

Note that Figure 4.1 is not drawn to scale. Furthermore, the relevant range is unrealistically large. The intent here is to emphasize the general shape of a cost behavior graph and not its exact position. Also, note that total variable costs plot as a straight line (linear), because the variable cost rate is assumed to be constant over the relevant range. We assume throughout the book that the variable cost rate is constant, and hence total variable costs are linear, at least within the relevant range. For most healthcare organizations in most situations, such an assumption is not unreasonable.

Before we leave this illustration of underlying cost structure, we should mention that fixed and variable costs represent two ends of the volume classification spectrum. Here, within the relevant range, the costs are either independent of volume (fixed) or directly related to volume (variable). A third classification, *semi-fixed costs*, falls in between the two extremes. To illustrate, assume that the actual relevant range of volume for the clinical laboratory is 15,000 to 20,000 tests. However, the laboratory's current workforce can only handle up to 17,500 tests per year, so an additional technician, at an annual cost of $35,000, would be required if volume exceeds that level. Now, labor costs are fixed from 15,000 to 17,500 tests and then again fixed at a higher level from 17,500 to 20,000 tests, but they are not fixed at the same level throughout the entire relevant range of 15,000 to 20,000 tests. Semi-fixed costs are fixed within ranges of volume, but there are multiple ranges of semi-fixed costs within the relevant range. To keep things manageable, we will not include semi-fixed costs in our examples in this book.

Semi-fixed costs
Costs that are fixed, but not at a single amount throughout the entire relevant range.

⑦ SELF-TEST QUESTIONS

1. Define the term "relevant range."

2. Explain the features and provide examples of fixed and variable costs.

3. How does time period affect the definition of fixed costs?

4. What is meant by underlying cost structure?

5. Sketch and explain a simple cost structure diagram similar to Figure 4.1.

6. What are semi-fixed costs?

4.4 Cost Classification II: Direct Versus Indirect (Overhead) Costs

The second major cost classification is by relationship to the unit being analyzed. Some costs—about 50 percent of a large healthcare organization's cost structure—are unique to the reporting subunit and hence usually can be identified with relative certainty. To illustrate, again think in terms of a hospital's clinical laboratory. Certain costs are unique to the laboratory; for example, the salaries and benefits for the technicians who work there and the costs of the equipment and supplies used to conduct the tests. These costs, which would not occur if the laboratory were closed, are classified as the **direct costs** of the department.

Unfortunately, direct costs constitute only a portion of the laboratory's total costs. The remaining resources used by the laboratory are **not** unique to the laboratory; the laboratory shares many resources of the hospital. For example, the laboratory shares the hospital's physical space as well as its infrastructure, which includes information systems, utilities, housekeeping, maintenance, medical records, and general administration. The costs not borne solely by the laboratory but shared by all of the hospital's departments are called **indirect (overhead) costs**.

Indirect costs, in contrast to direct costs, are more difficult to measure at the department level because they arise from shared resources—that is, if the laboratory were closed, the indirect costs would not disappear. Perhaps some indirect costs could be reduced, but the hospital still requires a basic infrastructure to operate its remaining departments. Note that the direct/indirect classification has relevance only at the subunit level. When the entire organization is considered, all costs are direct.

The two cost classifications (fixed/variable and direct/indirect) overlay one another. That is, fixed costs typically include both direct and indirect costs, while variable costs generally include only direct costs. For example, the fixed costs of a hospital laboratory include both labor (a direct cost) and facilities (an overhead cost) costs, but the variable costs (reagents and other supplies) are all direct costs. Conversely, direct costs usually include fixed and variable costs, while indirect costs typically include only fixed costs.

Although this mixing of cost classifications can give anyone a headache, the good news is that the classifications typically are used independent of one another.

(!) CRITICAL CONCEPT
Direct Versus Indirect (Overhead) Costs

In addition to their relationship to volume, costs can be classified by their relationship to the unit being analyzed. Those costs that are unique to a department, and hence would disappear if the department were abolished, are called direct costs. Costs incurred from the use of resources shared across the organization are classified as indirect (overhead) costs. For example, the costs of the supplies used by a hospital's emergency department are direct costs; they would disappear if the department were closed. But the costs of facilities (the space used) remain, so they represent overhead costs to the emergency department.

4.5 COST ALLOCATION

A critical part of cost measurement at the department level is the assignment, or allocation, of overhead costs. *Cost allocation* is a process within the organization whereby managers allocate the costs of one department to other departments. Because this process does not occur in a marketplace setting, no observable prices exist for the transferred services. Thus, cost allocation within a business must, to the extent possible, establish prices that mimic those that would be set under market conditions.

What costs within a healthcare organization must be allocated? Typically, the costs associated with the facilities and support personnel of the business, such as administrators, financial staffs, and housekeeping and maintenance personnel, must be allocated to those departments that generate revenues for the organization (generally, patient services departments). The allocation of support costs to patient services departments is necessary because there would be no need for support costs if there were no patient services departments. Thus, decisions regarding pricing and service offerings by the patient services departments must be based on the *total (full) costs* associated with each service, including both direct and overhead costs. Clearly, the proper allocation of overhead costs is essential to good decision making within healthcare organizations.

The goal of cost allocation is to assign all of the costs of an organization to the activities that cause them to be incurred. Ideally, healthcare managers track and assign costs by individual patient, physician, diagnosis, reimbursement contract, and so on. With complete cost data available in the organization's managerial accounting system, managers can make better decisions regarding how to control costs, what services should be offered, and how these services should be priced. Of course, the more data needed, the higher the costs of developing, implementing, and operating the system. As in all situations, the benefits associated with more accurate cost data must be weighed against the costs required to develop such data.

COST POOLS

To allocate costs, the first step is to identify the cost pools and drivers. Typically, a **cost pool** consists of all the direct costs of one support department. However, if the services of a single sup-

Cost allocation
The assignment (allocation) of overhead costs, such as financial services costs, to the patient services departments.

Total (full) costs
For purposes here, the sum of direct and indirect (overhead) costs. Thus, full costs include both direct and overhead costs.

CRITICAL CONCEPT
Cost Pool

A cost pool is a group of overhead costs to be allocated to the patient services departments. Typically, a cost pool consists of all of the direct costs of one overhead department. For example, the costs associated with the Housekeeping Department might constitute a cost pool. However, if an overhead department provides different types of support services, the direct costs of that department might be divided into several cost pools, one for each type of service supplied. For example, the Administrative Support Department might provide both human resources services and information technology services. If the patient services departments use these support services in varying proportions, the overhead department should be divided into two cost pools.

CRITICAL CONCEPT
Cost Driver

A cost driver is the basis for allocating a cost pool. For example, if the cost pool consists of the direct costs of the Housekeeping Department, then the cost driver might be the amount of space occupied by each patient services department. The theory here is that the greater the amount of square footage occupied by a patient services department, the greater the amount of housekeeping services required. Good cost drivers have two important attributes: (1) They are perceived by all involved as being fair, and (2) they promote organizational cost reduction. Put another way, good cost drivers allocate the greatest amount of overhead costs to those patient services departments that use the most overhead services and create incentives for department heads to use less overhead services.

port department differ substantially (in the sense that the patient services departments use different relative amounts), the costs of that support department may need to be separated into multiple pools.

For example, suppose a hospital's Financial Services Department provides two significantly different services: patient billing and managerial budgeting. Furthermore, assume that the Routine Care Department uses proportionally more patient billing services than the Laboratory Department does, but Laboratory proportionally uses more budgeting services than Routine Care does. In this situation, it would be best to create two cost pools for one support department. To do this, the total costs of Financial Services would be divided into a billing pool and a budgeting pool. Then, cost drivers would be chosen for each pool and the costs allocated to the patient services departments as described in the following sections.

COST DRIVERS

One of the most important steps in the cost allocation process is the identification of proper **cost drivers**. The theoretical basis for identifying cost drivers is the extent to which the costs from a pool actually vary as the value of the driver changes. For example, does a department with 10,000 square feet of space use twice the amount of housekeeping services as a department with only 5,000 square feet of space? The closer the relationship (correlation) between actual overhead resource expenditures at each patient services department and the value of the cost driver, the better the cost driver and hence the better the resulting cost allocations.

Good cost drivers possess two characteristics. The first is fairness—that is, do the cost drivers chosen result in an allocation that is equitable to the patient services departments? The second, and perhaps more important, characteristic is cost reduction—that is, do the cost drivers chosen create incentives for departments to use less overhead services? For example, inpatient department managers can do little to influence overhead cost allocations if the cost driver for administrative support is patient days. In fact, the action needed to reduce the overhead allocation—reduction in patient days—would likely lead to negative financial consequences for the organization. A good cost driver encourages patient services department managers to take overhead cost reduction actions that do not have negative implications for the organization.

THE ALLOCATION PROCESS

The steps involved in allocating overhead costs are summarized in Table 4.2, which illustrates how Prairie View Clinic allocated its housekeeping costs for the 2009 budget.

First, the cost pool must be established. In this case, the clinic is allocating housekeeping costs, so the cost pool is the projected total costs of the Housekeeping Department, $100,000.

Second, the best cost driver must be identified. After considerable investigation, Prairie View's managers conclude that the best cost driver for housekeeping costs is labor hours—that is, the number of hours of housekeeping services required by the clinic's departments is the measure most closely related to the actual cost of providing these services. The intent here, of course, is to pick the cost driver that provides the most accurate cause-and-effect relationship between the use of housekeeping services and the costs of the Housekeeping Department.

Step One: Determine the cost pool.

    The departmental costs to be allocated are for the Housekeeping Department, which has total budgeted costs of $100,000.

Step Two: Determine the cost driver.

    The best cost driver was judged to be the number of hours of housekeeping services provided. An expected total of 10,000 hours of such services will be provided to those departments that will receive the allocation.

Step Three: Calculate the allocation rate.

    $100,000 / 10,000 hours = $10 per hour of housekeeping services provided.

Step Four: Determine the allocation amount.

    Physical Therapy Department uses 3,000 hours of housekeeping services, so its allocation of Housekeeping Department overhead is $10 × 3,000 = $30,000.

TABLE 4.2
Prairie View Clinic: Allocation of Housekeeping Department Overhead to the Physical Therapy Department

Allocation rate
The numerical value
used to allocate a cost
pool to patient
services departments.
For example, $40 per
square foot of occupied
space.

Third, the allocation rate must be calculated. For 2009, Prairie View's managers estimate that Housekeeping will provide 10,000 hours of service to the departments that will receive the allocation. Now that the cost pool and cost driver have been defined and measured, the *allocation rate* is established by dividing the expected total overhead cost (the cost pool) by the expected total volume of the cost driver: $100,000 / 10,000 hours = $10 per hour of services provided. (Note that different allocation methods can identify different departments as the ones that will receive the allocation. In the example here, the relevant departments [the patient services departments] receive 10,000 hours of housekeeping service. If we had included the Financial Services Department in the allocation, the amount of service allocated might be 10,500 hours.)

Fourth, the allocation must be made to each department. To illustrate the allocation, consider Physical Therapy (PT), one of Prairie View's patient services departments. For 2009, PT is expected to use 3,000 hours of housekeeping services, so the dollar amount of housekeeping overhead allocated to PT is $10 × 3,000 = $30,000.

Other departments within the clinic will also use housekeeping services, and their allocations would be made in a similar manner. The $10 allocation rate per hour of services used is multiplied by the amount of each department's utilization of housekeeping services to obtain the dollar allocation. When all patient services departments are considered, the entire clinic is projected to use 10,000 hours of housekeeping services, so the total amount allocated must be $10 × 10,000 = $100,000, which is the amount in the cost pool. For any department, the amount allocated depends on both the allocation rate and the amount of overhead services utilized.

COST ALLOCATION METHODS

Mathematically, cost allocation can be accomplished in a variety of ways, and the method used is somewhat discretionary. No matter what method is chosen, all support department costs eventually must be allocated to the departments (primarily, patient services departments) that create the need for those costs.

Direct method
A cost allocation
method that allocates
overhead costs directly
to patient services departments and hence
does not recognize
services provided by
one support department to another.

The key differences among the methods are how support services provided by one department are allocated to other support departments. Figure 4.2 summarizes the three allocation methods. Prairie View Clinic has three support departments (Human Resources, Housekeeping, and Administration) and two patient services departments (Physical Therapy and Internal Medicine).

Under the *direct method*, shown in the top section of Figure 4.2, each support department's costs are allocated directly to the patient services departments that use the services. In the illustration, both Physical Therapy and Internal Medicine use the services of all three support departments, so the costs of each support department are allocated to both patient services departments. The key feature of the direct method, and the feature that makes it relatively simple to apply, is that none of the costs of providing sup-

FIGURE 4.2
Prairie View Clinic:
Alternative Cost
Allocation
Methods

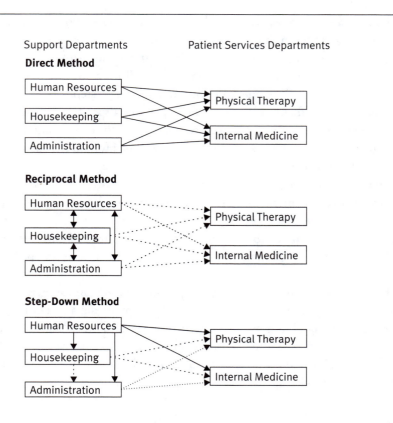

port services is allocated to other support departments. In effect, under the direct method, only the direct costs of the support departments are allocated to the patient services departments because no indirect costs have been created by intrasupport department allocations.

As shown in the center section of Figure 4.2, the *reciprocal method* recognizes the support department interdependencies among Human Resources, Housekeeping, and Administration, and hence the reciprocal method generally is considered to be more accurate and objective than the direct method. The reciprocal method derives its name from the fact that it recognizes all services that departments provide to and receive from other departments. The good news is that this method captures all of the intrasupport department relationships, so no information is ignored and no biases are introduced into the cost allocation process. The bad news is that the reciprocal method relies on the simultaneous solution of a series of equations representing the utilization of intrasupport department services. Thus, it is relatively complex, which makes explaining it to department heads difficult and implementing it costly.

Reciprocal method

A cost allocation method that fully recognizes all services provided from one support department to other support departments.

Step-down method
A cost allocation method that partially recognizes services provided from one support department to other support departments.

The *step-down method*, which is shown in the lower section of Figure 4.2, represents a compromise between the simplicity of the direct method and the complexity of the reciprocal method. It recognizes some of the intrasupport department effects that the direct method ignores, but it does not recognize the full range of interdependencies. The step-down method derives its name from the sequential, stair-step pattern of the allocation process, which requires that the allocation takes place in a specific sequence.

First, all the direct costs of Human Resources are allocated to both the patient services departments and the other two support departments. Human Resources is then closed out because all its costs have been allocated. Next, Housekeeping costs, which now consist of both direct and indirect costs (the allocation from Human Resources), are allocated to the patient services departments and the remaining support department—Administration. Finally, the direct and indirect costs of Administration are allocated to the patient services departments. The final allocation includes Human Resources, Housekeeping, and Administration costs because a portion of these support costs have been "stepped down" to Administration.

The critical difference between the step-down and reciprocal methods is that after each allocation is made in the step-down method, a support department is removed from the process. Even though Housekeeping and Administration provide support services back to Human Resources, these indirect costs are not recognized because Human Resources is removed from the allocation process after the initial allocation. Such costs are recognized in the reciprocal method.

(?) SELF-TEST QUESTIONS

1. What is the goal of cost allocation?

2. Under what conditions should a single overhead department be divided into multiple cost pools?

3. On what theoretical basis are cost drivers chosen?

4. What two characteristics make a good cost driver?

5. What are the four steps in the cost allocation process?

6. What are the three primary methods of cost allocation? How do they differ?

> **✳ INDUSTRY PRACTICE** The Cost Structures of Medical Practices
>
> Different healthcare organizations have different cost structures. Even within the same type of organization, cost structure differences occur. For example, medical practices that are hospital based, such as some radiology groups, tend to have low fixed costs (the hospital pays those). Conversely, other practices, such as cardiology, can have a great deal of diagnostic equipment and hence high fixed costs. In addition, the size of a practice will influence its underlying cost structure.
>
> Still, by examining the costs associated with a typical practice, we can get some feel for the cost structures involved. We have chosen a primary care practice to represent a typical medical practice. Because the costs involved in the practice are a function of the number of physicians in the practice, most of the data presented here are on a per physician basis.
>
> The average primary care practice has roughly five FTE physicians. (FTE stands for full-time equivalent, which adjusts for physicians who work only part time.) Each practice, on average, has two nonphysician providers, such as physician assistants and nurse practitioners, and a support staff of about 25. Thus, if we count the nonphysician providers as support staff for the physicians, each physician has more than five individuals working to support his or her patient services activities.
>
> Looking at costs, the total operating cost to support each physician is about $350,000, not including physician compensation. Of these costs, about $185,000 are labor costs, with the remaining costs devoted to facilities, equipment, malpractice insurance, and supplies. Thus, practice costs (again, excluding physician compensation) are about evenly split between labor and nonlabor components. Taking a closer look at support staff costs, about 61 percent of the labor costs are for clinical staff, 21 percent for front-office staff (receptionists and the like), and 18 percent for business-office staff (primarily coding, billing, and collections).
>
> On average, each primary care physician handles about 2,000 patients, who represent about 5,300 encounters (visits), during which the physician performs about 12,000 procedures. Thus, if we use patient visit as the unit of output (volume), the operating cost per visit averages out to be roughly $350,000 / 5,300 = $66 per visit. Unfortunately, the data do not break out fixed versus variable costs.
>
> *(Continued)*

(✱) **INDUSTRY PRACTICE** The Cost Structures of Medical Practices

However, variable costs, which consist mostly of administrative supplies (e.g., forms and letters) and medical supplies (e.g., rubber gloves, needles, vaccines, and dressings) are relatively small, say, $10 per visit. Thus, the underlying cost structure for an average primary care physician looks something like this:

Total costs = $297,000 + ($10 x Number of visits).

Here, the $297,000 represents the fixed costs of the practice (primarily facilities and labor), while the $10 represents the average cost of supplies consumed on each visit.

With this information, the support costs (on a per physician basis) can be estimated for different volumes. For example, the total cost to support 4,500 visits is $342,000, while the cost to support 5,500 visits is $352,000:

Total costs (4,500 visits) = $297,000 + ($10 x 4,500)
= $297,000 + $45,000
= $342,000

Total costs (5,500 visits) = $297,000 + ($10 x 5,500)
= $297,000 + $55,000
= $352,000.

In the next chapter, we expand this industry practice discussion to include revenues.

Note: This industry practice is based on data in Medical Group Management Association. 2006. *Performance and Practices of Successful Medical Groups*. Englewood, CO: MGMA.

Traditional costing methods

Traditional costing methods use the top-down approach to costing, wherein overhead costs are allocated "down" to patient services departments.

4.6 ACTIVITY-BASED COSTING

Our discussion thus far has focused on *traditional costing methods*. In essence, the traditional methods begin with costs at the department level. Then, the costs of support departments are allocated to the patient services departments. You can think of this approach as being top down (downstream), because organizational charts often show the support departments at the top and patient services departments at the bottom. Although traditional costing works well for estimating full costs at the department level, its usefulness for estimating the costs of activities within departments, such as individual tests, services, or diagnoses, is limited.

Activity-based costing (ABC) is a totally different approach to costing that uses an upstream approach to cost allocation. Its premise is that all costs within an organization stem from activities, hence its name. In ABC, because activities are considered to be the basic building blocks of costs, costs can be more easily assigned to individual patients, individual physicians, particular diagnoses, reimbursement contracts, managed care populations, and so on.

The steps required to implement ABC are as follows:

◆ Identify the relevant activities.

◆ Determine the cost of each activity, including equipment and supplies and both direct and overhead costs.

◆ Determine the cost drivers for the activity.

◆ Collect activity data for each service.

◆ Calculate the total cost of the service by aggregating activity costs.

> **⚠ CRITICAL CONCEPT**
> **Activity-Based Costing**
>
> Activity-based costing (ABC) is an alternative to traditional costing. For example, consider the costs associated with a particular service. To apply ABC costing, first identify the activities needed to provide the service. Next, estimate the cost of each activity. The sum of the activity costs, then, reflects the cost of providing that service. For example, the activities required to give a vaccination include check-in, administration of the shot, recording the treatment, and check-out. In ABC, the cost of each of these activities would be estimated (including supplies and overhead costs) and then summed to estimate the cost of a vaccination.

To illustrate ABC, suppose that there are seven activities performed at a family practice clinic: (1) patient check-in, including insurance verification; (2) preliminary assessment; (3) diagnosis; (4) treatment; (5) prescription writing; (6) patient check-out; and (7) third-party-payer billing. Furthermore, assume that the clinic has 10,000 visits annually split evenly between two services: A and B. (Before we go further, note that this example is highly simplified. Its purpose is merely to give you a flavor for how ABC works.)

Table 4.3 contains the initial data and allocation rate calculations. For example, the annual costs of patient check-in, consisting of clerical labor and supplies (direct costs) plus space and other overhead (indirect costs), are $50,000 to support 10,000 total visits, giving an allocation rate of $5 per visit. Also, the total (direct labor by a nurse and overhead) costs required to conduct the initial assessment is $75,000, spread over (5,000 visits × 5 minutes for A) + (5,000 visits × 10 minutes for B) = 25,000 + 50,000 = 75,000 minutes annually, giving an allocation rate of $1 per minute.

TABLE 4.3
ABC Illustration: Initial Data and Allocation Rate Calculation

Activity	Annual Costs	Cost Driver	Activity Data Service A	Service B	Total	Allocation Rate
Check-in	$ 50,000	Number of visits	5,000	5,000	10,000	$ 5.00
Assessment	75,000	Number of minutes per visit	5	10	75,000	1.00
Diagnosis	250,000	Number of minutes per visit	10	15	125,000	2.00
Treatment	450,000	Number of minutes per visit	10	20	150,000	3.00
Prescription	2,500	Number of drugs prescribed per visit	0.5	2.0	12,500	0.20
Check-out	50,000	Number of visits	5,000	5,000	10,000	5.00
Billing	150,000	Number of bills per visit	1.0	2.0	15,000	10.00
Total costs	$1,027,500					

TABLE 4.4
ABC Illustration: Final Aggregation of Activity Costs per Visit

Activity	Cost Driver	Rate	Service A Consumption	Cost	Service B Consumption	Cost
Check-in	Number of visits	$ 5.00	1	$ 5.00	1	$ 5.00
Assessment	Number of minutes	1.00	5	5.00	10	10.00
Diagnosis	Number of minutes	2.00	10	20.00	15	30.00
Treatment	Number of minutes	3.00	10	30.00	20	60.00
Prescription	Number of drugs	0.20	0.5	0.10	2.0	0.40
Check-out	Number of visits	5.00	1	5.00	1	5.00
Billing	Number of bills	10.00	1.0	10.00	2.0	20.00
Total cost per service				$75.10		$130.40

As shown in Table 4.4, the final step is to aggregate the activity costs for each service. Note that this is done on a per visit basis. For example, for Service A, the cost of check-in is 1 visit × $5.00 = $5.00, the cost of assessment is 5 minutes per visit × $1.00 = $5.00, and the cost of diagnosis is 10 minutes per visit × $2.00 = $20.00. Other activity costs for the two services are calculated in a similar manner.

The end result of summing the individual activity costs associated with each service is a total cost of $75.10 for Service A and $130.40 for Service B. The ability of the family practice to estimate the costs of its individual services allows the services to be priced properly (on the basis of costs). In addition, cost control is made easier because the activities, and hence resource expenditures, associated with each service have been clearly identified.

Note that the total annual costs of providing Service A are 5,000 visits × $75.10 = $375,500, while the total costs for Service B are 5,000 visits × $130.40 = $652,000. Because we only have two services in this simple example, the total costs of the practice are $375,500 + $652,000 = $1,027,500, which equals the total cost amount identified in Table 4.3.

ABC allows managers to estimate the costs of individual services, and hence provides managers with information that can be used in pricing and contract negotiations. However, the data and resource requirements to establish an ABC system far exceed those required for traditional costing. For this reason, traditional costing still dominates the scene, but ABC is becoming more prevalent as the need for better cost data becomes more important and providers invest in newer and more powerful managerial accounting systems.

(?) SELF-TEST QUESTIONS

1. What are the key differences between traditional and activity-based costing (ABC)?

2. Why does ABC hold so much promise for healthcare providers?

THEME WRAP-UP   COST STRUCTURE

What did Jen learn about the cost structure at Big Sky Dermatology Specialists? Well, first the good news. Because the practice is relatively small, with two dermatologists and support staff, it does not have a departmental organization. To think of it another way, the entire practice is a single department. Thus, Jen does not have to grapple with allocating overhead costs from one department to another. Certainly, the practice has both patient services functions and overhead functions, but all within a single organizational structure.

On the other hand, the practice does have both fixed and variable costs. In fact, finding a healthcare provider with either all fixed costs or all variable costs would be impossible, although as shown in the next chapter businesses can have an incentive to move their cost structures in one direction or the other.

After some research, Jen concluded that Big Sky's cost structure (not including physician compensation) can be expressed as follows:

$$
\begin{aligned}
\text{Total costs} &= \text{Fixed costs} + \quad \text{Total variable costs} \\
&= \text{Fixed costs} + (\text{Variable cost rate} \times \text{Volume}) \\
&= \$850,000 \quad + \quad (\$15 \times 10,000 \text{ visits}) \\
&= \$850,000 \quad + \quad \$150,000 \\
&= \$1,000,000.
\end{aligned}
$$

Furthermore, the relevant range for the number of visits is 8,000 to 12,000. Thus, if the number of visits were at the bottom of the range (8,000), total support costs would be

$$
\begin{aligned}
\text{Total costs} &= \$850,000 + (\$15 \times 8,000 \text{ visits}) \\
&= \$850,000 + \quad \$120,000 \\
&= \$970,000.
\end{aligned}
$$

But if the number of visits were at the top of the range (12,000), total support costs would equal

$$
\begin{aligned}
\text{Total costs} &= \$850,000 + (\$15 \times 12,000 \text{ visits}) \\
&= \$850,000 + \quad \$180,000 \\
&= \$1,030,000.
\end{aligned}
$$

With this knowledge of Big Sky's cost structure, the next job that Jen must tackle is to combine the practice's cost structure with its revenues to examine the practice's expected profitability. We will help Jen with that task in the next chapter.

KEY CONCEPTS

This chapter points out that managers rely on managerial accounting information to plan for and control a business's operations. A critical part of managerial accounting information is the measurement and allocation of costs. Here are the key concepts:

➤ Costs can be classified by their relationship to the *amount of services provided*. *Variable costs* are costs that are expected to increase and decrease with volume (patient days, number of visits, and so on), while *fixed costs* are costs that are expected to remain constant regardless of volume (within some *relevant range*).

➤ The relationship between cost and activity (volume) is called *underlying cost structure*.

➤ Costs can also be classified according to their relationship to the *unit being analyzed*. *Direct costs* are the unique (exclusive) resources used only by one unit of an organization, such as a department, and therefore are fairly easy to measure. *Indirect (overhead) costs*, in contrast, are inherently difficult to measure because they constitute a shared resource of the organization, such as administrative costs.

➤ *Cost allocation* is a critical part of the costing process because it addresses the issue of how to assign the costs of support activities to the revenue-producing (patient services) departments. The *goal* of cost allocation is to assign all costs of an organization to the activities that cause them to be incurred.

➤ A *cost pool* is a dollar amount of overhead services to be allocated. In general, a cost pool consists of the total costs of one support department. However, under some circumstances, it may be better to divide the costs of a single support department into multiple cost pools.

➤ A *cost driver* is the basis for making allocations from a cost pool. Cost drivers are chosen on the basis of their positive *correlation* with the amount of overhead services used by the patient services departments.

➤ A good cost driver will be perceived by department heads as being *fair* and will promote *cost reduction* within the organization.

➤ There are three primary *methods for cost allocation*: direct, reciprocal, and step down. Regardless of the allocation method, all costs eventually end up in the patient services departments.

➤ The *direct method* recognizes no intrasupport department services. Thus, support department costs are allocated exclusively to patient services departments.

➤ The *reciprocal method* recognizes all intrasupport department services. However, the reciprocal method is the most difficult to understand and to implement.

➤ The *step-down method* represents a compromise between the direct and reciprocal methods that recognizes some of the intrasupport department services.

➤ *Activity-based costing (ABC)* allocates costs on the basis of activities and hence aggregates costs from the basic components that create costs in the first place. ABC can estimate costs for individual patients, diagnoses, services, and so on, while traditional costing cannot (with any confidence) estimate costs below the department level. However, ABC requires a more sophisticated and costly managerial accounting information system.

This chapter contains a great deal of detail, but the most important concept to remember is that a sound cost estimation system is required for making good managerial decisions. We extend the discussion in Chapter 5, which covers pricing decisions and profit analysis.

END-OF-CHAPTER QUESTIONS

4.1 Explain the difference between fixed and variable costs.

4.2 a. What is meant by a business's underlying cost structure?
   b. Why is this information valuable to managers?

4.3 What cost structure creates economies of scale? Why?

4.4 What are the primary differences between direct and indirect (overhead) costs?

4.5 What is the goal of cost allocation?

4.6 a. What is a cost pool?
   b. What is a cost driver?
   c. How is the cost allocation rate determined?

4.7 Under what circumstances should an overhead department be divided into multiple cost pools?

4.8 Effective cost drivers, and hence the resulting allocation system, must have what two important attributes?

4.9 Briefly describe (illustrate) the cost allocation process.

4.10 a. What are the three primary methods of cost allocation?
      b. What are the differences among them?

4.11 Which is the better cost driver for a hospital's Financial Services Department — patient services department revenues or number of bills generated? Explain your rationale.

4.12 How does activity-based costing (ABC) differ from traditional costing?

END-OF-CHAPTER PROBLEMS

4.1 Assume that a radiology group practice has the following cost structure:

Fixed costs	$500,000	Variable cost per procedure	$25

Furthermore, assume that the group expects to perform 7,500 procedures in the coming year.
a. What is the group's underlying cost structure?
b. What are the group's expected total costs?
c. What are the group's estimated total costs at 5,000 procedures? At 10,000 procedures?
d. What is the average cost per procedure at 5,000, 7,500, and 10,000 procedures?

4.2 You are considering starting a walk-in clinic. Your financial projections for the first year of operations are as follows:

Number of visits	10,000	Utilities	$2,500
Wages and benefits	$220,000	Medical supplies	$50,000
Rent	$5,000	Administrative supplies	$10,000
Depreciation	$30,000		

Assume that all costs are fixed except supplies costs, which are variable.

a. What is the clinic's underlying cost structure?

b. What are the clinic's expected total costs?

c. What are the clinic's estimated total costs at 7,500 visits? At 12,500 visits?

d. What is the average cost per visit at 7,500, 10,000, and 12,500 visits?

4.3 General Hospital, a not-for-profit acute care facility, has estimated the following costs for its inpatient services:

Fixed costs $10,000,000   Variable cost per inpatient day $200

The hospital expects to have 15,000 inpatient days next year.

a. What is the hospital's underlying cost structure?

b. What are the hospital's expected total costs?

c. What are the hospital's estimated total costs at 12,500 inpatient days? At 17,500 patient days?

d. What is the average cost per patient day at 12,500, 15,000, and 17,500 patient days?

4.4 The Housekeeping Services Department of Ruger Clinic, a multispecialty practice in Toledo, Ohio, had $100,000 in direct costs during 2008. These costs must be allocated to Ruger's three revenue-producing patient services departments using the direct method. Two cost drivers are under consideration: patient services revenue and hours of housekeeping services used. The patient services departments generated $5 million in total revenues during 2008. To support these clinical activities, the departments used 5,000 hours of housekeeping services.

a. What is the value of the cost pool?

b. What is the allocation rate if (1) patient services revenue is used as the cost driver and (2) hours of housekeeping services are used as the cost driver?

4.5 Refer to Problem 4.4. Assume that the three patient services departments are Adult Services, Pediatric Services, and Other Services. The patient services revenue and hours of housekeeping services for each department are as follows:

Department	Revenue	Housekeeping Hours
Adult Services	$3,000,000	1,500
Pediatric Services	1,500,000	3,000
Other Services	500,000	500
Total	$5,000,000	5,000

a. What is the dollar allocation to each patient services department if patient services revenue is used as the cost driver?

b. What is the dollar allocation to each patient services department if hours of housekeeping support are used as the cost driver?

c. What is the difference in the allocation to each department between the two drivers?

d. Which of the two drivers is better? Why?

The following data pertain to Problems 4.6 through 4.8:

St. Benedict's Hospital has three support departments and four patient services departments. The direct costs to each of the support departments are:

General Administration	$2,000,000
Facilities	5,000,000
Financial Services	3,000,000

Selected data for the three support and four patient services departments are as follows:

Department	Patient Services Revenue	Space (Square Feet)	Housekeeping Labor Hours	Salary Dollars
Support:				
General Administration		10,000	2,000	$1,500,000
Facilities		20,000	5,000	3,000,000
Financial Services		15,000	3,000	2,000,000
Total		45,000	10,000	$6,500,000
Patient Services:				
Routine Care	$30,000,000	400,000	150,000	$12,000,000
Intensive Care	4,000,000	40,000	30,000	5,000,000
Diagnostic Services	6,000,000	60,000	15,000	6,000,000
Other Services	10,000,000	100,000	25,000	7,000,000
Total	$50,000,000	600,000	220,000	$30,000,000
Grand total	$50,000,000	645,000	230,000	$36,500,000

4.6 Assume that the hospital uses the direct method for cost allocation. Furthermore, the cost driver for General Administration and Financial Services is patient services revenue, while the cost driver for Facilities is space utilization.

a. What are the appropriate allocation rates?

b. Allocate the hospital's overhead costs to the patient services departments.

4.7 Assume that the hospital uses salary dollars as the cost driver for General Administration, housekeeping labor hours as the cost driver for Facilities, and patient services revenue as the cost driver for Financial Services. (The majority of the costs of the Facilities Department are devoted to housekeeping services.)

a. What are the appropriate allocation rates?

b. Allocate the hospital's overhead costs to the patient services departments.

c. Compare the dollar allocations with those obtained in Problem 4.6. Explain the differences.

d. Which of the two cost driver schemes is better? Explain your answer.

4.8 Now assume that $2 million of Financial Services costs are related to billing and managerial reporting and $1 million are related to payroll and personnel management activities.

a. Devise and implement a cost allocation scheme that recognizes that Financial Services has two widely different functions.

b. Is there any additional information that would be useful in completing Part a?

c. What are the costs and benefits to St. Benedict's of creating two cost pools for Financial Services?

4.9 Consider the following data for a clinical laboratory:

Activity	Annual Costs	Cost Driver	Activity Data			
			Test A	Test B	Test C	Test D
Receive specimen	$10,000	No. of tests	2,000	1,500	1,000	500
Equipment set-up	25,000	No. of mins. per test	5	5	10	10
Run test	100,000	No. of mins. per test	1	5	10	20
Record results	10,000	No. of mins. per test	2	2	2	4
Transmit results	5,000	No. of mins. per test	3	3	3	3
Total costs	$150,000					

a. Using ABC techniques, determine the allocation rate for each activity.

b. Now, using this allocation rate, estimate the total cost of performing each test.

c. Verify that the total annual costs aggregated from individual test costs equal the total annual costs of the laboratory given in the table above.

CHAPTER 5

PRICING DECISIONS AND PROFIT ANALYSIS

As you know from Chapters 3 and 4, Jen Latimer is the new manager at Big Sky Dermatology Specialists, a small group practice in Jackson, Wyoming. After reviewing the practice's revenue sources and examining its cost structure, Jen was ready to combine Big Sky's cost and revenue structures to get a feel for next year's profit potential. (Jen was accounting for all costs, except for physician compensation, so the "profit" projection was, in reality, the compensation available for the two physicians.)

Jen knew that the practice's profitability could be analyzed using a technique called profit analysis. (Accountants call this technique cost-volume-profit analysis.) She already identified the practice's cost structure. At an expected (base case) volume of 10,000 visits, total costs were forecasted to be $1,000,000:

$$
\begin{aligned}
\text{Total costs} &= \text{Fixed costs} + \text{Total variable costs} \\
&= \text{Fixed costs} + (\text{Variable cost rate x Volume}) \\
&= \$850,000 \ + (\$15 \text{ x } 10,000 \text{ visits}) \\
&= \$850,000 \ + \$150,000 \\
&= \$1,000,000.
\end{aligned}
$$

Now, Jen must fold in the revenue structure of the practice. This will give her the ability to analyze the impact of different volume assumptions on the practice's profitability. (In addition, she could analyze the impact of different revenue and cost assumptions.)

By the end of this chapter, you will have a better grasp of profit analysis and its benefit to healthcare managers. In addition, you, like Jen, will be able to examine Big Sky's profitability under varying assumptions of volume, costs, and revenues.

LEARNING OBJECTIVES

After studying this chapter, you will be able to

➤ Explain the difference between price setters and price takers.

➤ Differentiate full cost pricing from marginal cost pricing.

➤ Describe how target costing is used.

➤ Conduct profit analyses to learn the impact of volume changes on profitability and to determine breakeven points.

➤ Discuss the primary differences in profit analyses between fee-for-service and capitation reimbursement.

➤ Explain how revenue and cost structures affect a healthcare organization's risk.

5.1 INTRODUCTION

One of the most important uses of managerial accounting data is to establish a price for a particular service or, given a price, to determine whether or not the service will be profitable. For example, in a charge-based environment, healthcare managers must set prices on the services their organizations offer. Managers also must determine whether or not to offer volume discounts to valued payer groups, such as managed care plans or business coalitions, and how large these discounts should be.

After prices are set, managers can estimate revenues on the basis of volume estimates. Furthermore, the business's revenue structure (volumes coupled with reimbursements) can be combined with its cost structure to forecast profits under a wide range of operating assumptions. Having some knowledge of future profitability requirements, and the prices (and hence revenues) for attaining profitability, is critical for good financial decision making.

This chapter discusses pricing strategies and profit analysis. Along the way, it covers other important healthcare finance principles.

5.2 HEALTHCARE PROVIDERS AND THE POWER TO SET PRICES

Two extremes exist regarding the power of healthcare providers to set prices. At one extreme, providers have no power whatsoever and must accept the prices (reimbursement amounts) set by the marketplace. At the other extreme, providers can set any prices desired (but within reason), and payers must accept those prices. Clearly, few real-world markets for healthcare services support such extreme positions. Nevertheless, thinking in such terms can help healthcare managers better understand the pricing decisions they face.

PROVIDERS AS PRICE TAKERS

If a healthcare organization is one of many providers in a service area that has numerous fee-for-service purchasers (third-party payers), and if little distinguishes the services offered by different providers, then economic theory suggests that the prices are set by local supply-and-demand conditions. Furthermore, the actions of a single participant—whether a provider or payer—cannot influence the prices set in the marketplace. In such a perfectly competitive market, healthcare providers are said to be *price takers* because they are constrained by (or must accept) the prices set in the marketplace.

Few markets for healthcare services are perfectly competitive. But some payers—notably government payers and managed care plans with market power—can set reimbursement levels on a take-it-or-leave-it basis. In this situation, as in competitive markets, providers are price takers in the sense that they have very little influence over reimbursement rates. Because many markets either are somewhat competitive or are dominated by large payer groups, and because government payers cover a significant proportion of the population, most providers probably qualify as price takers for a large percentage of their revenue.

Price taker
A provider that has no power to influence the prices set by the marketplace.

As a general rule, providers that are price takers must take price as a given and concentrate managerial efforts on cost structure and utilization to ensure that their services are profitable. Thus, price takers are just as concerned about costs as are price setters.

From a purely financial perspective, a price-taking provider should offer all services with costs that are less than the given price, even when that price is reduced by discounting or other market actions. Although this approach to service decisions is obviously simplistic, it does raise an important issue: What costs are relevant to the decision at hand? To ensure long-term sustainability, prices must cover full (all) costs. However, prices that do not cover full costs may be acceptable for short periods, and it might be in the provider's best interests to do so.

PROVIDERS AS PRICE SETTERS

Price setter
A provider that has the power to set market prices for its services.

Healthcare providers with market dominance enjoy large market shares and hence exercise some pricing power. Within limits, such providers can decide what prices to set on the services offered. Furthermore, if a provider's services can be differentiated from others on the basis of quality, convenience, or another characteristic, the provider also has the ability, again within limits, to set prices on the differentiated services. Healthcare providers that have such pricing power are called *price setters*.

The situation would be much easier for healthcare managers if a provider's status as a price taker or a price setter were fixed for all payers for all services for long periods of time. Unfortunately, the healthcare market is ever changing, and hence providers can quickly move from one status to the other. For example, the merger of two healthcare providers may create sufficient market power to change two price takers (as separate entities) into one price setter (as a combined entity). Furthermore, providers can be price takers for some services (or some third-party payers or some geographic markets) and price setters for others.

⑦ SELF-TEST QUESTIONS

1. What is the difference between a price taker and a price setter?

2. Are healthcare providers generally either price takers or price setters exclusively? Explain your answer.

5.3 PRICE SETTING STRATEGIES

When providers are price setters, alternative strategies can be used to price healthcare services. Unfortunately, no single strategy is most appropriate in all situations. In this section, we discuss the two price setting strategies most frequently used by healthcare organizations.

FULL COST PRICING

Full cost pricing recognizes that to remain viable in the long run, healthcare organizations must set prices that recover all costs associated with operating the business. Thus, the full cost of a service—whether a patient day in a hospital, a visit to a clinic, a laboratory test, or the treatment of a particular diagnosis—must include the following: (1) the direct variable costs of providing the service, (2) the direct fixed costs, and (3) the appropriate share of the overhead expenses of the organization.

CRITICAL CONCEPT
Full Cost Pricing

In full cost pricing, prices are set to cover *all costs* associated with providing a particular service. Thus, the price must cover both direct and overhead costs. In addition, to truly cover all costs of doing business, including economic costs, the price must include a profit component. All providers, even not-for-profit ones, must earn a profit to ensure the ability to replace assets as needed, invest in new technologies, and expand facilities to meet growing community needs.

Because allocating overhead costs is complicated (see Chapter 4), the full costs of an individual service are difficult to determine with precision and hence have to be viewed as merely an estimate of the true costs. Nevertheless, in the aggregate, revenues must cover both direct and overhead costs, and hence prices in total must cover all costs of an organization.

Furthermore, all businesses need profits to survive in the long run. In not-for-profit businesses, prices must be set high enough to provide the profits needed to support asset replacement and to acquire new assets as needed to support volume growth and provide new technologies. In addition, for-profit providers must provide equity investors (owners) with a financial return on their investment. The bottom line here is that full cost pricing, to cover all costs, including economic costs, must cover all accounting costs plus a profit target.

MARGINAL COST PRICING

In economics, the *marginal cost* of an item is the cost of providing one additional unit of output, whether that output is a product or service. For example, suppose that a 150-bed hospital currently provides 40,000 patient days of care. Its marginal cost, based on inpatient day as the unit of service, is the cost of providing the 40,001th day of care. In this situation, fixed costs likely will not increase, so the marginal cost consists solely of the variable costs associated with an additional one-day stay.

In most situations, no additional labor costs would be involved. The marginal cost, therefore, consists of expenses such as laundry, food and expendable supplies, and any additional utility services consumed during that day. Obviously, the marginal cost associated with one additional patient day is far less than the full cost of that patient day, which must include all direct fixed and overhead costs plus a profit component.

Marginal cost
The cost of one additional unit of output. In an outpatient setting, the cost (typically only supplies) of one more patient visit.

> ⓘ **CRITICAL CONCEPT**
> Marginal Cost Pricing
>
> In marginal cost pricing, prices are set to cover only the marginal cost of providing the service. In general, this means the price covers just the variable costs. Marginal cost pricing is usually a temporary strategy, because it does not cover the full cost of providing services. Thus, it can only be sustained over the long run if the provider recoups the losses on the marginal-cost patients by charging another group more than full costs.

Many proponents of government programs such as Medicare and Medicaid argue that payments to providers should be made on the basis of marginal rather than full costs. The argument here is that some price above marginal cost is all that is required for the provider to "make money" on government-sponsored patients. By implication, nongovernmental payers would cover all fixed costs. However, what would happen if all payers for a particular provider set reimbursement rates based on marginal costs? If such a situation occurred, the organization would not recover its full costs, including both direct and overhead, and hence would ultimately fail.

Should any prices be set on the basis of marginal costs? In theory, the answer is no. For prices to be equitable, all payers should pay their fair shares in covering providers' total costs. Furthermore, if **marginal cost pricing** should be adopted, which payer(s) should receive its benefits by being charged lower prices? Should it be the government because it is taxpayer funded, or should it be the last payer to contract with the provider? There are no good answers to these questions. The easy way out, at least conceptually, is to require all payers to pay full costs and hence equitably share the burden of the organization's total costs.

Price shifting
The act of charging more than full costs to one set of patients to compensate for charging less to another set. Also called cross-subsidization.

However, as a practical matter, it may make sense for healthcare providers to occasionally use marginal cost pricing to attract a new patient group or to retain an existing group (gain or retain market share). To survive in the long run, however, businesses must earn revenues that cover their full costs. Thus, marginal cost pricing must be a temporary measure, or the organization must overcharge other payers for services (compared to full cost) to make up for the losses on patients who are undercharged. This situation is called *price shifting (or cross-subsidization)*.

Historically, price shifting was used to support services that were not self-supporting, such as emergency care, teaching and research, and indigent care. Without price shifting strategies, many providers would not have been able to offer a full range of services. Payers were willing to accept price shifting because the additional burden was not excessive. Today, however, overall healthcare costs have risen to the point where the major purchasers of healthcare services are not willing to support the costs associated with providing services to others, and hence purchasers are demanding prices that cover only the true costs of the covered populations. Payers believe (perhaps rightly so) that they do not have the moral responsibility to fund healthcare services for others.

5.4 TARGET COSTING

Target costing is a management strategy that helps providers deal with situations in which they are price takers. Target costing assumes that the amount received for a service is fixed, and subtracts the desired profit on that service to obtain the target cost level. If possible, management will reduce the full cost of the service to the target level, with a goal of continuous cost reduction, which will eventually push costs below the target. Essentially, target costing backs into the cost at which a healthcare service must be provided in the long run to attain a given profitability target.

> **(!) CRITICAL CONCEPT**
> Target Costing
>
> Target costing is a strategy used by price takers. In essence, the price (reimbursement rate) is assumed to be fixed, and the goal is to create a cost structure for that service that allows the provider to make a profit. Target costing forces managers to focus on costs, rather than prices, as the key to profitability. Thus, it leads managers to examine factors that are within their control (costs) as opposed to factors that are, for the most part, uncontrollable (prices).

Perhaps the greatest value of target costing lies in the fact that it forces managers to take seriously the prices set by external forces; that is, it recognizes that the purchasers of healthcare services are not concerned whether or not prices are based on the underlying costs of the services provided. Thus, to ensure financial survival, providers must attain cost structures compatible with the revenue stream. Providers that cannot lower costs to the level required to make a profit ultimately fail.

Profit analysis combines data on costs, volume, and prices to estimate the profitability of organizations, departments, or services. Profit analysis is important in planning for the future. Specifically, it allows managers to see how profitability is affected by changes in cost, volume, and price assumptions. In essence, profit analysis is used to conduct "what if" analyses— What if volume is lower than expected? What if prices are higher than anticipated? What if costs are higher than forecasted? and so on. The answers to these, and similar, questions provide managers with insights into the organization's financial future.

5.5 PROFIT ANALYSIS

Profit analysis is a technique often used to analyze the effects of volume changes on profit. (Accountants often refer to this technique as cost-volume-profit [CVP] analysis.) In addition, profit analysis can be used to examine the effects of alternative assumptions regarding costs and prices. Such information is useful as managers evaluate future courses of action regarding pricing and the introduction of new services.

BASIC DATA

Table 5.1 presents the estimated annual costs for Atlanta Clinic, a large primary care practice, for 2009. These costs are based on the clinic's best (most likely) estimate of volume: 75,000 visits. The most likely estimate often is called the *base case*, so the data in Table 5.1 represent the clinic's base case cost forecast. Expected total costs for 2009 are $7,080,962. Because these costs support 75,000 visits, the forecasted base case average cost per visit is $7,080,962 / 75,000 = $94.41.

TABLE 5.1
Atlanta Clinic: Forecasted Cost Data for 2009 (based on 75,000 patient visits)

	Variable Costs	Fixed Costs	Total Costs
Salaries and Benefits:			
Management and supervision	$ 0	$ 928,687	$ 928,687
Coordinators	442,617	598,063	1,040,680
Specialists	0	38,600	38,600
Technicians	681,383	552,670	1,234,053
Clerical/administrative	71,182	58,240	129,422
Social Security taxes	89,622	163,188	252,810
Group health insurance	115,924	211,081	327,005
Professional fees	325,489	383,360	708,849
Supplies	313,283	231,184	544,467
Utilities	74,000	45,040	119,040
Allocated costs	0	1,757,349	1,757,349
Total	$2,113,500	$4,967,462	$7,080,962

Focusing solely on total costs does not provide the clinic's managers with much information regarding potential alternative financial outcomes for 2009. Total cost information is necessary and useful, but the detailed breakdown in Table 5.1 gives the clinic's managers more insight into the possible financial outcomes for 2009 than is possible with a total cost focus.

Table 5.1 categorizes the clinic's total costs of $7,080,962 into two components: total variable costs of $2,113,500 and total fixed costs of $4,967,462. As you know, these cost amounts are fundamentally different. The total fixed costs of $4,967,462 must be borne by the clinic regardless of actual volume, as long as it stays within the *relevant range* of 70,000–80,000 visits. However, total variable costs of $2,113,500 apply only to a volume of 75,000 patient visits. If the actual number of visits realized in 2009 is less than or greater than 75,000, total variable costs will be less than or greater than $2,113,500. (Of course, this is the primary reason that costs are classified as fixed and variable in the first place.)

To conduct a profit analysis, it is necessary to express variable costs on a per unit (variable cost rate) basis. For Atlanta Clinic, the implied variable cost rate is $2,113,500 / 75,000 visits = $28.18 per visit. Thus, the clinic's total costs at any volume within the relevant range can be calculated as follows:

Total costs = Fixed costs + Total variable costs
            = $4,967,462 + ($28.18 × Number of visits).

This equation, the clinic's *underlying cost structure* (or cost behavior model), shows that total costs depend on volume. To illustrate use of this model, consider three potential volumes for 2009: 70,000, 75,000, and 80,000 patient visits:

Volume = 70,000:
Total costs = $4,967,462 + ($28.18 × 70,000)
            = $4,967,462 + $1,972,600 = $6,940,062.

Volume = 75,000:
Total costs = $4,967,462 + ($28.18 × 75,000)
            = $4,967,462 + $2,113,500 = $7,080,962.

Volume = 80,000:
Total costs = $4,967,462 + ($28.18 × 80,000)
            = $4,967,462 + $2,254,400 = $7,221,862.

When an organization's costs are expressed in this way, it is easy to see that higher volume leads to higher total costs.

Atlanta Clinic's underlying cost structure is plotted in Figure 5.1. (To simplify the graph, we assume that the relevant range extends to zero visits.) Fixed costs are

Base case
In profit analysis, the scenario (outcome) that is expected (most likely) to occur.

Relevant range
The range of output (volume) over which the organization's cost structure holds.

Underlying cost structure
The relationship between volume and an organization's total costs. Also called cost behavior model.

FIGURE 5.1

Atlanta Clinic: Profit Analysis Graph

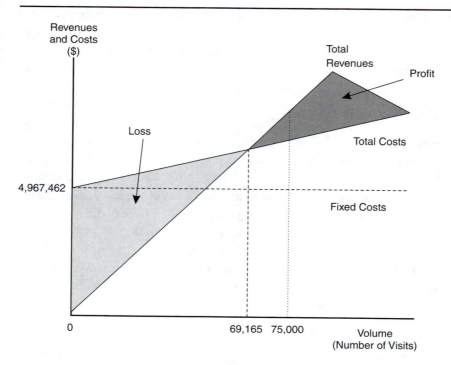

shown as a horizontal dashed line and total costs are shown as an upward-sloping solid line with a slope (rise over run) equal to the variable cost rate: $28.18 per visit. Total variable costs are represented by the vertical distance between the total costs line and the fixed costs line.

Note that Atlanta Clinic's financial manager does not literally write out a check for $28.18 for each visit, although there may be examples of variable costs in which this is the case. Rather, the clinic's cost structure indicates that the clinic uses certain resources that its managers have defined as inherently variable, and the best estimate of the value of such resources, on average, is $28.18 per visit.

To complete the profit analysis graph, a revenue component must be added to the cost structure. For 2009, the clinic expects revenues, on average, to be $100 per patient visit. Total revenues are plotted on Figure 5.1 as an upward-sloping solid line starting at the origin and having a slope of $100 per visit. If there were no visits, total revenues would be zero; at one visit, total revenues would be $100; at ten visits, total revenues would be $1,000; at 75,000 visits, total revenues would be $7,500,000; and so on. Note that the vertical dashed line is drawn at the point where total revenues equal total costs and the vertical dotted line is drawn at the base case volume estimate, 75,000 visits. We examine the significance of these two vertical lines in later sections.

THE PROJECTED P&L STATEMENT

To begin their profit analysis, Atlanta Clinic's managers would forecast profit given the base case assumptions on costs, volume, and prices. Such a forecast is called a **profit and loss (P&L) statement**. P&L statements, as with all managerial accounting data, are developed for specific purposes and hence can be formatted to best fit the situation at hand.

Atlanta Clinic's base case projected P&L statement is shown in Table 5.2. The bottom line projects Atlanta's 2009 profit using base case (most likely estimate) values for costs, volume, and prices. Note that the format of a P&L statement for CVP analysis purposes distinguishes between variable and fixed costs, whereas P&L statements for other purposes may not make this distinction. Also, note that the projected P&L statement contains a line labeled "total contribution margin." This concept is discussed in the next section.

> **(!) CRITICAL CONCEPT**
> Profit and Loss (P&L) Statement
>
> A P&L (pronounced P and L) statement is a listing of revenues, expenses, and profit (revenues minus expenses). There are numerous formats for P&L statements, depending on the specific purpose of the statement. For example, for use in profit analysis, costs must be broken out as fixed and variable. Note that P&L statements can be constructed for the entire organization, a department, or a service. Also, P&L statements can contain historical data, which report what has happened in the past, or forecasted data, which express expectations about the future.

The projected P&L statement used in profit analysis contains four variables; three of the variables are assumed and the fourth is calculated. In Table 5.2, the assumed variables are expected volume (75,000 visits), expected price ($100 per visit), and expected costs (as defined by the clinic's cost structure). Profit, the fourth variable, is calculated on the basis of the three assumed variables.

The base case projected P&L statement in Table 5.2 represents only one point on the graphical model in Figure 5.1. This point is shown by the dotted vertical line at a volume of 75,000 patient visits. Moving up along this dotted line, the distance from the X-axis to the horizontal line represents the $4,967,462 fixed costs. The distance from the fixed costs line to the total costs line represents the $2,113,500 total variable costs. The distance between the total costs line and the total revenues line represents the $419,038 profit. Of course, the graph in Figure 5.1 is not drawn to scale and hence cannot be used to develop numerical data. Rather,

Total revenues ($100 × 75,000)	$7,500,000
Total variable costs ($28.18 × 75,000)	2,113,500
Total contribution margin ($71.82 × 75,000)	$5,386,500
Fixed costs	4,967,462
Profit	$ 419,038

TABLE 5.2

Atlanta Clinic: 2009 Base Case Projected P&L Statement (based on 75,000 patient visits)

Contribution margin is defined as the amount of per unit revenue that is available to cover fixed costs and contribute to profitability. It is the average revenue per unit of service minus the variable cost per unit of service (variable cost rate). The idea here is that if we strip the variable costs off of revenue, we will be left with the amount available per unit of output to cover fixed costs. Once fixed costs are covered, any additional contribution margin amounts flow directly to profit.

To illustrate, consider your custom pen business (which we set up in Chapter 4). The pens cost you $1.75 a pop, but you had to pay someone $50 to design the logo. The contribution margin on each pen is Per unit revenue − Variable cost rate. If you sell the pens for $3 each, the contribution margin is $3.00 − $1.75 = $1.25. Thus, each pen sold will contribute $1.25 to cover the $50 fixed costs. After you sell 40 pens, you will have recouped the $50 fixed costs (40 x $1.25 = $50), so all sales after the first 40 create profits for your custom pen enterprise.

Total contribution margin is the sum of the contribution margins of all units sold. Assume that you sell 50 pens. With a contribution margin of $1.25 per pen, the total contribution margin is 50 x $1.25 = $62.50. The first $50 of the total contribution margin is needed to cover your fixed costs of $50, so the remaining $12.50 flows to profit. Thus, at a volume of 60 pens, your profit is $12.50.

it provides the clinic's managers with a pictorial representation of the clinic's projected profitability.

CONTRIBUTION MARGIN

The base case projected P&L statement in Table 5.2 introduces the concept of **contribution margin,** which is defined as the difference between per unit revenue and per unit variable cost (variable cost rate). In this illustration, the contribution margin is $100.00 − $28.18 = $71.82. What is the inherent meaning of this contribution margin value of $71.82? The contribution margin appears to be a type of "profit" because it is calculated as revenue minus costs.

However, because none of the fixed costs of providing service have been included in the calculation, it is not profit. Rather, because only variable costs have been stripped out, the contribution margin is the dollar amount of per visit revenue available to cover Atlanta Clinic's fixed costs. Only after fixed costs are fully covered does the contribution margin begin to contribute to profit.

With a contribution margin of $71.82 on each of the clinic's 75,000 visits, the projected base case **total contribution margin** for 2009 is $71.82 × 75,000 = $5,386,500, which is sufficient to cover the clinic's fixed costs of $4,967,462 and then provide a $5,386,500 − $4,967,462 = $419,038 profit. After fixed costs have been covered, any additional visits contribute to the clinic's profit at a rate of $71.82 per visit.

1. Construct a simple P&L statement like the one in Table 5.2, and discuss its elements.

2. Sketch and explain a simple diagram to match your table.

3. Define and explain the use of contribution margin and total contribution margin.

5.6 BREAKEVEN ANALYSIS

Breakeven analysis is applied in many different situations. Generically, breakeven analyses are used to determine the value of a given input variable (such as volume, costs, or price) that produces some minimum desired result (typically some profit amount). For example, a laboratory might break even (make zero profit) on a particular type of blood test if the reimbursement for that test is $23. Or, given a reimbursement amount, the laboratory might break even if it conducts 1,050 tests.

Although the breakeven analysis discussed here is actually part of profit analysis, the concept is important enough to deserve its own section. For now, we will use breakeven analysis to estimate the volume at which a business, department, or service becomes financially self-sufficient.

To complicate matters slightly, there are two different definitions of breakeven volume. *Accounting breakeven* is defined as the volume needed to produce zero profit. In other words, it is the volume that produces revenues equal to total accounting costs. Alternatively, *economic breakeven* is defined as the volume needed to produce some target profit level. In other words, it is the volume that creates revenues equal to total accounting costs plus the desired profit amount.

As mentioned in the previous section, the P&L statement format used for profit analysis is a four-variable model. When the focus is profit, the three assumed variables are costs, volume, and price, while profit is calculated. When the focus is volume breakeven, the same four variables are used, but profit is now assumed to be known while volume is the unknown (calculated) value.

To illustrate **volume breakeven**, the projected P&L statement presented in Table 5.2 can be expressed in equation form as shown here:

$$\text{Total revenues} - \text{Total variable costs} - \text{Fixed costs} = \text{Profit}$$
$$(\$100 \times \text{Volume}) - (\$28.18 \times \text{Volume}) - \$4,967,462 = \text{Profit}.$$

At accounting breakeven the clinic's profit equals zero, so the breakeven equation can be rewritten this way:

$$(\$100 \times \text{Volume}) - (\$28.18 \times \text{Volume}) - \$4,967,462 = \$0.$$

CRITICAL CONCEPT
Breakeven Analysis

Breakeven analysis has many applications in healthcare finance. In the context of profit analysis, breakeven analysis involves finding the value of an input variable that produces zero profit (or some profit target). For example, a nursing home might break even when it has 55 residents (out of 70 beds). Or a family practice might break even when it has 10,000 patient visits annually. Breakeven analysis is also applied to variables other than volume. For example, a home health agency might break even if its per visit costs are $70 or less. Or a radiology group might break even if its reimbursement averages at least $25 per reading. Note that breakeven can be defined in two ways. It can be based either on accounting costs alone or on accounting costs plus a profit target.

Total contribution margin
Contribution margin multiplied by volume, or the amount of total revenues over some time period available to cover fixed costs.

Accounting breakeven
Accounting breakeven occurs when all accounting costs are covered (zero profitability).

Economic breakeven
Economic breakeven occurs when all accounting costs plus a profit target are covered.

Volume breakeven can be estimated using a very simple equation:

(Contribution margin x Volume) – Fixed costs = $0 (or some profit target).

To illustrate, what is the accounting breakeven volume of your custom pen business? Remember that the pens cost $1.75 a piece; plus, you had to pay a $50 fee for the logo. Also, you plan to sell the pens for $3.00 each. Under these assumptions, the contribution margin is $3.00 – $1.75 = $1.25 and the breakeven point is 40 pens:

$$(\$1.25 \times Volume) - \$50 = \$0$$
$$\$1.25 \times Volume = \$50$$
$$Volume = \$50/\$1.25$$
$$= 40.$$

As an alternative, breakeven could be defined as meeting some profit target. For example, assume you wanted to make $100 on your pen business. The breakeven volume now is 120 pens:

$$(\$1.25 \times Volume) - \$50 = \$100$$
$$\$1.25 \times Volume = \$150$$
$$Volume = \$150/\$1.25$$
$$= 120.$$

Rearranging the terms so that only the terms related to volume appear on the left side produces this equation:

$$(\$100 \times Volume) - (\$28.18 \times Volume) = \$4,967,462.$$

Using basic algebra, the two terms on the left side can be combined because volume appears in both. The end result is this:

$$(\$100 - \$28.18) \times Volume = \$4,967,462$$
$$\$71.82 \times Volume = \$4,967,462.$$

The left side of the breakeven equation now contains the contribution margin, $71.82, multiplied by volume. Thus, the clinic will break even when the total contribution margin equals fixed costs. Solving the equation for volume results in a breakeven point of $4,967,462 / $71.82 = 69,165 visits. Any volume greater than 69,165 visits produces an accounting profit for the clinic, while any volume less than 69,165 results in a loss.

The logic behind the breakeven point is this: Each patient visit brings in $100, of which $28.18 is the variable cost to treat the patient. This leaves a $71.82 contribution margin from each visit. If the clinic sets the contribution margin aside for the first 69,165 visits in 2009, it would have $4,967,430, which is enough (except for a small rounding difference) to cover its fixed costs. Once the clinic exceeds breakeven volume, each visit's contribution margin flows directly to profit. If the clinic achieves its base case volume estimate of 75,000 visits, the 5,835 visits above the breakeven point result in a total profit of 5,835 × $71.82 = $419,070, which matches the profit (again except for a rounding difference) shown on the clinic's projected income statement in Table 5.2.

On a profit analysis graph such as Figure 5.1, breakeven occurs at the intersection of the total revenues line and total costs line. This point is indicated by a vertical dashed line drawn at a volume of 69,165 visits. Before even one patient walks in the door, the clinic has already committed to $4,967,462 in fixed costs. Because the total revenues line is steeper than the total variable costs line (and hence the total costs line), as volume increases total revenues eventually catch up to the clinic's cost structure. Any volume to the right of the breakeven point, which is shown as a dark-shaded area, produces a profit; any volume to the left, which is shown as a light-shaded area, results in a loss.

This breakeven analysis contains two important assumptions:

1. The price or set of prices for different types of patients and different payers is independent of volume. In other words, volume increases are not attained by lowering prices, and price increases are not met with volume declines.

2. Costs can be reasonably subdivided into fixed and variable components, and the breakeven volume falls within the relevant range.

Breakeven analysis is often performed in an iterative manner. After the breakeven volume is calculated, managers must determine whether the resulting volume can realistically be achieved at the price assumed in the analysis. If the price appears to be unreasonable for the breakeven volume, a new price has to be estimated and the breakeven analysis repeated. Likewise, if the cost structure used for the calculation appears to be unrealistic at the breakeven volume, operational and cost assumptions should be changed and the analysis repeated.

Instead of asking how many visits are needed for accounting breakeven, Atlanta Clinic's managers may ask how many visits are needed to achieve a $100,000 profit or, for that matter, any other profit level. By building a profit target into the breakeven analysis, the focus is now on economic breakeven. The clinic will have a $419,038 profit if it has 75,000 visits, and it will have no profit if it has 69,165 visits. Thus, the number of visits required to achieve a $100,000 profit target (economic breakeven) is somewhere between 69,165 and 75,000. In fact, the number of visits required is 70,558:

$$\text{(Contribution margin} \times \text{Volume)} - \text{Fixed costs} = \text{Profit target}$$
$$(\$71.82 \times \text{Volume}) - \$4,967,462 = \$100,000$$
$$\$71.82 \times \text{Volume} = \$5,067,462$$
$$\text{Volume} = 70,558.$$

? SELF-TEST QUESTIONS

1. What is the purpose of breakeven analysis?

2. What is the equation for volume breakeven?

3. Why is breakeven analysis often conducted in an iterative manner?

4. What is the difference between accounting and economic breakeven?

5.7 MARGINAL ANALYSIS

Now assume that a new payer, Peachtree Managed Care (PMC), makes a proposal to Atlanta Clinic's managers. PMC would like the clinic to provide primary healthcare services to its 1,500 enrollees. The best estimate is that these individuals would add 5,000 visits to the clinic's base case forecast of 75,000. However, PMC wants a discount of 40 percent from current pricing. Thus, the net price (and revenue) for their new patients would be, on average, $60 per visit instead of the undiscounted $100 that is received on current patients. If the clinic refuses, PMC will take its business elsewhere.

At first blush, PMC's proposal appears to be unacceptable. First and foremost, $60 is less than the full cost of providing service, which was determined previously to be $94.41 per visit at a volume of 75,000. Thus, Atlanta would lose roughly $94.41 − $60 = $34.41 per visit on PMC's patients. (This is only a rough estimate because the average cost per visit decreases as the number of patient visits increases.) However, before the clinic's managers reject PMC's proposal, they must examine it in more detail using a technique called **marginal analysis**.

Although each new (marginal) visit from the contract brings in only $60, compared with $100 on the clinic's other contracts, the marginal cost is the variable cost rate of $28.18. (Remember that marginal cost is the cost of the next unit sold.) The clinic's $4,967,462 in fixed costs will be incurred whether PMC's offer is accepted or rejected, so these costs are not relevant to the decision. Because the contribution margin on the new contract is $60 − $28.18 = $31.82 per visit (a positive amount), each visit will contribute to the clinic's recovery of fixed costs and ultimately flow to profit. Thus, the offer must be seriously considered.

Note that this conclusion is based on the assumption that the relevant range of volumes is from 70,000 to 80,000 visits, and hence the current level of fixed costs can support the added volume of 5,000 visits. If the contract were expected to add 10,000 visits, then perhaps new (marginal) fixed costs would be incurred. In this situation, the marginal cost of each new visit would be $28.18 plus some additional per visit fixed cost, which would change the numbers used in the analysis.

> ### ⓘ CRITICAL CONCEPT
> Marginal Analysis
>
> Marginal analysis is used to analyze the impact of adding volume to an existing base. For example, assume you have sold 40 of your pens at $3.00 each, but now a classmate offers to buy 20 more at $2.00 a piece. The total cost of 60 pens, based on a $1.75 cost of each pen and a $50 up-front charge, is (60 x $1.75) + $50 = $155. Thus, the cost per pen is $155/60 = $2.58, so you might be inclined to say no to the offer. But the $50 charge has already been paid, so the marginal cost to you of each pen is the variable cost rate of $1.75. The contribution margin on each of the 20 pens is $2.00 − $1.75 = $0.25, so each pen sold would contribute that amount to your bottom line. Unless there are other issues to consider, you should take your classmate's offer.

To verify the positive impact of the proposal, consider the P&L statement in Table 5.3. Here, we have combined the existing 75,000 patient visits with the additional 5,000 visits, for a total of 80,000. The revenues had to be split between the two patient groups because of the price difference. However, the cost structure is assumed to hold, so it is the same, except for the fact that 80,000 visits are now expected. The end result is that the clinic's profit is now expected to be $578,138 instead of the $419,038 shown in Table 5.2 for the base case (75,000 visits).

Note that the additional profit expected from the new contract is $578,138 − $419,038 = $159,100. We could have arrived at this result more easily by merely noting that each of the 5,000 new visits has a contribution margin of $31.82, so the total contribution margin is expected to be 5,000 × $31.82 = $159,100. Because the existing 75,000 patient visits are more than sufficient to cover fixed costs, the entire amount of the additional contribution margin flows to profit.

What should the clinic's managers do? If PMC's proposal is accepted, the clinic is expected to make an additional $159,100 in profit, so it appears to be a "no brainer" to accept the proposal. However, acceptance may have unintended consequences.

The clinic's other payers will undoubtedly learn about the new contract with reduced payments and will want to renegotiate their own contracts with the same, or an even greater, discount. Such a reaction could result in discounts being offered to current payers, which could result in the clinic losing more money on current patients than it gains on new patients. If that outcome were anticipated, the clinic's managers would be better off saying "no" to the offer.

Perhaps Atlanta Clinic can negotiate with PMC and reach a compromise on the size of the discount. The quantitative analysis required to make the decision is relatively easy, but the qualitative issues are more complex. Unfortunately, most financial decision making is like that.

Undiscounted revenue ($100 × 75,000)	$7,500,000
Discounted revenue ($60 × 5,000)	300,000
Total revenues	$7,800,000
Total variable costs ($28.18 × 80,000)	2,254,400
Total contribution margin	$5,545,600
Fixed costs	4,967,462
Profit	$ 578,138

TABLE 5.3

Atlanta Clinic: 2009 Projected P&L Statement (based on 75,000 visits at $100 and 5,000 visits at $60)

1. What is the impact of a discounted contract on revenues, fixed costs, total variable costs, and the breakeven point?

2. Describe marginal analysis.

3. Can qualitative issues come into play in marginal analysis? Give an example.

(✱) INDUSTRY PRACTICE Costs and Revenues of Medical Practices

The Industry Practice box in Chapter 4 discusses the average cost structure of a primary care practice. Because practice costs (and revenues) are a function of the number of physicians in the practice, the data presented are on a per physician basis.

On average, each physician handles about 2,000 patients, who make about 5,300 encounters (visits) during which the physician performs about 12,000 procedures. In addition, each physician requires $350,000 in operating (support) costs. If we use patient visit as the unit of output (volume), the operating cost per visit averages out to be about $350,000 / 5,300 = roughly $66 per visit.

Unfortunately, the data do not break out fixed versus variable costs. However, variable costs, which consist mostly of administrative supplies (e.g., forms and letters) and medical supplies (e.g., rubber gloves, needles, vaccines, dressings) are relatively small, say, $10 per visit. With this assumption, the underlying cost structure for an average primary care practice looks like this:

Total costs = $297,000 + ($10 x Number of visits).

On average, primary care physicians generate roughly $550,000 of revenues per physician. Thus, the per physician P&L statement, assuming 5,300 visits, can be expressed as follows:

Total revenues	$550,000
Total variable costs ($10 x 5,300)	53,000
Total contribution margin	$497,000
Fixed costs	297,000
Profit	$200,000

Of course, the "profit" here represents the primary care physician's compensation.

To convert the average per physician P&L statement to an equation format, note that the average revenue per visit is $550,000 / 5,300 = $103.77. Thus,

$$\text{Total revenues} - \text{Total variable costs} - \text{Fixed costs} = \text{Profit}$$
$$(\$103.77 \times \text{Volume}) - (\$10 \times \text{Volume}) - \$297,000 = \text{Profit}.$$

So, at 5,300 visits, the profit per physician is

$$(\$103.77 \times 5,300) - (\$10 \times 5,300) - \$297,000 = \text{Profit}$$
$$\$550,000 - \$53,000 - \$297,000 = \$200,000.$$

Of course, this is the same profit (physician compensation) as calculated in the P&L statement. The advantage of the equation format is that we can now estimate profit at different volume levels. For example, assume that the volume is only 5,000 visits per physician, instead of the 5,300 visits forecast. With fewer visits, the profit (and hence physician compensation) falls to $171,850:

$$(\$103.77 \times 5,000) - (\$10 \times 5,000) - \$297,000 = \text{Profit}$$
$$\$518,850 - \$50,000 - \$297,000 = \$171,850.$$

But with more visits (say, 5,600), the profit (and hence physician compensation) rises to $228,112:

(Continued)

INDUSTRY PRACTICE Costs and Revenues of Medical Practices

($103.77 x 5,600) − ($10 x 5,600) − $297,000 = Profit

$581,112 − $56,000 − $297,000 = $228,112.

This analysis confirms that fee-for-service reimbursement creates a powerful incentive for clinicians to see as many patients as possible.

Note: This industry practice is based on information in Medical Group Management Association. 2006. *Performance and Practices of Successful Medical Groups.* Englewood, CO: MGMA.

5.8 PROFIT ANALYSIS IN A CAPITATED ENVIRONMENT

As a review of profit analysis, consider how the analysis changes when a provider operates in a capitated environment. Although capitation is used less today than it was, say, 10 years ago, a discussion of capitation provides an excellent review of profit analysis and highlights the basic differences between capitation and fee-for-service reimbursement methods.

To begin, assume that Atlanta Clinic's current payer is the Alliance, a local business coalition. The Alliance is paying the clinic $7,500,000 to provide services for an expected 75,000 visits, but the amount is capitated. Although the clinic's projected total revenues remain the same (see Table 5.2), the situation is actually quite different. The $7,500,000 that the Alliance is paying is not explicitly tied to the amount of services provided by the clinic. Rather, it is tied to the size of the employee group (covered population).

Under capitation, the clinic is taking on the additional risk associated with the amount of services provided. If the total costs of services delivered by the clinic exceed the premium revenue (paid monthly on a per member basis), the clinic will suffer the financial consequences. However, if the clinic can efficiently manage the healthcare of the population served, it will be the economic beneficiary.

How might the clinic's managers evaluate whether or not the $7,500,000 revenue attached to the contract is adequate? To do the analysis, the managers need two critical pieces of information: cost information and utilization information. The clinic already has the cost information—the full cost per visit is expected to be $94.41 (at a volume of 75,000 visits), with an underlying cost structure of $28.18 per visit in variable costs and $4,967,462 in fixed costs. For its *actuarial information*, the managers estimate that the Alliance will have a covered population of 18,750 members, with an expected utilization rate of four visits per member per year. Thus, the total number of visits expected is 18,750 × 4 = 75,000.

Actuarial information
Data (including utilization data on the covered population) regarding the financial risks associated with insurance programs.

The revenues expected from this contract—$7,500,000—exceed the expected costs of serving this population, which are 75,000 visits multiplied by $94.41 per visit, or $7,080,750. Thus, this contract is expected to generate a profit of $419,250, which, not surprisingly, is the same as the original base case fee-for-service result (except for a rounding difference); see Table 5.2.

GRAPHICAL VIEW BASED ON UTILIZATION

Figure 5.2 contains a graphical profit analysis for the capitation contract that is constructed similar to the fee-for-service graph shown in Figure 5.1—that is, the horizontal axis shows volume as measured by number of visits, while the vertical axis shows revenues and costs. Also shown is the same underlying cost structure of $4,967,462 in fixed costs, coupled with a variable cost rate of $28.18. One significant difference exists, however. Instead of being upward sloping, the total revenues line is horizontal, which shows that total revenue is $7,500,000 regardless of volume as measured by the number of visits.

The flat revenue line in Figure 5.2 tells managers that revenue is being driven by something other than the volume of services provided. Under capitation, revenue is driven by the per member premium payment and number of *enrollees*.

Enrollee

A member of a managed care plan. Or, more general, an individual that has (is enrolled in) a health insurance plan.

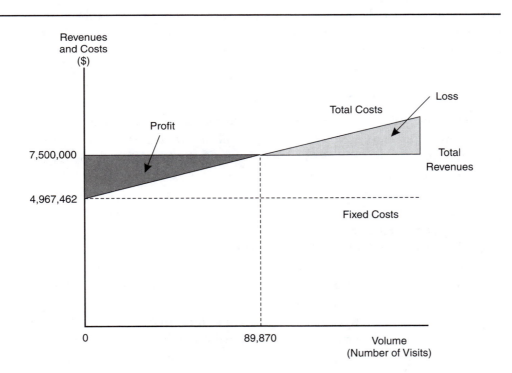

FIGURE 5.2

Atlanta Clinic: Profit Analysis Based on Number of Visits

Also, note the difference between the revenue and fixed cost lines. Atlanta Clinic has a constant spread of $7,500,000 - $4,967,462 = $2,532,538 to work with in providing for the healthcare of this population for the period of the contract. If total variable costs equal $2,532,538, the clinic breaks even; if total variable costs exceed $2,532,538, the clinic loses. Thus, to make a profit, the number of visits must be less than $2,532,538 / $28.18 = 89,870. If everyone at the clinic does not understand the inherent utilization risk under capitation, the clinic could find itself in serious financial trouble. On the other hand, if all of the clinic's managers and clinicians understand and manage this utilization risk, a handsome reward may result.

The key feature of capitation is the reversal of the profit and loss portions of the graph. To see this, compare Figure 5.1 with Figure 5.2. The fact that profits occur at lower volumes under capitation differs from what will happen under the fee-for-service environment. It is obvious, however, when one recognizes that the contribution margin, on a per visit basis, is Revenue per visit – Variable cost per visit = $0 – $28.18 = -$28.18. With a negative contribution margin, each additional visit increases costs by $28.18 without bringing in additional revenue.

From a purely financial perspective, the obvious response to capitation is to provide minimal services (reduce utilization) because doing so generates the greatest profit, at least in the short run. Of course, the clinic would have trouble renewing the contract in subsequent years, and patients may become more ill (and costly to the practice) if only minimal service is provided, so this course of action is neither appropriate nor feasible. Still, its implications are at the heart of concerns expressed by critics of managed care about the incentives to withhold patient care inherent in a capitated environment.

GRAPHICAL VIEW BASED ON MEMBERSHIP

Figure 5.2 is like Alice (of *Alice in Wonderland*) peering through the looking glass and finding that everything is reversed. The key to this problem is that the horizontal axis does not measure the volume to which revenues are related; that is, the horizontal axis in Figure 5.2 has number of visits on the horizontal axis, just as if Atlanta Clinic were reimbursed on a fee-for-service basis. Because it is now selling both healthcare services and insurance, the appropriate horizontal axis measure is the number of members (enrollees).

Figure 5.3 recognizes that membership, rather than the amount of services provided, drives revenues. With number of members on the horizontal axis, the total revenues line is no longer flat; revenues only look flat when they are considered relative to the number of visits. The revenue earned by the clinic is actually $7,500,000 / 18,750 = $400 per member; as membership increases, so do revenues.

The cost structure can easily be expressed on a membership basis as well. Fixed costs are no problem within the relevant range; they are inherently volume insensitive, whether volume is measured by number of visits or by members. Thus, Figure 5.3 shows fixed costs as the same flat, dashed line as before. However, the variable cost rate based on number of

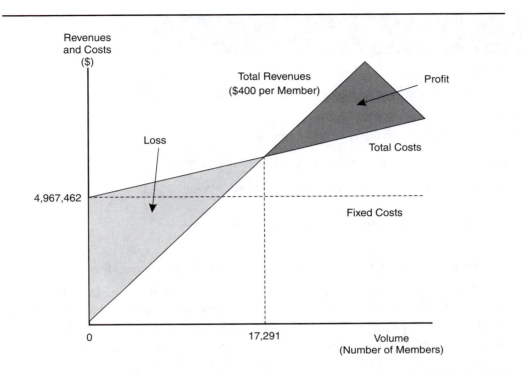

FIGURE 5.3
Atlanta Clinic:
Profit Analysis
Based on Number
of Members

enrollees is not the same as the variable cost rate based on number of visits. Per member variable cost must be estimated from two other factors: the variable cost rate of $28.18 per visit and the expected utilization of four visits per year. The combination of the two is 4 × $28.18 = $112.72, which is the clinic's expected variable cost per member.

Expressed on a per member basis, the contribution margin is now Revenue per member – Variable cost per member = $400 – $112.72 = $287.28, rather than the -$28.18 when volume is based on number of visits. With a positive contribution margin, additional members translate to additional profitability.

Under capitation, utilization is a component of the variable cost rate and hence total variable costs. Thus, utilization management becomes an important cost control tool. If both utilization and per visit costs can be reduced, the clinic can reap greater benefits (profits) than is possible under fee-for-service reimbursement. Of course, control of fixed costs is always financially prudent, regardless of the type of reimbursement.

Also, in a capitated environment revenues are driven by the number of members rather than the amount of services provided. Thus, capitation contracts must bring in a large number of enrollees. A large number of enrollees increases revenues to providers and reduces risk. (If there is a small number of members, only a few high-utilization enrollees can create costs that exceed the total revenues from that payer.)

5.9 THE IMPACT OF COST STRUCTURE ON FINANCIAL RISK

The financial risk of a healthcare provider, at least in theory, is minimized by having a cost structure that "matches" its revenue structure. To illustrate, consider a clinic with all payers using fee-for-service reimbursement, which means revenues are directly related to volume. If the clinic's cost structure consisted of all variable costs (no fixed costs), then each visit would incur costs but also create revenues. Assuming that the per visit revenue amount exceeds the variable cost rate (the per visit cost), the clinic would lock in a profit on each visit. The total profitability of the clinic would be uncertain, as it is tied to volume, but the ability of the clinic to generate a profit would be guaranteed.

To illustrate, if Atlanta Clinic's costs were all variable, then its variable cost rate at 75,000 visits would be $94.41. Thus, the contribution margin would be $100 − $94.41 = $5.59, and because there are no fixed costs to cover, that amount would flow directly to profit on every visit (even the first one). Of course, the amount of profit would be uncertain as it depends on the volume, but the clinic could not lose money.

At the other extreme, consider a clinic that is totally capitated. In this situation, assuming a fixed number of covered lives, the clinic's revenue stream is fixed regardless of volume. Now, to match the revenue and cost structures, the clinic must have all fixed (no variable) costs. If the annual fixed revenue exceeds annual fixed costs, the clinic has a guaranteed profit at the end of the year, assuming that volume does not increase beyond the relevant range.

Applying this concept to Atlanta Clinic, if its $7,080,962 in total costs at 75,000 visits were all fixed, and it received $7,500,000 in capitated revenues, it would lock in a profit of $419,038. Volume could be higher or lower than 75,000, but the profit would remain the same.

In both illustrations, the key to minimizing risk (ensuring a predictable profit) is to create a cost structure that matches the revenue structure: variable costs for fee-for-service revenues and fixed costs for capitated revenues. Of course, "real-world" problems occur when a provider tries to implement a cost structure that matches its revenue structure. First, few providers are reimbursed solely on a fee-for-service or capitated basis; most providers face a mix of reimbursement methods. Still, most providers are either predominantly fee for service or predominantly capitated.

Second, providers do not have complete control over their cost structures. Providers cannot create cost structures with all variable or all fixed costs. Nevertheless, a manager can take actions to make the existing cost structure more compatible with the revenue structure (has less risk). For example, assume a medical group practice is reimbursed almost exclusively on a per procedure basis. To minimize financial risk, the practice can take such actions as pay physicians on a per procedure basis and use per procedure leases for diagnostic equipment. The greater the proportion of variable costs in the practice's cost structure, the lower its financial risk.

(?) SELF-TEST QUESTIONS

1. Explain this statement: To minimize financial risk, match the cost structure to the revenue structure.

2. What cost structure would minimize risk if a provider had all fee-for-service reimbursement? If it were entirely capitated?

3. What are the real-world constraints on creating matching cost structures?

THEME WRAP-UP PROFIT ANALYSIS

Jen concluded that Big Sky's cost structure (not including physician compensation) could be expressed as follows:

$$
\begin{aligned}
\text{Total costs} &= \text{Fixed costs} + \text{Total variable costs} \\
&= \text{Fixed costs} + (\text{Variable cost rate} \times \text{Volume}) \\
&= \$850,000 + (\$15 \times 10,000 \text{ visits}) \\
&= \$850,000 + \$150,000 \\
&= \$1,000,000.
\end{aligned}
$$

By analyzing the practice's revenues, she determined that each patient visit brings in, on average, $160. Thus, the base case P&L statement looks like this:

Total revenues ($160 x 10,000)	$1,600,000
Total variable costs ($15 x 10,000)	150,000
Total contribution margin	$1,450,000
Fixed costs	850,000
Profit	$ 600,000

Here, the profit represents the amount available for compensation to the two dermatologist owners.

The profit analysis for Big Sky can be expressed in this equation format:

Total revenues – Total variable costs – Fixed costs = Profit
($160 x Volume) – ($15 x Volume) – $850,000 = Profit.

This permits Jen to analyze profitability under different assumptions. For example, at 9,000, 10,000 (base case), and 11,000 visits:

($160 x 9,000) – ($15 x 9,000) – $850,000 = Profit
$1,440,000 – $135,000 – $850,000 = $455,000.

($160 x 10,000) – ($15 x 10,000) – $850,000 = Profit
$1,600,000 – $150,000 – $850,000 = $600,000.

($160 x 11,000) – ($15 x 11,000) – $850,000 = Profit
$1,760,000 – $165,000 – $850,000 = $745,000.

The higher the volume, the greater the amount available for physician compensation.
Profit analysis also allows Jen to vary inputs other than volume. Suppose the variable cost rate is actually $20 rather than $15. Under that assumption, and assuming the base case volume of 10,000 visits, profit falls from $600,000 to $550,000.

($160 x 10,000) – ($20 x 10,000) – $850,000 = Profit
$1,600,000 – $200,000 – $850,000 = $550,000.

It should be obvious to you, and Jen, that she now has an important tool to help plan for and manage Big Sky's future.

KEY CONCEPTS

Managers rely on managerial accounting information to help make pricing decisions and to conduct profit analyses. Here are the key concepts:

➤ *Price takers* have to accept, more or less, the prices set in the marketplace for their services, including the prices set by government insurers.

➤ *Price setters* provide services that can be differentiated from others, either by market share, quality, or other differences, such that they have the ability to set the prices on some or all of their services.

➤ *Full cost pricing* permits businesses to recover all costs, including both fixed and variable and direct and indirect, while *marginal cost pricing* typically recovers only variable costs.

➤ *Target costing* is a concept that takes the prices paid for healthcare services as a given and then determines the cost structure necessary for financial success given the prices set.

➤ *Profit analysis,* sometimes called *cost-volume-profit (CVP) analysis*, is an analytical technique to determine the effects of volume changes on revenues, costs, and profit.

➤ A *projected profit and loss (P&L) statement* is a profit forecast that uses estimated values for volume, price, and costs.

➤ *Breakeven analysis* is used to estimate the volume needed (or the value of some other variable) for the organization to break even in profitability.

➤ *Accounting breakeven* occurs when revenues equal accounting costs, while *economic breakeven* occurs when revenues equal accounting costs *plus* some profit target.

➤ *Contribution margin* is the difference between unit price and the *variable cost rate*, or per unit revenue minus per unit variable cost. Thus, contribution margin is the per unit dollar amount available to cover an organization's fixed costs and then to contribute to profits.

➤ In *marginal analysis*, the focus is on the incremental (marginal) profitability associated with increasing (or decreasing) volume.

➤ A *capitated environment* dramatically changes the situation for providers vis-à-vis a fee-for-service environment. In essence, a capitated provider takes on the insurance function and hence bears *utilization risk*.

➤ The keys to success in a capitated environment are to (1) manage (reduce) utilization and (2) increase the number of members covered.

➤ To minimize financial risk, a provider should strive to attain a cost structure that matches its revenue structure.

Our coverage of managerial accounting continues in Chapter 6 with a discussion of planning and budgeting.

END-OF-CHAPTER QUESTIONS

5.1 a. Using a hospital to illustrate your answer, explain the difference between a price setter and a price taker.

b. Can most providers be classified strictly as price setters or price takers?

5.2 Explain the essential differences between full cost and marginal cost pricing strategies.

5.3 What would happen financially to a healthcare organization over time if its prices were set at either full costs or marginal costs?

5.4 What is cross-subsidization (price shifting)?

5.5 a. What is target costing?

b. Suppose a hospital was offered a capitation rate for a covered population of $40 per member per month. Briefly explain how target costing would be applied in this situation.

5.6 a. What is profit (CVP) analysis?

b. Why is it so useful to healthcare managers?

c. What is a profit and loss (P&L) statement?

5.7 a. Define contribution margin.

b. What is its economic meaning?

5.8 a. Write out and explain the equation for volume breakeven.

b. What is the difference between accounting and economic breakeven?

5.9 What are the critical differences in profit analysis when conducted in a capitated environment versus a fee-for-service environment?

5.10 How does a provider's incentive differ when it moves from a fee-for-service to a capitated environment?

5.11 a. What cost structure is best when a provider is capitated? Explain.

b. What cost structure is best when a provider is reimbursed primarily by fee-for-service payers? Explain.

END-OF-CHAPTER PROBLEMS

5.1 Assume that the managers of Fort Winston Hospital are setting the price on a new outpatient service. Here are the relevant data estimates:

Variable cost per visit	$5.00
Annual direct fixed costs	$500,000
Annual overhead allocation	$50,000
Expected annual utilization	10,000 visits

a. What per visit price must be set for the service to break even? To earn an annual profit of $100,000?

b. Repeat Part a, but assume that the variable cost per visit is $10.

c. Return to the data given in the problem. Again repeat Part a, but assume that direct fixed costs are $1,000,000.

d. Repeat Part a assuming both a $10 variable cost and $1,000,000 in direct fixed costs.

5.2 The Audiology Department at Randall Clinic offers many services to the clinic's patients. The three most common, along with cost and utilization data, are as follows:

Service	Variable Cost per Service	Annual Direct Fixed Costs	Annual Number of Visits
Basic examination	$5	$50,000	3,000
Advanced examination	7	30,000	1,500
Therapy session	10	40,000	500

a. What is the fee schedule for these services, assuming that the goal is to cover only variable and direct fixed costs?

b. Assume that the Audiology Department is allocated $100,000 in total overhead by the clinic, and the department director has allocated $50,000 of this amount to the three services listed above. What is the fee schedule assuming that these overhead costs must be covered? (To answer this question, assume that the allocation of overhead costs to each service is made on the basis of number of visits.)

c. Assume that these services must make a combined profit of $25,000. Now, what is the fee schedule? (To answer this question, assume that the profit requirement is allocated in the same way as overhead costs.)

5.3 Allied Laboratories is combining some of its most common tests into one-price packages. One such package will contain three tests that have the following variable costs:

	Test A	Test B	Test C
Disposable syringe	$3.00	$3.00	$3.00
Blood vial	0.50	0.50	0.50
Forms	0.15	0.15	0.15
Reagents	0.80	0.60	1.20
Sterile bandage	0.10	0.10	0.10
Breakage/losses	0.05	0.05	0.05

When the tests are combined, only one syringe, form, and sterile bandage will be used. Furthermore, only one charge for breakage/losses will apply. Two blood vials are required and reagent costs will remain the same (reagents are required for all three tests).

a. As a starting point, what is the price of the combined test assuming marginal cost pricing?

b. Assume that Allied wants a contribution margin of $10 per test. What price must be set to achieve this goal?

c. Allied estimates that 2,000 of the combined tests will be conducted during the first year. The annual allocation of direct fixed and overhead costs total $40,000. What price must be set to cover full costs? What price must be set to produce a profit of $20,000 on the combined test?

5.4 Consider the CVP graphs below for two providers operating in a fee-for-service environment:

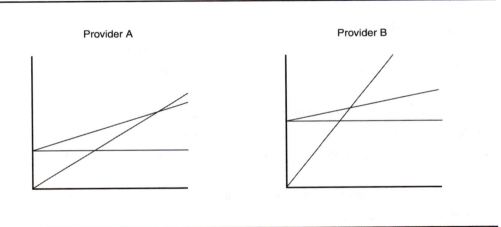

Provider A   Provider B

a. Assuming the graphs are drawn to the same scale, which provider has the greater fixed costs? The greater variable cost rate? The greater per unit revenue?

b. Which provider has the greater contribution margin?

c. Which provider needs the higher volume to break even?

d. How would the graphs change if the providers were operating in a discounted fee-for-service environment? In a capitated environment?

5.5 Consider the data in the following table for three independent healthcare organizations:

	Revenues	Total Variable Costs	Fixed Costs	Total Costs	Profit
a.	$2,000	$1,400	?	$2,000	?
b.	?	1,000	?	1,600	$2,400
c.	4,000	?	$600	?	400

Fill in the missing data indicated by question marks.

5.6 Assume that a radiology group practice has the following cost structure:

Fixed costs	$500,000
Variable cost per procedure	25
Charge (revenue) per procedure	100

Furthermore, assume that the group expects to perform 7,500 procedures in the coming year.

a. Construct the group's base case projected P&L statement.

b. What is the group's contribution margin? What is its breakeven point?

c. What volume is required to provide a pretax profit of $100,000? A pretax profit of $200,000?

d. Sketch out a CVP analysis graph depicting the base case situation.

e. Now, assume that the practice contracts with one HMO, and the plan proposes a 20 percent discount from charges. Redo questions a, b, c, and d under these conditions.

5.7 General Hospital, a not-for-profit acute care facility, has the following cost structure for its inpatient services:

Fixed costs	$10,000,000
Variable cost per inpatient day	200
Charge (revenue) per inpatient day	1,000

The hospital expects to have a patient load of 15,000 inpatient days next year.

a. Construct the hospital's base case projected P&L statement.

b. What is the hospital's breakeven point?

c. What volume is required to provide a profit of $1,000,000? A profit of $500,000?

d. Now, assume that 20 percent of the hospital's inpatient days come from a managed care plan that wants a 25 percent discount from charges. Should the hospital agree to the discount proposal?

5.8 You are considering starting a walk-in clinic. Your financial projections for the first year of operations are as follows:

Revenues (10,000 visits)	$400,000
Wages and benefits	220,000
Rent	5,000
Depreciation	30,000
Utilities	2,500
Medical supplies	50,000
Administrative supplies	10,000

Assume that all costs are fixed except supply costs, which are variable. Furthermore, assume that the clinic must pay taxes at a 30 percent rate.
   a. Construct the clinic's projected P&L statement.
   b. What number of visits is required to break even?
   c. What number of visits is required to provide you with an after-tax profit of $100,000?

5.9 Grandview Clinic has fixed costs of $2 million and an average variable cost rate of $15 per visit. Its sole payer, an HMO, has proposed an annual capitation payment of $150 for each of its 20,000 members. Past experience indicates that the population served will average two visits per year.
   a. Construct the base case projected P&L statement on the contract.
   b. Sketch two CVP analysis graphs for the clinic—one with number of visits on the X axis, and one with number of members on the X axis. Compare and contrast these graphs with the one in Problem 5.6 d.
   c. What is the clinic's contribution margin on the contract? How does this value compare with the value in Problem 5.6 b?
   d. What profit gain can be realized if the clinic can lower per member utilization to 1.8 visits?

CHAPTER 6

PLANNING AND BUDGETING

THEME SET-UP ACTUAL VERSUS EXPECTED RESULTS

The Sumter County Organization for Rural Needs (SCORN) delivers low-cost healthcare services to residents of the county's rural areas. SCORN relies on volunteers to offer high-quality healthcare to people without health insurance and those who have insurance but find the organization's location more convenient than other alternatives. In 2008, more than 50 physicians, dentists, nurse practitioners, and other clinical professionals volunteered their services, providing more than $1.5 million of patient care.

One part of SCORN's operations is the dental clinic, whose services include pediatric dentistry, extractions, fillings, crowns, and dentures. Although the dentists are all volunteers, the support staff consists of volunteers, paid part-timers, partially paid workers, and one full-time, paid employee.

At the end of 2008, Mark Mason, SCORN's director, created this budget for the dental clinic's 2009 annual and first-quarter expenses:

	Annual 2009	First Quarter 2009
Coordinator compensation	$ 53,334	$13,334
Hygienists compensation	28,164	7,041
Assistants compensation	103,877	25,969
Office staff compensation	38,047	9,512
Clinical supplies	40,000	10,000
Office supplies	2,000	500
Equipment maintenance	5,000	1,250
Utilities	6,000	1,500
Telephone	3,600	900
Total	$280,022	$70,006

In early April 2009, SCORN's accountant provided Mark with the actual expenses for the dental clinic for the first quarter (January-March):

Coordinator compensation	$12,855
Hygienists compensation	8,614
Assistants compensation	27,443
Office staff compensation	8,470
Clinical supplies	9,344
Office supplies	529
Equipment maintenance	1,250
Utilities	1,355
Telephone	793
Total	$70,653

Mark must compare what has happened in the first quarter with what was expected to happen. Then, he must determine problem areas and take action to ensure that, at the close of 2009, actual expenses are in line with those projected at the beginning of the year.

By the end of this chapter, you will know more about the planning and budgeting process. In addition, you, like Mark, will be able to judge how well the dental clinic is sticking to its expense budget.

LEARNING OBJECTIVES

After studying this chapter, you will be able to

➤ Describe the overall planning process and the key components of the financial plan.

➤ Discuss briefly the format and use of several types of budgets.

➤ Differentiate between a simple budget and a flexible budget.

➤ Create a simple operating budget.

➤ Explain how variance analysis is used in the budgeting process.

6.1 INTRODUCTION

Planning and budgeting play a critical role in the finance function of all healthcare organizations. In fact, one could argue (and usually win) that planning and budgeting are the most important of all finance-related tasks.

Planning encompasses the overall process of preparing for the future. Because of its importance to organizational success, most healthcare managers, especially at large organizations, spend a great deal of time on activities related to planning.

Budgeting is one part of the planning process. Managers use a set of budgets to tie together planning and control functions. In general, organizational plans focus on the long-term big picture, whereas budgets address the details of both planning for the immediate future and, through the control process, ensuring that current performance is consistent with organizational goals.

This chapter explores the planning process and the way budgets are used within healthcare organizations. In particular, we focus on how managers can use variance analysis (what has happened versus what was expected to happen) to exercise control over current operations.

Planning
The process of preparing for the future.

Budgeting
The creation and use of financial forecasts to plan for and control a business's operations.

6.2 STRATEGIC PLANNING

Financial plans and budgets are developed within the framework of the business's overall **strategic plan**. Thus, we begin our discussion with an overview of strategic planning.

MISSION STATEMENT

The *mission statement,* which is the guiding light for the strategic plan, defines the organization's overall purpose and reason for existence. The mission may be defined either specifically or generally, but it must describe what the organization does and for whom. For example, an investor-owned diagnostic imaging center might state that its mission is "to provide our patients with state-of-the-art diagnostic services at the lowest possible cost, which will also maximize benefits to our employees and owners."

Normally, mission statements for not-for-profit businesses are stated in different terms. The reality of competition in the healthcare industry, however, forces all businesses, regardless of ownership, to operate in a manner consistent with financial viability. To illustrate a not-for-profit mission statement, consider the following statement of Bayside Memorial Hospital:

> (!) **CRITICAL CONCEPT**
> Strategic Plan
>
> A business's strategic plan is a statement of where the business is now, where it wants to be in the future, and how it intends to get there. A comprehensive strategic plan contains many elements, including the mission, values, and vision statements as well as goals and objectives. One way to think of a strategic plan is See-Think-Develop. In other words, *see* the current situation, *think* about where the organization wants to be, and *develop* plans to get there.

Mission statement
A statement that defines the overall purpose of the organization.

The mission of Bayside Memorial Hospital is to

◆ Provide comprehensive, state-of-the-art patient services.

◆ Emphasize caring and other human values in the treatment of patients and in relations with employees, medical staff, and community.

◆ Provide employees and medical staff with maximum opportunities to achieve their personal and professional goals.

VALUES STATEMENT

Values statement
A statement of the core beliefs that underlie the culture of the organization.

The *values statement* represents the core beliefs that define the culture of an organization. In general, this statement contains a brief list of the basic beliefs that underlie the culture of the organization.

Bayside Memorial Hospital believes in the following values:

◆ To treat everyone with respect and dignity.

◆ To be compassionate in comfort and care.

◆ To do the right thing at the right time for the right reason.

◆ To achieve excellence and ensure quality.

You can get a good feel for Bayside's organizational culture from this list, which plays an important role in constructing the remainder of the strategic plan.

VISION STATEMENT

Vision statement
A statement that describes the desired position of the business at a future point in time.

The *vision statement* usually is a single-sentence description of the organization's desired position in a future point in time—say, ten years. The intent is to provide a single goal that motivates managers, employees, and the medical staff. Bayside's vision statement is "to be the regional leader in providing state-of-the-art compassionate care in a humanistic environment."

In addition to providing basic guidance regarding management and employee behavior at Bayside, the mission, values, and vision statements provide managers with a framework for establishing specific goals and objectives.

CORPORATE GOALS

Although the mission, values, and vision statements articulate the general philosophy and approach of the organization, they do not provide managers with specific operational goals.

Corporate goals set forth the outcomes from operations, usually qualitative, that management strives to attain. These goals should be changed over time as conditions change, and they should be challenging yet realistically achievable. Corporate goals occasionally conflict with each other, and when they do, senior managers have to make judgments regarding which ones should take precedence.

> **Corporate goals**
> Specified goals, including financial, that an organization strives to attain. Generally, corporate goals are qualitative.

Bayside divides its corporate goals into the following five major areas:

1. *Quality and customer satisfaction:*
   - To make quality performance the goal of each employee.

   - To be recognized by our patients as the provider of choice in our market area.

   - To rapidly identify and resolve areas of patient dissatisfaction.

2. *Medical staff relations:*
   - To identify and develop timely channels of communication among all members of the medical staff, management, and board of directors.

   - To respond in a timely manner to all medical staff concerns brought to the attention of management.

   - To make Bayside Memorial Hospital a more desirable location to practice medicine.

   - To develop strategies to enhance the mutual commitment of the medical staff, administration, and board of directors for the benefit of the hospital's stakeholders.

   - To provide the highest-quality, most cost-effective medical care through a collaborative effort among the medical staff, administration, and board of directors.

3. *Human resource management:*
   - To be recognized as the customer service leader in our market area.

   - To develop and manage human resources to make Bayside Memorial Hospital the most attractive location to work in our market area.

4. *Financial performance:*
   - To maintain a financial condition that permits us to be highly competitive in our market area.

♦ To develop the systems necessary to identify inpatient and outpatient costs by unit of service.

5. *Health systems management:*

♦ To be a leader in applied technology based on patient needs.

♦ To establish new services and programs in response to patient needs.

♦ To be in the forefront of electronic medical records technology.

CORPORATE OBJECTIVES

Corporate objectives
Quantitative targets that an organization sets to meet its corporate goals.

Once an organization has defined its corporate goals, it must develop corporate objectives to help achieve those goals. *Corporate objectives* generally are quantitative in nature, such as specifying a target market share, a target volume growth rate, or a target profitability measure. Furthermore, the extent to which corporate objectives are met is commonly the basis of managers' performance compensation (bonuses and the like).

To illustrate, consider Bayside's financial performance goal of maintaining a financial condition that permits the hospital to be highly competitive in its market area. The following objectives are tied to that goal. (The financial measures listed here are explained in detail in Chapter 13.)

♦ To maintain or exceed the hospital's current 4.3 percent operating margin.

♦ To maintain the hospital's debt ratio in the range of 35 to 40 percent.

♦ To maintain the hospital's liquidity at a minimum of 2.0 as measured by the current ratio.

♦ To increase fixed asset utilization, as measured by the fixed asset turnover ratio, to 1.5.

Corporate objectives give managers precise targets to shoot for. But the objectives must support the business's goals and must be chosen carefully so that they are challenging yet attainable in a reasonable period of time.

? SELF-TEST QUESTIONS

1. Briefly describe the nature and use of the following corporate planning tools:
   a. Mission statement

(?) SELF-TEST QUESTIONS

    b. Values statement

    c. Vision statement

    d. Corporate goals

    e. Corporate objectives

2. Why do managers at all levels need to be familiar with the organization's strategic plan?

6.3 OPERATIONAL PLANNING

Operational planning provides a road map for executing the business's strategic plan. The key document here is the **operating plan,** which contains the detailed guidelines for meeting corporate objectives. In other words, the operating plan provides the "how to" or perhaps the "how we expect to" portion of an organization's overall plan for the future.

    Operating plans can be developed for any time horizon, but most firms use a five-year horizon. Thus, the term "five-year plan" is often used in place of operating plan. In a five-year plan, the plans are most detailed for the first year, with each succeeding year's plan becoming less specific.

    Table 6.1 outlines the key elements of Bayside Memorial Hospital's five-year plan, with an expanded section for the financial plan (Chapter 7.C

> **(!) CRITICAL CONCEPT**
> Operating Plan
>
> An operating plan is a schedule of events and a list of responsibilities for meeting the goals and objectives laid out in the strategic plan. The operating plan ensures that everyone knows what needs to get done by when and provides a means to coordinate and track progress. Operating plans are more detailed than strategic plans. In fact, too much detail in the strategic plan can obscure the overall vision of the organization. Often, operating plans are constructed to cover a five-year period, so they are also called five-year plans. Typically, the plans for the first year are laid out in great detail, while the plans for the following years are increasingly less specific.

of the table). A full five-year plan outline requires several pages, but the one in Table 6.1 provides insights into such a plan's format and contents. Note that the first two chapters of the operating plan are drawn from Bayside's strategic plan.

    For Bayside, much of the financial planning function takes place at the department level, with technical assistance from the marketing, planning, and financial staffs. Large businesses undertake the planning process at the divisional level. Each division has its own mission and goals as well as objectives and budgets designed to support the goals. When consolidated, division-level plans constitute the overall corporate plan.

Financial plan

That portion of the oper-
ating plan that focuses
on the finance function.

Section 1 of the *financial plan* (Chapter 7.C of the Table 6.1 operating plan) is the analysis of current financial condition, which in turn provides the basis, or starting point, for the remaining sections of the financial plan. (Insights into financial condition analysis are presented in Chapter 13.)

Section 2 lists planned investments in land, buildings, and equipment (the capital budget) along with how these investments will be financed. (Capital investment decisions are discussed in Chapters 9 and 10, and business financing is covered in Chapter 8.)

Section 3 provides overall guidance on day-to-day financial operations. (Many aspects of financial operations are discussed in Chapter 7.)

Section 4 focuses on budgeting and control, laying out financial goals at the micro level (e.g., by division, contract, or diagnosis) and the mechanisms used to manage operations through frequent comparisons with actual results. In essence, this section contains the budgets that provide the benchmarks that line managers should be striving to attain throughout the year.

Much of the information from the first four sections feeds into the forecasted financial statements contained in Section 5. (Financial statements are covered in Chapters 11 and 12.) The forecasted statements allow managers to see the financial implications of the five-year plan. If the financial statements do not meet managerial goals for financial performance, then the initial operating plan must be modified to create the desired financial results.

? SELF-TEST QUESTIONS

1. What is the primary difference between strategic and operating plans?

2. What is the most common time horizon for operating plans?

3. Briefly describe the contents of a typical financial plan.

4. What is the primary difference between Sections 2 and 3 of the financial plan?

6.4 INTRODUCTION TO BUDGETING

Budgeting entails the entire process of constructing and using budgets, which are detailed plans for obtaining and using resources during a specified period of time. In general, budgets rely heavily on revenue and cost estimates, so the budgeting process applies many of the concepts presented in Chapters 4 and 5.

Managers must think of budgets not as accounting tools but as managerial tools. Budgets are more important to managers than to accountants because budgets provide the means to plan and communicate operational expectations within an organization. Every manager must be aware of the plans made by other managers and by the organization as a whole, and budgets are a way to communicate these plans. The budgeting process and the resultant final budget allow senior managers to allocate financial resources.

Planning, communication, and allocation are important purposes of the budgeting process, but perhaps the greatest value of budgeting is that it establishes financial

⚠ **CRITICAL CONCEPT**
Budgeting

Budgeting can be defined simply as "planning for how much money you have and how it is spent." The purpose of budgeting for large business enterprises is essentially the same as budgeting for families (or individuals). However, the complexities in large organizations with many subunits make the budgeting process difficult and time consuming. Budgeting plays an important role in businesses because it is the primary tool for senior managers both to establish performance goals and to monitor operations to ensure that those goals are met.

benchmarks for control. When compared to actual results, budgets provide managers with feedback about the financial performance of a department, a service, a contract, or the organization as a whole. Such comparisons help managers evaluate the performance of individuals, departments, product lines, reimbursement contracts, and so on.

Finally, budgets inform managers about what needs to be done to improve performance. When actual results fall short of those specified in the budget, managers must identify the areas that caused the subpar performance. In this way, managerial resources can be brought to bear on those areas of operations that offer the most promise for financial improvement.

The information developed by comparing actual results with expected (planned) results (the control process) is useful in improving the overall accuracy of the planning process. Managers want to meet budget targets, and hence most managers will think long and hard when those targets are being developed.

❓ SELF-TEST QUESTIONS

1. What is budgeting?

2. What are its primary purposes and benefits?

6.5 BUDGETING DECISIONS

Managers must make several decisions regarding the budgeting process, including these three most important ones: (1) general approach to the process, (2) timing of the budget(s), and (3) the forecast basis.

GENERAL APPROACH

Because budgets affect virtually everyone in the organization, and individuals' reactions to the budgeting process can have considerable influence on an organization's overall effectiveness, it is wise to carefully plot how the budgeting process takes place.

In the *bottom-up approach*, budgets are developed first by department or program managers. Presumably, such individuals are most knowledgeable about the needs of their respective departments or programs. Next, the department budgets are submitted to the finance department for review and incorporation into the organizational budget, which then must be approved by senior management. Unfortunately, the aggregation of department budgets often results in an organizational budget that is not financially feasible. In such cases, the department budgets are sent back for revision to the initial preparers (managers). This starts a negotiation process aimed at creating a budget that is acceptable to all parties, or at least to as many parties as possible.

A more authoritarian approach to budgeting is the *top-down approach*, in which little negotiation takes place between department and senior managers. Here, the budget is developed by the finance staff and then, after approval by senior management, sent to department managers for implementation. Department managers may have some input into the process, but not nearly as much as in the bottom-up approach.

The top-down approach has the advantages of being relatively expeditious and reflecting top management's perspective from the start. However, because it limits involvement and communication, the top-down approach often results in less commitment among department managers and employees than does the bottom-up approach. Most people will perform better and make greater attempts to achieve budgetary goals if they have played a prominent role in setting those goals. The idea of participatory budgeting is to involve as many managers, and even other employees, as possible in the budgeting process.

TIMING

Virtually all healthcare organizations have annual budgets, which set the standards for the coming year. The problem with an annual cycle is that it does not allow managers to detect adverse trends quickly. Thus, most organizations also have quarterly budgets, while many have monthly or even weekly budgets.

Not all budget types or subunits within an organization have to use the same timing pattern. Additionally, many organizations prepare budgets for one or more *out years*, which are more closely aligned with financial planning than with operational control.

FORECAST BASIS

Traditionally, healthcare organizations have used the conventional approach to budgeting as the forecast basis. In this approach, the previous budget is used as the starting point for creating the new budget. Each line on the old budget is examined, and then adjustments are made to reflect changes in circumstances.

Under **conventional (incremental) budgeting**, many budget changes are applied more or less equally across departments and programs. For example, wages and salaries might be assumed to increase at the same inflation rate for all departments and programs within an

Bottom-up approach
A budgeting system where budgets originate at the department or program level and then are aggregated and approved by senior managers.

Top-down approach
A budgeting system where the finance staff prepares the budget for senior management approval, after which it is sent to department and program heads for implementation.

Out year
A future year beyond the next budget year.

organization. In essence, conventional budgeting assumes that prior budgets are valid (make sound economic sense), so it focuses on determining the adjustments (typically minor) that must be made to account for changes in the operating environment.

As its name implies, **zero-based budgeting** starts with a clean slate. Thus, departments begin with a budget of zero. Department managers must fully justify every line item (i.e., employee, piece of equipment, amount of space allocated, inventory, and the like) on the basis of expected volume. In effect, departments and programs must justify their contribution (positive or negative) to the organization's financial condition each budget period. In some situations, department and program managers must create budgets that show the impact of alternative funding (resource allocation) levels. Senior management, then, can use this information to make rational decisions about where cuts could be made in the event of financial constraints.

Conceptually, zero-based budgeting is superior to conventional budgeting, but the managerial resources required for zero-based budgeting far exceed those required for conventional budgeting. Zero-based budgeting is most useful at organizations facing reimbursement constraints, because such providers are forced to implement cost-control efforts on a more or less continuous basis.

As a compromise to bearing the full costs of zero-based budgeting, some healthcare organizations use conventional budgeting annually but then use a zero-based budget on a less-frequent basis—say, every five years. An alternative way to reduce budgeting costs is to use the conventional approach on 80 percent of the budget each year and the zero-based approach on 20 percent. Then, over every five-year period, the entire budget will be subjected to zero-based budgeting. This approach takes advantage of the benefits of zero-based budgeting without allowing it to consume more resources than it is worth.

> ### (!) CRITICAL CONCEPT
> #### Conventional Versus Zero-Based Budgeting
>
> Conventional (incremental) budgeting is based on the assumption that the previous year's budget accurately reflects the true (minimum) costs and (maximum) revenues of the organization. Thus, relatively minor changes are made to the current year's budget to reflect any changes in circumstances, such as increased labor rates. In zero-based budgeting, each budget unit starts with a clean slate, and all costs and revenues must be justified and created from scratch. Conventional budgeting is less costly to perform, but any inaccuracies and inefficiencies existing in such a budget tend to reoccur year after year. Zero-based budgeting is more time consuming and hence costly, but usually it produces a more realistic, and hence effective, budget.

(?) SELF-TEST QUESTIONS

1. What is the difference between the bottom-up and top-down budgeting approaches?

2. What time periods are used in budgeting?

3. What are the primary differences between conventional and zero-based budgets?

6.6 BUDGET TYPES

Although an organization's immediate financial expectations are expressed in a document called the budget (or master budget), in most organizations "the budget" is actually composed of several components whose contents and format are dictated by the business's structure and by managerial preferences. That said, several types of budgets are used either formally or informally at virtually all healthcare organizations.

REVENUE BUDGET

The starting point for the budgeting process is the volume forecast. Unfortunately, volume forecasting can be difficult and complex. (See the Industry Practice box.) Detailed information from the volume estimate feeds into the *revenue budget*, which combines volume and reimbursement data to develop revenue forecasts. Planners at Bayside Memorial Hospital consider the hospital's pricing strategy for managed care plans, conventional fee-for-service contracts, and private-pay patients as well as trends in inflation and third-party payer reimbursement, all of which affect operating revenues.

> **Revenue budget**
> A listing of the expected revenues of an organization, usually on a monthly, quarterly, and annual basis and broken out by department, service, and payer.

The result is a compilation of operating revenue forecasts by service, both in the aggregate—for example, inpatient revenue—and on an individual diagnosis or procedure basis. The individual diagnosis and procedure forecasts are summed and then compared with the aggregate service group forecasts. Differences are reconciled, and the result is an operating revenue forecast for the hospital as a whole, but with breakdowns by service categories and by individual diagnoses and procedures.

In addition to operating revenues, other revenues (e.g., contributions, interest income on investments, rental receipts on medical office buildings) must be forecasted. Note that in all revenue forecasts, timing is important. Thus, the revenue budget must forecast not only the amount of revenue but also the time it is expected to occur—typically by month, quarter, and year.

EXPENSE BUDGET

Like the revenue budget, the *expense budget* is driven by the volume of services provided. Here, the focus is on the costs of providing services. Similar to the revenue budget, the expense budget is a compilation of expense forecasts by department, service, and individual diagnosis or procedure.

> **Expense budget**
> A listing of the expected expenses of an organization, usually by department and service, and further broken down into components such as facilities, labor, and supplies.

The expense budget typically is divided into labor and nonlabor components. Labor expenses include salaries, wages, and fringe benefits, including travel and education. Nonlabor components include expenses associated with such items as depreciation, leases, utilities, and administrative and medical supplies. Expenses normally will be broken down into fixed and variable components. (As discussed later in this chapter, cost structure information is required if an organization uses flexible budgeting techniques.)

To get a better feel for the complexities of volume forecasting, consider the procedures followed by Bayside Memorial Hospital.

First, Bayside managers divide the demand for services into four major groups: inpatient, outpatient, ancillary, and other services. Second, they plot volume trends in each of these areas over the past five years, and they make a first approximation forecast, assuming a continuation of past trends. Third, the managers forecast the level of population growth and disease trends. For example, how much will the aged-65-or-older population in the hospital's service area grow? These forecasts are used to develop volume by major diagnoses and to differentiate between normal services and critical care services.

Fourth, Bayside's managers analyze the competitive environment. Consideration is given to such factors as the hospital's inpatient and outpatient capacities, its competitors' capacities, and new services or service improvements that either Bayside or its competitors might institute. Fifth, they consider the effect of the hospital's planned pricing actions on volume. For example, does the hospital have plans to raise outpatient charges to boost profit margins or to lower charges to gain market share and use excess capacity? If such actions are expected to affect volume forecasts, these forecasts must be revised to reflect the expected impact. Marketing campaigns and changes in managed care plan contracts also affect volume, so probable developments in these areas must be considered.

The consequences can be serious if the hospital's volume forecast is off the mark. If the market for any particular service expands more than Bayside has expected and planned for, the hospital will not be able to meet its patients' needs. Potential patients will end up going to competitors, and Bayside will lose market share and perhaps miss a major opportunity. However, if Bayside's projections are overly optimistic, it could end up with too much capacity, which means higher-than-necessary costs because of excess facilities and staff.

Interestingly, Bayside recently revised its entire budgeting process. Previously, the process was spreadsheet driven and took more than five months to complete. There was constant concern that the paper budget would not be completed in time to be presented at the September board of trustees meeting, which was the

---

traditional approval date. Once the annual budget was approved, six more weeks was required to break down the budget into monthly and quarterly budgets and to distribute the reports to department managers.

Bayside currently uses proprietary software that creates the budget electronically. This system reduced the budget cycle by two months, or about 40 percent. The budget now is integrated with the hospital's financial reporting system, which means feedback (and hence control) is available on a continuous basis. The result is more efficiency in budget preparation, more confidence in the budget process, and streamlined reporting with easy online access for both department and senior managers.

OPERATING BUDGET

For large organizations, the **operating budget** is a combination of the revenue and expense budgets. Small businesses, on the other hand, may not prepare formal revenue and expense budgets, but rather use the data directly to prepare a single operating budget. Because the operating budget focuses on revenues and expenses, and hence profits, it can be thought of as a forecasted profit and loss (P&L) statement. Operating budgets can be, and are, prepared at multiple levels within organizations. Thus, operating budgets are prepared for entire organizations, departments, service lines, payers, and at any other level that makes sense for managerial monitoring and control.

(!) **CRITICAL CONCEPT**
Operating Budget

An operating budget uses underlying data, such as volume, reimbursements, and labor requirements, to forecast revenues, expenses (costs), and profits. Operating budgets are prepared at multiple levels within organizations and for specific services and contracts. These budgets typically are prepared on a monthly, quarterly, and annual basis. For most organizations, operating budgets are the primary focus of the budgeting process because they focus on a key financial indicator—profitability.

For budgeting purposes, departments often are classified as cost centers or profit centers. *Cost centers* are organizational subunits, typically departments, that incur costs but do not directly generate revenues. For example, the overhead units in a hospital, such as facilities and finance departments, are cost centers. Managers of cost centers are held responsible only for the costs of running their departments.

Cost center
A subunit within an organization that incurs costs but generates no revenues.

Profit (revenue) center
A subunit within an organization that both generates revenues and incurs costs, and hence creates profits.

Profit (revenue) centers are organizational subunits that generate revenues as well as costs, so their managers can be held accountable for profitability. Note, however, that profit center managers typically have more control over costs than over revenues. (In reality, their ability to control indirect, or overhead, costs also is limited. See Chapter 4 for a discussion of overhead cost allocation.) In a hospital, examples of revenue centers include routine care, outpatient, and emergency departments.

(?) SELF-TEST QUESTIONS

1. What are some of the budget types used within healthcare organizations?

2. What is the difference between a cost center and a profit center? Give examples of each in a hospital setting.

Operating Budget Illustration

Table 6.2 contains the 2008 operating budget for Carroll Clinic, a small primary care practice. Most operating budgets are more complex than this illustration, which has purposely been kept simple for ease of discussion.

As with most financial forecasts, the starting point for this operating budget, which was developed in late 2007, is patient volume. A volume projection gives managers a starting point for making revenue and cost estimates. Part I of Table 6.2 shows that Carroll Clinic's expected patient volume for 2008 comes from two sources: Payer A and Payer B. In total, the clinic's patient base is expected to produce 9,000 + 12,000 = 21,000 visits.

Part II contains reimbursement data. The clinic's net collection for each visit averages $100 from Payer A and $90 from Payer B. (Both payers reimburse the clinic on a fee-for-service basis.) Of course, some visits will generate greater revenues, and some will generate less. The patients that visit the clinic are essentially the same in demographics, diagnoses, and treatment, regardless of payer. However, Payer B has been more aggressive in negotiating discounts from charges, and hence it pays, on average, $10 less per visit than does Payer A.

Part III focuses on costs. Supplies expense, the bulk of which is inherently variable in nature, is expected to total $315,000 for the year. Examples include forms, rubber gloves, syringes, medications, bandage materials, and a host of other medical expendables. Because these supplies will support 21,000 visits, their average cost per visit is $315,000 / 21,000 = $15.

To support the forecasted 21,000 visits, the clinic is expected to incur labor costs of $1,035,000. Thus, labor costs are expected to average $1,035,000 / 21,000 = $49.29 per visit. However, labor costs are predominantly fixed costs, so the per visit amount is not as

I.	*Volume (Number of Visits)*	
	Payer A	9,000
	Payer B	12,000
	Total	21,000
II.	*Reimbursement (Per Visit)*	
	Payer A	$ 100
	Payer B	$ 90
III.	*Costs*	
	Variable Costs:	
	Supplies	$ 315,000
	Fixed Costs:	
	Labor	$1,035,000
	Overhead	500,000
	Total	$1,535,000
IV.	*Forecasted P&L Statement*	
	Revenues:	
	Payer A	$ 900,000
	Payer B	1,080,000
	Total revenues	$1,980,000
	Variable costs	$ 315,000
	Fixed costs	1,535,000
	Total costs	$1,850,000
	Profit	$ 130,000

TABLE 6.2

Carroll Clinic: 2008 Operating Budget

meaningful as the $15 per visit supplies cost. Finally, the clinic is expected to incur $500,000 of overhead costs in 2008, primarily for contract support (e.g., accounting, billing, collections) and facilities expenses (e.g., rent, housekeeping, utilities).

Part IV contains the budgeted (forecasted) 2008 P&L statement, the heart of the operating budget. Total revenues for the clinic are forecasted to be ($100 × Number of Payer A visits) + ($90 × Number of Payer B visits) = ($100 × 9,000) + ($90 × 12,000) = $900,000 + $1,080,000 = $1,980,000. If the actual number of visits is more or less than 21,000 in 2008, the resulting revenues will be different from the $1,980,000 forecast. The difference between the projected revenues of $1,980,000 and projected total costs of $315,000 + $1,535,000 = $1,850,000 produces a budgeted profit of $130,000.

The true purpose of the operating budget is to set financial goals for the clinic. In effect, the operating budget can be thought of as a contract between the organization and its managers and employees. Thus, the $130,000 profit forecast becomes the overall profit benchmark for Carroll Clinic in 2008, and the clinic's managers and employees will be held accountable for the revenues and expenses needed to meet the budget.

6.7 VARIANCE ANALYSIS

Variance
In accounting, the difference between what is expected to happen and what actually happens.

In accounting, a *variance* is the difference between an actual, or realized, value and the budgeted value. Note that the accounting definition of variance is not the same as the statistical definition, although both meanings connote a difference from some base value. Thus, **variance analysis** is an examination and interpretation of what has actually happened versus what was expected to happen. If the budget is based on realistic expectations, variance analysis can provide managers with useful information. Variance analysis does not provide all the answers, but it does help managers ask the right questions.

Variance analysis is essential to the managerial control process. Actions taken in response to variance analysis often have the potential to dramatically improve the operations and financial performance of the organization. For example, many variances are more or less controllable by managerial actions, so managers can take steps to avoid unfavorable variances in the future.

The primary goal of variance analysis should not be to assign blame for unfavorable results. Rather, it should be to uncover the cause of operational problems so that they can be avoided, or at least minimized, in the future. Even if the variances are beyond managerial control, their identification is still important to the well-being of the organization. For example, it may be necessary to tighten controllable costs to offset unfavorable variances in areas that are beyond managerial control.

Here we consider two approaches to variance analysis: simple variance analysis and flexible variance analysis.

> ⓘ **CRITICAL CONCEPT**
> Variance Analysis
>
> Variance analysis involves comparing what was expected to happen with what has actually happened. A budget yields no value if it is not used as a benchmark for financial performance. If budget benchmarks are not met, managers must identify the shortcomings and, more important, must take actions to ensure that the shortcomings are corrected and hence do not occur in future budgets. Furthermore, variance analysis of monthly and quarterly budgets should lead to operational changes that will help the organization meet annual goals when short-term performance lags behind expectations.

SIMPLE VARIANCE ANALYSIS

Consider Table 6.3. Here, we combined Carroll Clinic's 2008 operating budget (shown in Table 6.2) with the actual results for 2008. Then, we calculated both dollar (or visit) and percentage variances.

		Simple Budget	Actual Results	Variance Dollar Visit	%
I.	**Volume (Number of Visits)**				
	Payer A	9,000	10,000	1,000	11.1%
	Payer B	12,000	11,500	(500)	(4.2)
	Total	21,000	21,500	500	2.4
II.	**Reimbursement (Per Visit)**				
	Payer A	$100	$105	$5	5.0%
	Payer B	$ 90	$ 85	($5)	(5.6)
III.	**Costs**				
	Variable Costs:				
	Supplies	$ 315,000	$ 320,000	($ 5,000)	(1.6%)
	Fixed Costs:				
	Labor	$1,035,000	$1,050,000	($ 15,000)	(1.4)
	Overhead	500,000	550,000	(50,000)	(10.0)
	Total	$1,535,000	$1,600,000	($ 65,000)	(4.2)
IV.	**Forecasted P&L Statement**				
	Revenues:				
	Payer A	$ 900,000	$1,050,000	$ 150,000	16.7%
	Payer B	1,080,000	977,500	(102,500)	(9.5)
	Total revenues	$1,980,000	$2,027,500	$ 47,500	2.4
	Variable costs	$ 315,000	$ 320,000	($ 5,000)	(1.6)
	Fixed costs	1,535,000	1,600,000	(65,000)	(4.2)
	Total costs	$1,850,000	$1,920,000	($ 70,000)	(3.8)
	Profit	$ 130,000	$ 107,500	($ 22,500)	(17.3)

TABLE 6.3

Carroll Clinic: 2008 Simple Budget Variance Analysis

Standard

In variance analysis, the budgeted (expected) value established at the beginning of the budget period.

As explained earlier, variance analysis involves comparing two amounts, with the variance being the difference between the values. For example, if at the beginning of the year, a hospital expected to make a profit of $2 million, but actual results were a profit of $2.2 million, the variance would be a positive $0.2 million or $200,000.

The budgeted value, in this case $2 million of profits, is often called the *standard*, because that is the profit goal of the hospital (the standard to be reached) as expressed in the budget. In general, variances are calculated so that positive amounts signify "good" or desirable results, while negative amounts are "bad" results. As discussed in the following paragraphs, all variances are calculated in more or less the same way.

To begin a simple variance analysis on Carroll Clinic, consider the profit reported in Part IV of Table 6.3. We start here because this is the most important single line on the operating budget. The profit variance was -$22,500, calculated as Actual value – Budgeted value = $107,500 – $130,000 = -$22,500. In words, the clinic's 2008 profitability was $22,500 below standard, or $22,500 less than expected. Although this negative variance should generate concern, a more detailed analysis is required to determine the underlying causes.

Perhaps the first question that the clinic's management would want answered is this: Is the loss (relative to expectations) caused by a revenue shortfall, cost overruns, or both? To answer this question, we must examine the revenue and cost variances. The total revenues variance was Actual value – Budgeted value = $2,027,500 – $1,980,000 = $47,500, meaning that revenues were $47,500 greater than budgeted. Thus, all else the same, profits should be $47,500 greater than standard.

But the total cost variance was a negative $70,000, so costs were $70,000 greater than budgeted. (Budgeted value – Actual value = $1,850,000 – $1,920,000 = -$70,000. Note that we had to reverse the calculation to show that higher costs are bad, and hence create a negative variance.)

With revenues $47,500 greater than budgeted and costs $70,000 greater than budgeted, the net result is an impact of $47,500 + (-$70,000) = -$22,500, which means a shortfall in profits of $22,500. Of course, this is the profit variance reported in Table 6.3. But, by breaking down the profit variance into its revenue and cost components, it is readily apparent that the major cause of the clinic's poor financial performance in 2008 was that costs were too high.

In fact, we can go further in the analysis. Note that volume variance is a positive 500, meaning that volume exceeded expectations by 500 visits. Because the clinic's two payers use fee-for-service reimbursement, increased volume would lead to higher revenues, all else the same. But, in Carroll Clinic's case, Payer A had higher-than-expected per visit reimbursement (a positive $5 variance), while Payer B had lower-than-expected reimbursement (a negative $5 variance). Payer A, with higher-than-expected average reimbursement, had its volume increase, while Payer B, with lower-than-expected average reimbursement, had its visits decrease. The net result is total revenues that were higher than budgeted.

Finally, note that all cost categories (supplies, labor, and overhead) had negative variances, meaning that all costs were greater than planned. However, the clinic's volume was greater than expected (by 500 visits), and higher volume typically leads to higher costs.

The real question here is whether or not the higher costs were justified by the higher volume. To answer this question, we must construct another budget—the flexible budget.

FLEXIBLE VARIANCE ANALYSIS

To be of maximum use, variance analysis must be approached systematically. The starting point is the initial approved budget unadjusted for differences between planned and actual volumes, which we have called a *simple budget*. However, at the end of a budget period, actual volume will not likely equal budgeted volume, so it would be useful to know whether the variances are caused by volume forecast errors or some other factors.

Simple budget
The original budget, unadjusted for actual volume.

A better explanation to what is driving the variances can be given by a **flexible budget**, which is the initial budget adjusted to reflect the actual volume achieved in the budget period. Essentially, a flexible budget is an after-the-fact device that tells managers what the results would have been under the volume level actually attained, assuming all other simple (initial) budget assumptions are held constant. A flexible budget permits a more detailed analysis than is possible in a simple budget variance analysis. However, a flexible budget requires the identification of fixed costs and variable costs and hence places a larger burden on the organization's managerial accounting system.

To illustrate flexible variance analysis, consider Carroll Clinic's 2008 simple budget, contained in Table 6.3. The profit projection—$130,000—is predicated on specific volume assumptions: 9,000 visits from Payer A and 12,000 visits from Payer B. At the end of the year, the clinic's managers will compare actual profits with budgeted profits. The problem is that it is highly unlikely that actual profits will be based on 21,000 visits.

Table 6.4 is similar to Table 6.3, except that in this table the budget standard is the flexible budget rather than the simple budget. The flexible budget reflects projected revenues and costs at the actual volume, as opposed to the projected volume, but it incorporates all other assumptions that went into the simple budget. By analyzing these new variances, Carroll Clinic's managers can gain additional insights into why the clinic ended the year with a loss (as compared to budget).

> **⚠ CRITICAL CONCEPT**
> Flexible Budget
>
> A flexible budget is one that is created after the budget period has elapsed. It is based on all of the assumptions, except volume, inherent in the simple budget. In other words, the flexible budget reflects the actual volume coupled with all other original assumptions. For example, assume that a hospital has a payer that is expected to provide 1,000 patient days at a per diem reimbursement rate of $900. Thus, the simple budget would show 1,000 x $900 = $900,000 in revenues from this payer. However, when the year is over, this payer actually had 1,100 patient days at a per diem reimbursement rate of $925, for actual revenues of 1,100 x $925 = $1,017,500. The flexible budget would show revenues from this payer as 1,100 x $900 = $990,000, because the flexible budget reflects the actual volume along with all other original assumptions. By creating a flexible budget, managers are able to identify whether variances stemmed from managerial factors or from volume forecast errors.

TABLE 6.4

Carroll Clinic:
2008 Flexible
Budget Variance
Analysis

		Flexible Budget	Actual Results	Variance Dollar Visit	%
I.	Volume (Number of Visits)				
	Payer A	10,000	10,000		
	Payer B	11,500	11,500		
	Total	21,500	21,500		
II.	Reimbursement (Per Visit)				
	Payer A	$ 100	$105	$5	5.0%
	Payer B	$ 90	$ 85	($5)	(5.6)
III.	Costs				
	Variable Costs:				
	Supplies	$ 322,500	$ 320,000	$ 2,500	0.8%
	Fixed Costs:				
	Labor	$ 1,035,000	$1,050,000	($ 15,000)	(1.4)
	Overhead	500,000	550,000	(50,000)	(10.0)
	Total	$ 1,535,000	$1,600,000	($ 65,000)	(4.2)
IV.	Forecasted P&L Statement				
	Revenues:				
	Payer A	$ 1,000,000	$1,050,000	$ 50,000	5.0%
	Payer B	1,035,000	977,500	(57,500)	(5.6)
	Total revenues	$ 2,035,000	$2,027,500	($ 7,500)	(0.4)
	Variable costs	$ 322,500	$ 320,000	$ 2,500	0.8
	Fixed costs	1,535,000	1,600,000	(65,000)	(4.2)
	Total costs	$ 1,857,500	$1,920,000	($ 62,500)	(3.4)
	Profit	$ 177,500	$ 107,500	($ 70,000)	(39.4)

Note that the volumes listed in Part I of Table 6.4 are the same in both the Flexible Budget and Actual Results columns, and hence there are no variances. This occurs because actual volumes are used to create the flexible budget.

The flexible budget maintains the simple budget assumptions of Revenues = ($100 × Number of Payer A visits) + ($90 × Number of Payer B visits). However, the flexible budget flexes (adjusts) revenues (and costs) to reflect actual volume levels. Thus, in the Part IV Flexible Budget column, Total revenues = ($100 × 10,000) + ($90 × 11,500) = $1,000,000 + $1,035,000 = $2,035,000, which reflects the initial assumptions regarding reimbursement along with actual volumes.

On the cost side, fixed costs are presumably unaffected by volume changes (within the relevant range), but budgeted variable costs reflect actual volume of 21,500 visits: 21,500 × $15 = $322,500, where $15 is the assumed variable cost rate in the simple budget.

The flexible budget can be described as follows. The $2,035,000 in total revenues is what the clinic would have expected at the start of the year if the volume estimates had been 10,000 visits for Payer A and 11,500 for Payer B. In addition, the total variable costs of $322,500 in the flexible budget are the costs that Carroll would have expected for 21,500 total visits. By definition, the fixed costs should be the same, within a reasonable range, no matter what the volume level. On net, the $177,500 shown on the bottom line of the flexible budget represents the profit expected given the initial assumed revenue, cost, and volume relationships, coupled with the actual volume.

Now, let's examine the variances. The profit variance of -$70,000 tells us that, after adjusting for the actual volume, the clinic's profit was $70,000 less than expected. Thus, the situation is actually worse than that indicated by the simple variance analysis. In effect, greater volume should have led to greater profit, but that did not happen.

To understand why, take a look at the revenue variances. Payer A has a $50,000 positive variance, while Payer B has a negative $57,500 variance. Because these variances have already been adjusted for actual volume, these variances solely reflect reimbursement changes. In fact, higher reimbursement from Payer A and lower reimbursement from Payer B (as compared to original expectations) created these variances. On net, revenues were $7,500 less than expected, given actual volume. In essence, the lower reimbursement per visit from Payer B more than offset the higher reimbursement from Payer A.

Now let's change our focus to the cost side. Table 6.4 tells us that the variable cost variance (which solely reflects supplies costs) was $2,500. Because this is a positive (good) variance, supplies costs were $2,500 less than expected after adjusting for actual volume. Thus, Carroll Clinic's personnel actually did a good job of managing supplies in spite of the negative variance reported in Table 6.3.

On the fixed-cost side, the variance analysis remains unchanged between Tables 6.3 and 6.4. Because fixed costs are not affected by volume, the simple and flexible budget amounts are the same, and hence the variance analysis is the same.

FINAL COMMENTS ON VARIANCE ANALYSIS

The Carroll Clinic example presented here is meant to illustrate variance analysis techniques; it is not a complete analysis. A complete analysis would encompass many more variances. Furthermore, at most organizations, variance analysis is conducted at the department level, as well as at other sublevels such as service lines, and by the organization as a whole. Nevertheless, the Carroll Clinic example is sufficient to give you an idea of the variance analysis process and its benefits to the organization.

Variance analysis helps managers identify the factors that cause actual profits to be different from those expected. If profits are higher than expected, managers can see why and try to exploit even further those factors in the future. If profits are lower than expected, managers can identify the causes and embark on a plan to correct the deficiencies.

Large healthcare organizations have made significant improvements in their use of variance analysis. The benefit of expanding the level of detail is that it allows managers to isolate and presumably rectify problem areas. Fortunately, the marginal cost of obtaining such detailed information is lower now than ever because information technology initiatives are creating managerial accounting systems that generate large amounts of data that support budgeting and cost-control efforts.

(?) SELF-TEST QUESTIONS

1. What are some of the key assumptions required to prepare an operating budget?

2. Why is the budgeted P&L statement so important?

3. What is variance analysis, and what is its value to healthcare providers?

4. What is the difference between a simple budget and a flexible budget?

THEME WRAP-UP ACTUAL VERSUS EXPECTED RESULTS

As mentioned in the Theme Set-Up, Mark Mason, SCORN's director, needed to compare the dental clinic's actual first quarter 2008 expenses against those budgeted. Here's how he did the variance analysis:

	First Quarter Budget	Actual Results	Variance Dollar	Variance Percentage
Coordinator compensation	$ 13,334	$12,855	$479	3.6%
Hygienists compensation	7,041	8,614	(1,573)	(22.3)
Assistants compensation	25,969	27,433	(1,464)	(5.6)
Office staff compensation	9,512	8,470	1,042	11.0
Clinical supplies	10,000	9,344	656	6.6

Office supplies	500	529	(29)	(5.8)
Equipment maintenance	1,250	1,250	0	0
Utilities	1,500	1,355	145	9.7
Telephone	900	793	107	11.9
Total	$70,006	$70,643	($637)	(0.9%)

The dental clinic ended the first quarter with a negative total expense variance of $637, which means costs were $637 greater than budgeted. This represents a difference of less than 1 percent. Considering the difficulties in forecasting, Mark believes that overall the dental clinic's staff did a good job of managing expenses.

However, the individual cost item results are not all rosy. The compensation for hygienists and assistants was significantly over budget; in fact, the cost for hygienists was 22.3 percent over budget. Mark needs to look into these line items more closely to make sure they do not get out of control.

Of course, this variance analysis is only for a small portion of the dental clinic's overall budget, which in itself is only one component of SCORN's organizational budget. Still, this illustration gives you an idea of how budgeting and variance analysis is done by one healthcare provider.

KEY CONCEPTS

This chapter covers two important managerial activities—planning and budgeting. Budgets allow healthcare managers to plan for and set expectations for the future, assess financial performance on a timely basis, and ensure that operations are carried out in a manner consistent with expectations. Here are the key concepts:

➤ *Planning* encompasses the overall process of preparing for the future, while *budgeting* is the accounting process that ties together planning and control functions.

➤ The *strategic plan*, which provides broad guidance for the future, is the foundation of any organization's planning process.

➤ The *operating plan*, often called the *five-year plan*, contains more detailed information than does the strategic plan.

➤ The *financial plan* is the portion of the operating plan that deals with financial matters.

➤ *Budgeting* provides a means for communication and coordination of organizational expectations as well as allocation of financial resources. In addition, budgeting establishes benchmarks for control.

➤ The *conventional (incremental) approach* to budgeting uses the previous budget as the basis for constructing the new budget. *Zero-based budgeting* begins each budget as a clean slate, and hence all entries have to be justified each budget period.

➤ *Bottom-up budgeting*, which begins at the subunit level, encourages maximum involvement by department or program managers. Conversely, *top-down budgeting*, which is less participatory, communicates senior management's views.

➤ There are several types of budgets, including the *revenue budget*, *expense budget*, and *operating budget*. The *operating budget* sets the profit target for the budget period.

➤ A *variance* is the difference between a budgeted (planned) value, or *standard*, and the actual (realized) value. *Variance analysis* examines differences between budgeted and actual amounts with the goal of finding out why things went either badly or well.

➤ The budget created at the beginning of a budget period is called a *simple budget*. When this budget is recast to reflect the actual volume of patients treated, leaving all other assumptions unchanged, the result is a *flexible budget*.

In Chapter 7, we discuss some of the techniques used to manage operations.

END-OF-CHAPTER QUESTIONS

6.1 Why are planning and budgeting so important to an organization's success?

6.2 Briefly describe the planning process. In your description, include summaries of strategic, operating, and financial plans.

6.3 Describe the components of a financial plan.

6.4 How are the revenue, expense, and operating budgets related?

6.5 a. What are the advantages and disadvantages of conventional budgeting and zero-based budgeting?

  b. What organizational characteristics create likely candidates for zero-based budgeting?

6.6 If you were the CEO of Bayside Memorial Hospital, would you advocate a top-down or bottom-up approach to budgeting? Explain your rationale.

6.7 What is variance analysis?

6.8 Explain the relationship between a simple budget and a flexible budget.

END-OF-CHAPTER PROBLEMS

6.1 Consider the following 2008 data for Newark General Hospital (in millions of dollars):

	Simple Budget	Flexible Budget	Actual Results
Revenues	$4.7	$4.8	$4.5
Costs	4.1	4.1	4.2
Profit	0.6	0.7	0.3

  a. Calculate and interpret the two profit variances.
  b. Calculate and interpret the two revenue variances.
  c. Calculate and interpret the two cost variances.
  d. How are the variances related?

6.2 Here are the budgets of Brandon Surgery Center for the most recent historical quarter, in thousands of dollars:

	Simple	Flexible	Actual
Number of surgeries	1,200	1,300	1,300
Patient revenue	$2,400	$2,600	$2,535
Salary expense	$1,200	$1,300	$1,365
Non-salary expense	$600	$650	$585
Profit	$600	$650	$585

The center assumes that all revenues and costs are variable and hence tied directly to patient volume.

a. Explain how each amount in the flexible budget was calculated. (Hint: Examine the simple budget to determine the relationship of each budget line to volume.)

b. Determine the variances for each line of the P&L statement, both in dollar terms and in percentage terms.

c. What do the results in Part b tell Brandon's managers about the center's operations for the quarter?

6.3 Refer to Carroll Clinic's 2008 operating budget contained in Table 6.2. Instead of the actual results reported in Table 6.3, assume the results reported below:

Carroll Clinic: New 2008 Results

I.   *Volume (Number of Visits)*

Payer A	11,000
Payer B	12,000
Total	23,000

II.   *Reimbursement (Per Visit)*

Payer A	$95
Payer B	$95

III. *Costs*

Variable Costs:

Supplies $350,000

Fixed Costs:

Labor	$1,000,000
Overhead	500,000
Total	$1,500,000

IV. Forecasted P&L Statement

Revenues:

Payer A	$1,045,000
Payer B	1,140,000
Total revenues	$2,185,000
Variable costs	$ 350,000
Fixed costs	1,500,000
Total	$1,850,000
Profit	$ 335,000

a. What are the profit, revenue, and cost variances based on the simple (Table 6.2) budget?

b. Construct Carroll's flexible budget for 2008.

c. What are the profit, revenue, and cost variances based on the flexible budget?

d. Interpret your results. In particular, focus on the differences between the variance analysis here and the Carroll Clinic illustration presented in the chapter.

6.4 Again refer to Carroll Clinic's 2008 operating budget contained in Table 6.2. Instead of the actual results reported in Table 6.3 or listed in Problem 6.3, assume these results:

Carroll Clinic: New 2008 Results

I. Volume (Number of Visits)

Payer A	8,500
Payer B	11,000
Total	19,500

II. Reimbursement (Per Visit)

Payer A	$90
Payer B	$80

III. Costs

Variable Costs:	
Supplies	$ 320,000
Fixed Costs:	
Labor	$1,050,000
Overhead	550,000
Total	$1,600,000

IV. Forecasted P&L Statement

Revenues:	
Payer A	$ 765,000
Payer B	880,000
Total revenues	$1,645,000
Variable costs	$ 320,000
Fixed costs	1,600,000
Total	$1,920,000
Profit	($ 275,000)

a. What are the profit, revenue, and cost variances based on the simple (Table 6.2) budget?

b. Construct Carroll's flexible budget for 2008.

c. What are the profit, revenue, and cost variances based on the flexible budget?

d. Interpret your results. In particular, focus on the differences between the variance analysis here and the Carroll Clinic illustration presented in the chapter and in Problem 6.3.

CHAPTER 7

MANAGING FINANCIAL OPERATIONS

THEME SET-UP REVENUE CYCLE MANAGEMENT

Big City Medical Center is a major not-for-profit healthcare system. It operates five hospitals with roughly 2,000 beds and a physician staff of more than 2,000. It has total revenues that top $1 billion stemming from almost 100,000 inpatient stays and more than 600,000 outpatient visits.

In 2007, Big City's senior management recognized that the system had a big problem with its revenue cycle: It could not quickly bill and collect the amounts due from its third-party payers. Like all healthcare providers, Big City must pay its employees, buy medical supplies, and run the facilities where patient services are given. Thus, it must pay its bills at more or less the same time (or even before) it provides services. After the services are provided, it bills for the services but does not collect the bulk of its revenues until some time later. In 2007, Big City was waiting about 60 days, on average, to collect from third-party payers.

With annual revenues of $1 billion, Big City bills, on average, about $2.7 million per day ($1,000,000,000/365). Thus, with 60 days' worth of bills outstanding, the system must carry

$2.7 x 60 = $162 million of receivables. With no money collected to pay the costs of providing these services, Big City must finance (borrow) roughly the amount of revenues that it is owed. The average hospital collects its bills in about 50 days, so Big City was not doing well in this measure of financial condition.

Recognizing the problem, Big City hired a consulting company to help shorten the amount of time it takes to collect from payers. After several meetings with Big City's senior management, the consultants offered several suggestions to improve Big City's financial operations, including the measures used to monitor the revenue cycle.

As you read this chapter, you will gain an understanding of what the revenue cycle is and how managers use metrics to monitor and control operations. Then, at the end, you will learn what the consultants recommended to improve Big City's billing and collections procedures.

LEARNING OBJECTIVES

After studying this chapter, you will be able to

➤ Describe the revenue cycle and its importance to healthcare managers.

➤ Explain how receivables are created and managed.

➤ Discuss in general terms how businesses manage cash and marketable securities.

➤ Relate the basics of inventory management.

➤ Understand how managers monitor and control operations.

7.1 INTRODUCTION

In previous chapters, our discussion generally focused on how to estimate costs and profits and how to use this information to plan for the future. This chapter covers a different element of healthcare finance—the management of day-to-day financial operations.

Unlike cost and profit estimation and planning for the future, the management of day-to-day financial operations is highly dependent on the specific type of provider organization (hospital versus medical practice versus nursing home). Thus, we treat this topic in somewhat generic terms. Our discussion begins with the revenue cycle and receivables management and continues to the management of two related items: cash and inventories.

It is not enough to merely establish a sound framework for financial operations. Good managers ensure that financial operations continue to run smoothly even when factors, both internal and external, create turbulence in the environment. For the most part, clinical operations are monitored and controlled by the budgeting process, while financial operations are monitored and controlled using a set of metrics (measures) that define good performance. This chapter concludes with a brief discussion of several of these metrics. Our intent here is not to make you an expert, but rather to provide some insights into financial operations and how they are monitored.

7.2 THE REVENUE CYCLE AND RECEIVABLES MANAGEMENT

One of the hottest topics in healthcare finance today, especially among hospitals, is the revenue cycle, which arises because most healthcare providers do not get paid at the same time services are rendered. Providers incur cash costs for facilities, supplies, and labor but do not receive immediate payment to cover those costs. In fact, both hospitals and medical practices, on average, have to wait about 50 days to collect from third-party payers.

The revenue cycle concept is not new, but it is gaining increased emphasis as it becomes harder and harder to maintain profitability in today's healthcare environment. One element of the revenue cycle (and perhaps the most important) is the management of receivables—that is, the management of monies owed to a provider (predominantly by third-party payers). Because receivables management is a critical part of the revenue cycle, these topics are discussed together.

THE REVENUE CYCLE

Generally, the **revenue cycle** is defined as the set of recurring business activities and related information processing necessary to bill for and collect the revenues due for services provided. More pragmatically, the revenue cycle at provider organizations should ensure that patients are properly categorized by payment obligation, that correct and timely billing takes place, and that the correct payment is promptly received.

The revenue cycle stems from the fact that healthcare businesses must provide (and hence bear the costs of) services up front but do not get paid for those services until some time later. Essentially, the revenue cycle consists of activities associated with gathering patient financial information, billing for services rendered, and then collecting payment on those bills. The process begins when a patient walks in the door (or perhaps even before) and ends when the organization has the cash reimbursement in hand. The shorter the time it takes to complete the revenue cycle, the better it is financially for the provider. At large providers, many people in different functional areas are involved in the revenue cycle. Furthermore, the process is complicated by the fact that most providers must deal with multiple third-party payers, each of which may use different billing formats and pay according to different contractual arrangements. Proper management of the revenue cycle usually requires a significant investment in information technology to support the billing and collections functions.

Revenue cycle activities typically are broken down into four phases on the basis of when they occur: (1) those that occur before the service is provided, (2) those that are simultaneous with the service, (3) those that occur afterward, and (4) those activities that are continuous. Here are some examples of revenue cycle activities listed by phase:

Before-Service Activities:

◆ *Preservice insurance verification*. Here, the insurance status of the patient is identified immediately after the outpatient visit (or inpatient stay) is scheduled. The idea here is to ensure that the patient actually has the insurance indicated when the appointment was made.

◆ *Precertification (if necessary)*. If the insurance verification indicates that the payer requires *precertification*, it should be done immediately. Without precertification for services that require it, the provider runs the risk of having the claim (bill) denied even though the services were provided.

Precertification
An insurer's authorization indicating its willingness to pay for a particular service.

◆ *Preservice patient financial counseling*. Before the service, the patient should be counseled regarding both the payer's and patient's responsibilities regarding payment. It is not fair to present a large bill to an unsuspecting patient after the service is rendered.

At-Service Activities:

◆ *Time of service verification*. The patient's insurance status should be checked at the time of service to ensure that no changes have occurred since the initial verification. The time of service verification should be done with both the patient and the payer.

◆ *Service documentation/claims production*. The services provided should be documented in a way that facilitates correct claims submission. The documentation process should ensure that (1) the services provided are coded in accordance with the payer's claim system, (2) the code reflects the highest legitimate reimbursement amount, and (3) the claim will be formatted in accordance with payer guidelines and will contain all required information.

After-Service Activities:

◆ *Claims submission.* The claim should be submitted to the payer as quickly as possible after the service is rendered. However, speed should not take precedence over accuracy because incomplete and inaccurate billing accounts for a large proportion of late payments.

◆ *Third-party follow-up.* If payment is not received within 30 days, a follow-up should be sent.

◆ *Denials management. Claims denial* by third-party payers is one of the major impediments to prompt reimbursement. Typically, most denials are caused by improper precertification and incomplete or erroneous claims submission. Prompt claims resubmission is essential to good revenue cycle management.

Claims denial
The refusal of a third-party payer to honor a submitted bill (claim).

◆ *Payment receipt and posting.* When the reimbursement is received, it must be properly deposited and credited. This activity ends the revenue cycle.

Continuous Activities:

◆ *Monitoring.* Once the revenue cycle activities are identified and timing goals are set for each activity, the provider should implement a system of metrics (key indicators) to ensure that these goals are being met.

◆ *Review and improvement.* The key indicators that monitor the revenue cycle must be continually reviewed with the goals of correcting any deficiencies and constantly striving to improve the process.

The revenue cycle requires constant attention, because the external factors that influence the cycle are constantly changing. Also, problems that occur at any point in the cycle tend to have ripple effects. That is, a problem that occurs early in the cycle can create additional problems at later points in the cycle. For example, failure to obtain required precertification can lead to claims denial, which at best means delayed payment and at worst no payment at all.

The ability of healthcare providers to convert services rendered into cash is critical to their financial performance. Problems in the revenue cycle lead to lost and late payments, both of which degrade provider revenues and hence financial condition. You can think of the provider as giving an interest-free loan to the payer that covers the costs of the services rendered. The faster the loan is repaid, the better for the lender (provider).

RECEIVABLES MANAGEMENT

Because healthcare services are provided before payment is received, healthcare providers extend credit to patients (in reality, the credit typically is extended to third-party payers). The monies owed for each service rendered create an **account receivable** for the provider. (The recording of accounts receivable on a provider's financial statements will be discussed in Chapter 12.) A provider's receivables accumulate over time as more and more services are provided. Eventually, however, the patient or third-party payer will pay the account, at which time the provider will receive cash and its receivables balance will decline. The management of receivables is the most critical part of the revenue cycle, so it warrants a separate discussion.

The Accumulation of Receivables

The total amount of accounts receivable outstanding at any given time is determined by two factors: patient volume and the average length of time between service and collection. For example, suppose Home Infusion provides an average of ten home health visits a day at an average reimbursement of $100 per visit, for $1,000 in average daily billings. Assuming 250 workdays a year, the company's annual billings total Average daily billings × Number of days = $1,000 × 250 = $250,000.

At Home Infusion, all services are paid for by only two third-party payers: Payer A, which pays for half of the billings 15 days after the service is provided, and Payer B, which pays for the other half of total billings in 25 days. Home Infusion's **average collection period (ACP)**, also called days in patient accounts receivable, is 20 days.

$$ACP = (0.5 \times 15 \text{ days}) + (0.5 \times 25 \text{ days}) = 20 \text{ days}.$$

Thus, on average, it takes Home Infusion 20 days from the time that a service is provided to receive payment for that service.

Assuming a constant uniform rate of services provided, and hence billings, Home Infusion will have, at any given point in time, $20,000 of receivables outstanding. We know this because the receivables are building up at a rate of $1,000 per day, and it will take 20 days to collect them.

You can think of it this way. Assume Home Infusion just started operations, so it will provide and bill for $1,000 of services on Day 1, Day 2, Day 3, and so on. These billings will accumulate for 20 days, at which point $20,000 of billings have accumulated.

On Day 21, the $1,000 owed for Day 1 services is collected. After Day 21, the company will collect $1,000 per day but, at the same time, provide another $1,000 of services that will add to billings. The amount of billings outstanding (the receivables) thus will stabilize at $20,000.

What is the financial implication of carrying $20,000 in receivables? The $20,000, for the most part, represents the cost of the home health services rendered: salaries, supplies, and so on, which have to be paid either before or as the services are provided. Thus, the funds required to pay the bills associated with the services must be obtained elsewhere until the receivables are collected. Home Infusion uses a bank loan to pay the bills (finance the receivables), which has an interest rate of 8 percent. Thus, over a year, the firm must pay the bank roughly $0.08 \times \$20,000 = \$1,600$ in interest to finance (carry) its $20,000 receivables balance. (We use the term roughly here because Home Infusion's cost of providing $20,000 worth of services is somewhat less than $20,000 because it earns a profit on each visit.)

> ### ⓘ CRITICAL CONCEPT
> #### Average Collection Period
>
> The average collection period, commonly called days in patient accounts receivable, is the average time that it takes a provider to collect for services rendered. For example, the average collection period for hospitals today is about 50 days. That means hospitals, on average, have to wait 50 days from the time a service is provided until payment is received. The best hospitals (top 10 percent) collect in about 35 days, while the worst (bottom 10 percent) wait about 75 days. Of course, some portion of the payment (the copay) often is collected when the service is rendered, and some patients are self-pay. Still, the bulk of a provider's revenues comes from third-party payers, which cause much of the delay between services and payment.

Monitoring the Receivables Position

If a receivable is never collected, the revenue is never received. Thus, healthcare managers must closely monitor receivables to ensure that they are being collected in a timely manner and to uncover any deterioration in the quality of receivables. (Receivables quality is a measure of the likelihood that the receivables will be collected.) Early detection can help managers take corrective action before the situation has a significant negative impact on the organization's financial condition.

One way to monitor receivables is to compare the organization's ACP to the industry average ACP. For example, if the home health industry ACP is 22 days and Home Infusion's ACP is 20 days, then Home Infusion's collections department is doing a better-than-average job.

Note, however, that even though Home Infusion's payers are, on average, paying faster than the 22-day industry average, Payer A pays in 15 days while Payer B takes 25 days. Thus, the firm's collections department should take a hard look to see if the ACP of the 25-day payer can be reduced to the industry average, or even to the 15 days of the other payer.

Why is it so important to minimize a business's ACP? To illustrate, assume that Home Infusion's ACP was 25 days, and hence its receivables balance was $25,000. Assuming an 8 percent cost of financing (carrying) its receivables, the annual carrying cost to Home Infusion is about 0.08 × $25,000 = $2,000. But, at its actual ACP of 20 days, its carrying costs are roughly only 0.08 × $20,000 = $1,600. Thus, by reducing its ACP by five days, Home Infusion reduced its receivables carrying costs by about $400 annually.

No big deal, you may say. True, but now consider a large hospital with $100 million in receivables and a 60-day ACP, which implies average daily billings of $100 million / 60 days = $1.67 million. A reduction of ACP by five days would reduce the receivables balance to $1.67 million × 55 days = $91.85 million, or by about $8 million. Assuming the same 8 percent cost of carrying receivables, the savings would roughly amount to a substantial 0.08 × $8,000,000 = $640,000. In addition, the hospital would receive a one-time cash flow of $8 million as the receivables balance is reduced. It should be apparent that immediate cash flow as well as large savings can be obtained by reducing a business's ACP, and hence its receivables balance. This is the driving force behind revenue cycle management—the faster the bills for services rendered are produced and collected, the better.

A second tool for monitoring receivables is the *aging schedule*, which breaks down a business's receivables by age of account. Aging schedules are important to good receivables management for two reasons. First, the longer it takes to collect receivables, the greater the cost of carrying (financing) those receivables. Thus, aging schedules that show a large percentage of "old" accounts imply high carrying costs. Second, accounts that are long past due often become "problem" accounts, meaning that they end up not being collected and hence are written off as bad debts.

To illustrate, Table 7.1 contains the December 31, 2008, aging schedules of two home health companies: Home Infusion and Home Care. Both firms offer the same services and show the same total receivables balance. However, Home Infusion's aging schedule indicates that it is collecting its receivables faster than Home Care is. Only 50 percent of Home Infusion's receivables are more than ten days old, while Home Care has 55 percent of its receivables in the over-ten-days category. More important, Home Care has receivables that are more than 30 days old, and even some that are more than 40 days old. Based on an industry ACP of 22 days, Home Care's managers should be concerned both about the efficiency of the firm's collections effort and the ability of the late payers to actually make the payments due.

The bottom line here is that management of a provider's receivables is important. Providers need to collect as fast as they can for services they render. We have just scratched the surface here. Furthermore, we have focused on third-party payment. In general, providers also have to worry about collecting directly from patients, either the entire amount for uninsured patients or the copayment (or coinsurance) amount for insured patients.

Aging schedule

A table that expresses a business's accounts receivable in increments according to how long it takes to collect each account.

| Age of | Home Infusion | | Home Care | |
Account (Days)	Value of Account	Percentage of Total Value	Value of Account	Percentage of Total Value
0–10	$10,000	50%	$ 9,000	45%
11–20	7,500	38	5,000	25
21–30	2,500	12	3,000	15
31–40	0	0	2,000	10
Over 40	0	0	1,000	5
Total	$20,000	100%	$20,000	100%

TABLE 7.1
Aging Schedules for Two Home Health Companies

(?) SELF-TEST QUESTIONS

1. What is the revenue cycle?

2. What are the four phases of activities that make up the cycle?

3. Why is proper management of the revenue cycle critical to the financial performance of healthcare providers?

4. Explain how a firm's receivables balance is built up over time and why there are costs associated with carrying receivables.

5. Briefly discuss two means by which a firm can monitor its receivables position.

(*) INDUSTRY PRACTICE Managing Hospital Receivables

Although the general principles of receivables management discussed in this chapter are applicable to all providers, hospitals (especially large ones) face unique problems. The most obvious problem is the complexities in billing that result from having to deal with a large number of governmental and private insurers that use

(Continued)

⊛ **INDUSTRY PRACTICE** Managing Hospital Receivables

different payment methodologies. To deal with these complexities, hospitals have to maintain large staffs of specialists just to manage billing and collections.

To illustrate the problem, consider the following data on the receivables mix for the hospital industry:

Payer	Percentage of Total Accounts Receivable
Medicare	30.2
Commercial insurers	19.5
Medicaid	14.0
Self-pay	13.4
HMO/PPO	9.7
Blue Cross	8.1
TRICARE (CHAMPUS)	5.1
Total	100.0

There are multiple payers within many of the categories listed here, so the number of individual insurers can easily run into the hundreds. It is easy to imagine the problems that arise when dealing with a large and diverse collection of payers.

The data below provide information on how long it takes hospitals to collect receivables:

Average Collection Period (Days in Patient Accounts Receivable):

Percentile	Average Collection Period (Days)
10th	35.9
25th	43.8
Median	53.0
75th	63.5
90th	78.4

⊛ INDUSTRY PRACTICE Managing Hospital Receivables

Aggregate Aging Schedule:

Age of Account (Days)	Percentage of Total Accounts Receivable
0–30	42.5
31–60	21.4
61–90	11.2
91–120	7.8
Over 120	17.1
Total	100.0

Hospitals clearly have some difficulty collecting bills in a timely manner. On average, collecting a receivable takes a little more than 50 days. However, this number has decreased in recent years as hospital managers have become increasingly aware of the costs associated with carrying receivables and as electronic billing and collections have become more prevalent. In spite of the positive trend, about 25 percent of receivables still are more than 90 days old. In addition, about 6 percent of patient bills are never paid at all, with about 3 percent being charged off as bad debt losses (patients and insurers that have the ability to pay but do not) and 3 percent going to charity (indigent) care.

To help providers collect from managed care plans in a timely fashion, many states have enacted prompt-payment laws, which require payers to pay within a mandated time period or face penalties. For example, New York State requires that all undisputed claims by providers be paid by managed care plans within 45 days of receipt. If prompt payment is not made, fines are assessed.

Note: This industry practice is based on data in the following publications: *Hospital Accounts Receivable Analysis* (updated quarterly). Frederick, MD: Aspen Publishers; *Comprehensive Performance Report* (published annually). Eden Prairie, MN: Ingenix; "Uncompensated Care Fact Sheet, 2007." Chicago: American Hospital Association.

7.3 CASH MANAGEMENT

Although the management of a provider's revenue cycle focuses on receivables, it could not be optimized without good management of the business's cash and inventories. In the next two sections, we introduce some concepts used by providers to manage cash and inventories.

Liquidity
The ability of a business to meet its cash obligations as they become due.

Businesses need cash, which includes both actual cash on hand and cash held in commercial checking accounts, to pay for labor and materials, to buy facilities and equipment, to pay taxes (if applicable), to service (pay interest on) debt, and so on. In essence, maintaining sufficient cash ensures a business's *liquidity*, which means having the ability to meet its cash obligations as they become due. A business that is illiquid cannot meet its payment obligations, and hence its operations suffer.

However, cash is a nonearning asset; it provides no tangible return (does not earn interest). (Commercial checking accounts for businesses, except the very smallest, do not pay interest.) Thus, the goal of cash management is to minimize the amount of cash on hand but, at the same time, have enough to meet the business's immediate cash obligations.

The value of careful cash management depends on the current level of interest rates. For example, in the early 1980s, with short-term interest rates higher than 15 percent, businesses were devoting a great deal of care to cash management. Today, with short-term interest rates under 5 percent, the value of cash management is reduced. Clearly, larger businesses, with larger cash balances, can better afford to hire the personnel necessary to maintain tight control over their cash positions.

Because cash management is an element of business operations in which economies of scale are present, banks have placed considerable emphasis on developing and marketing these services. Thus, banks can generally provide cash management services to smaller businesses at lower costs than such businesses would incur if operating in-house cash management systems.

FLOAT MANAGEMENT

A well-run business has more money in its checking account than the balance shown on its checkbook. **Float** is defined as the difference between the balance shown on the bank's records and the balance on the business's checkbook. Because float can be thought of as an interest-free loan from the bank, the larger the float the better. (Personal float is also a good idea. Perhaps the best way to obtain personal float is to use a credit card to make purchases and then to pay the full amount of the credit card bill each month before the due date. In effect, the credit card company is providing you with an interest-free loan for the amount of purchases made that month, and hence extending float.)

To illustrate float, assume that Gainesville Clinic writes, on average, checks in the amount of $5,000 each day. (As the checks are written, the amounts are deducted from the checkbook balance at the clinic.) It takes six days for these checks to be mailed, delivered, deposited, and cleared, and hence for the amounts to be reflected on bank's records. This will cause the clinic's own checkbook to show a balance that is 6 × $5,000 = $30,000 less than the balance at the bank.

Now assume that the clinic receives checks in the amount of $5,000 daily, but it loses four days while the checks are processed by the business office, deposited in the clinic's bank account, and cleared by the banking system. Because of the delay in depositing and clearing the checks, the clinic's balance at the bank is 4 × $5,000 = $20,000 less than that on its checkbook.

The clinic's overall float, then, is a combination of the incoming and outgoing check float components. The bank balance is $30,000 more than the checkbook because of checks writ-

> ⓘ **CRITICAL CONCEPT**
> Float
>
> Float is the difference between the checking account balance at the bank and the balance shown on the business's checkbook. For example, if a business has a bank balance of $75,000 and its checkbook shows a balance of $50,000, the business has $25,000 of float. Float is created when checks received by a business are processed by the banking system faster than checks that are written by the business. Float can be thought of as an interest-free loan from the bank. Thus, the larger the float, the better for the business.

ten, but $20,000 less because of checks deposited. On net, its balance at the bank is $10,000 larger than the balance on its checkbook, so Gainesville Clinic's float is $10,000.

A firm's float is a function of its ability to speed up collections on checks received and to slow down collections on checks written. Efficient businesses go to great lengths to (1) speed up the processing of incoming checks, thus putting the funds to work faster and (2) stretch out their own payments as long as possible (without engaging in unethical or illegal practices).

MARKETABLE SECURITIES MANAGEMENT

Many businesses hold temporary portfolios of securities called **marketable securities** (or short-term investments or near-cash). In practice, cash and marketable securities management cannot be separated because management of one implies management of the other. There are two primary reasons for holding marketable securities:

1. They serve as an interest-earning substitute for cash balances.

2. They are used to hold funds that are accumulated to meet a specific large near-term obligation, such as a tax payment, a construction project, or a new equipment purchase.

In general, the key characteristic sought in marketable securities investments is safety. Thus, most healthcare managers are willing to give up some return to ensure that

> ## ⓘ CRITICAL CONCEPT
> Marketable Securities
>
> Marketable securities are short-term investments held by businesses in lieu of cash. The idea here is that cash (including commercial checking accounts) earns no interest. Thus, as little cash as possible should be held—only that necessary to meet immediate needs. Any excess cash should be invested in safe, short-term securities, such as money market funds or Treasury securities. By doing so, businesses convert a nonearning asset (cash) into an earning asset (securities). Of course, the amount earned on marketable securities depends on the prevailing level of interest rates. Still, some return is better than no return.

funds are available, in the amounts expected, when needed. Large businesses, with large amounts of surplus cash, often directly own securities such as Treasury bills or negotiable certificates of deposit.

Conversely, smaller businesses are more likely to invest excess cash with a bank or with a money market mutual fund because a small firm's volume of investment simply does not warrant its hiring specialists to manage a marketable securities portfolio. Interest rates on mutual funds are somewhat lower than rates on direct investments of equivalent risk because of management fees. However, for smaller companies, net returns may well be higher on mutual funds because no in-house management expense is required.

> ## ❓ SELF-TEST QUESTIONS
>
> 1. What is float?
>
> 2. How do firms use float to increase cash management efficiency?
>
> 3. Why do firms hold marketable securities portfolios?
>
> 4. How do the cash management practices of large and small businesses differ?

7.4 INVENTORY MANAGEMENT

Inventory management involves the ordering, receipt, storage, and payment of supplies, including clinical supplies (e.g., tongue depressors) and office supplies (e.g., consent forms). Inventories are an essential part of virtually all healthcare operations. Inventory levels depend heavily on volume—the greater the amount of services provided, the greater the need for supplies, both clinical and administrative. At many organizations, inventory management is called either supply chain management or materials management. (To those who work in this field, each of these terms has a slightly different meaning. For most of us, they connote the same thing—managing a business's inventories.)

Perhaps the greatest problem in inventory management is the fact that inventories must be acquired ahead of time: The necessity of forecasting volume before establishing inventory levels makes inventory management a difficult task. Also, because errors in inventory levels can lead either to catastrophic consequences for patients or to excessive inventory costs, inventory management in healthcare organizations is as important as it is difficult.

Each item of inventory can be thought of as having two components. The first is a *base stock*, which is designed to meet forecasted volume. For example, a clinic might stock 100 test strips for prothrombin time testing, which is used to assess how long it takes for blood to clot. Regarding resupply, it takes one week to order and receive the strips, and the clinic expects to use 25 strips each week. Thus, the clinic orders the strips when 25 (one week's supply) remain and receives the resupply order as the last strips on hand are being used.

On top of the base stock, the clinic holds ten additional test strips to meet any unexpected

> ### ⚠ CRITICAL CONCEPT
> Inventory Management
>
> Inventory management involves the ordering, receipt, storage, and payment of supplies. The process starts with the decision about how many items to keep on hand and ends when the supplies are used to provide services and are ultimately paid for by patients or third-party payers. Inventories are expensive to buy and to carry (keep on hand). Furthermore, some inventory items, such as drugs and reagents, have limited shelf lives (become unusable if not used by a certain date). For example, according to the manufacturer, Bayer Aspirin has a shelf life of two years. Thus, the goal of inventory management, like cash management, is to have enough usable items on hand, but not too many.

usage increases or delays in receiving base stock reorders. These additional inventory items are called the *safety stock*. (Note that the same concept could be applied to cash management.) The idea of a safety stock is based on the fact that a *stockout*, which means that an item is not available, can be a matter of life or death for a provider's patients.

In large organizations, inventory management requires close coordination among patient services, purchasing, and finance departments. The patient services department is generally the first to spot changes in demand. These changes must be worked into the purchasing and operating schedules, and the financial manager must arrange any financing needed to support inventory buildups. Improper communication among departments, poor volume forecasts, or both can lead to disaster.

The key to good inventory management is information technology. Without information systems that support inventory management, the control system will become bogged down with slow-moving hard-copy data. To illustrate, most healthcare businesses now employ computerized inventory control systems. The computer starts with an inventory count in memory. As withdrawals are made, they are recorded in the computer, and the inventory balance is revised. When the point is reached that items must be reordered, the computer automatically places the order, and when the new items are received, the recorded balance is increased.

A good inventory management system must be dynamic. A large provider stocks thousands of different items of inventory. The usage of these various items can increase or decrease separately from rising or falling aggregate utilization of services. As the usage rate for an individual item begins to rise or fall, the inventory management system must adjust to avoid running short or having excessive, and potentially unusable, items. If the change in the usage rate appears to be permanent, then the base inventory level should be recom-

Base stock
The amount of inventory held to meet expected usage.

Safety stock
The amount of inventory, above the base stock, held to meet unexpected usage increases or delays in receipt of reorders.

Stockout
The situation in which a needed inventory item is not available.

Just-in-time system
An inventory manage-
ment approach where
the inventory arrives
just a short time before
it is used, as opposed
to sitting on the shelf
for long periods.

**Stockless inventory
system**
A system where the
supplier delivers small
quantities of inventory
directly to the using de-
partments. This system
is a refinement of the
just-in-time system.

**Consigned inventory
system**
A system in which the
supplier owns and man-
ages the inventory until
it is consumed (used).

puted, the safety stock should be reconsidered, and the computer model used in the control process should be reprogrammed.

A relatively new approach to inventory management, called the *just-in-time system*,
is gaining popularity in all industries, including healthcare. To illustrate, consider Bayside
Memorial Hospital, which consumes large quantities of medical supplies each year. A few
years ago, the hospital maintained a 25,000-square-foot warehouse to hold its medical supplies. However, as cost pressures mounted, the hospital closed its warehouse and converted
to a just-in-time system.

The process began with daily deliveries to the hospital's loading dock, where the
supplies were sorted and taken to smaller storerooms within the hospital. But after a few
years, the system was converted to a *stockless inventory system*. Now, the supplier fills orders
in exact, sometimes small, quantities and delivers them directly to departmental storage cab-
inets inside the hospital, including those in the operating rooms and nursing floors.

Bayside's managers estimate that the stockless system has saved the hospital about
$1.5 million a year since it was instituted, including $350,000 from staff reductions and
$650,000 from inventory reductions. Additionally, the hospital has converted space pre-
viously used as storerooms to patient care and other cash-generating uses. The distributors
that offer stockless inventory systems typically add 3 percent to 5 percent service fees, but
many hospitals still can realize savings on total inventory costs.

As stockless inventory systems become more prevalent in hospitals, more and more
hospitals are relying on outside contractors who assume both inventory management and
supplier roles. In effect, hospitals are beginning to outsource inventory management. For
example, some hospitals are experimenting with an inventory management program in
which the supplier delivers supplies just as in a stockless system. But the supplier owns the
products until they are used by the hospital, at which time the hospital pays for the items.
Such an approach is called a *consigned inventory system*.

In addition to reducing inventories, outside inventory managers often are better at
ferreting out waste than are their in-house counterparts. For example, an inventory management company found that one hospital was spending $600 for products used in open-
heart surgery, while another was spending only $420. Because there was no meaningful
difference in the procedure or outcomes, the higher-cost hospital was able to convince the
surgeons to change the medical devices used in the surgery and to pocket the difference.

(?) SELF-TEST QUESTIONS

1. Why is good inventory management important to a firm's success?

2. What is the difference between a base stock and a safety stock?

3. Describe some recent trends in inventory management by healthcare providers.

7.5 MONITORING OPERATIONS

Thus far in this chapter, we have discussed many concepts related to managing financial operations. An important part of any healthcare manager's job is to ensure that the day-to-day operations of the business run smoothly and meet performance expectations. For the most part, this is accomplished by monitoring a set of *metrics* that measure various aspects of performance, including financial performance. When the metric fails to meet organizational standards, action is taken to correct the operational deficiency.

Metric
A value used to assess one element of performance.

Providers typically use a large number of metrics to monitor operations. Furthermore, many of the specific metrics used depend on the nature of the healthcare business. For example, the hospital metric to measure inpatient volume is number of days; but for a medical practice, the volume metric is number of visits.

To give you a better appreciation of how managers monitor both clinical and financial operations, several commonly used operational metrics are defined and illustrated in this section. We are just scratching the surface here. For a more comprehensive list, see the Health Administration Press Book Companion website at ache.org/books/Finance Fundamentals.

VOLUME METRICS

One of the major concerns of managers is patient volume. After all, providers typically have a large investment in land, buildings, and equipment and hence have to generate the number of patients necessary to cover the fixed costs of treatment.

A declining patient volume means falling revenue, which ultimately will have to be offset by decreasing costs. At first, labor and inventory costs will be cut, but if the volume decline is large, managers will have to consider shedding facilities. An increasing volume means just the opposite. Inventories and labor will have to be added and perhaps plans for new facilities to handle the expected additional volume will need to be developed. Thus, the measurement of volume is critical to good management.

Inpatient Volume

For hospitals, *occupancy rate* measures the extent of utilization of inpatient facilities. Because facilities costs are incurred on all assets, whether used or not, higher occupancy spreads these costs over more patients and hence increases per patient profitability. To illustrate this metric, consider Riverside Memorial Hospital, which on one day in 2008 had 261 inpatients in its 450 beds. Thus, its occupancy rate was 58 percent:

Occupancy rate
The proportion (percentage) of hospital beds occupied.

$$\text{Occupancy rate} = \text{Number of inpatients/Number of beds}$$
$$= 261/450 = 0.58 = 58\%.$$

To interpret operating and financial metrics, managers compare the value against some standard as well as track the metric over time. The industry average occupancy rate for all hospitals is 46 percent. Thus, Riverside has a higher occupancy rate and hence is using its inpatient assets more productively than the average hospital. Furthermore, Riverside's occupancy rate has been climbing slowly over time, which is a good sign for the hospital. (The top 10 percent of hospitals have an occupancy rate of more than 68 percent, so Riverside has a way to go to be among the best.)

Note, however, that we have measured occupancy rate for only one day. Day-to-day fluctuations in volume are important indicators of seasonal volume changes. Once Riverside's managers identify seasonal utilization patterns, they can better plan for and manage their inpatient operations.

In addition to monitoring daily inpatient volume, Riverside's managers will track occupancy on a weekly, monthly, quarterly, and annual basis. All in all, utilization metrics are important to the efficient management of any healthcare provider.

Outpatient Volume

One could just record the number of outpatient visits, which would be the volume measure for hospital outpatient departments, clinics, and medical practices. In a similar manner, we could have measured inpatient volume by the number of occupied beds. However, neither of these metrics provide much information, because they do not account for the scale (capacity) of the organization. Thus, we used occupancy rate to measure inpatient utilization.

Number of visits per physician
The volume of an outpatient facility on a per physician basis.

For outpatients, especially at medical practices, one common measure of volume is the *number of visits per physician*. This measure can be more easily compared to other organizations (which typically are different sizes) or over time as physician staffing changes.

Assume that Medford Family Practice has five physicians and a total of 26,987 patient visits in 2008. Thus, the annual number of visits per physician is 5,397:

$$\text{Number of visits per physician} = \text{Number of visits/Number of physicians}$$
$$= 26{,}987/5 = 5{,}397.$$

The average volume for primary care physician practices is 5,090 visits per physician, so Medford is doing better than the average practice in using its physician resources. However, practices considered by the Medical Group Management Association to be top performers have more than 7,000 visits per physician, so Medford should consider actions to increase volume.

If the practice has unmet demand (e.g., long appointment wait times), perhaps it should add support personnel to enable the physicians to be more productive. Or, if the practice has an insufficient number of patients, it may consider instituting an aggressive marketing program or cutting the number of personnel.

PATIENT CHARACTERISTIC METRICS

In addition to raw volume, healthcare managers must have other information about the organization's patients. For example, in a hospital setting, what proportion of patients use outpatient services as opposed to being inpatients? Also, what proportion of patients is insured by Medicare, Medicaid, commercial insurers, and others?

A host of measures defines the characteristics of a provider's patients. Clearly, this is important information, because patient characteristics define the nature of the services required and the reimbursement methods used.

Patient (Outpatient/Inpatient) Mix

Hospitals typically offer both inpatient and outpatient services. Historically, outpatient services were regarded to be more profitable than inpatient services. However, comparative profitability between inpatient and outpatient services is highly dependent on overhead allocation amounts and the organization being analyzed, so it is difficult to make universal judgments.

Outpatient revenue percentage
Outpatient revenues as a percentage of total revenues.

The *outpatient revenue percentage* measures the percentage of total revenues that stem from outpatient services. Riverside has $163,832,000 in total revenues composed of $40,092,000 in outpatient revenues and $123,740,000 in inpatient revenues, for an outpatient revenue percentage of 24.5 percent:

$$\text{Outpatient revenue percentage} = \text{Outpatient revenues/Total revenues}$$
$$= \$40{,}092{,}000/\$163{,}832{,}000 = 24.5\%.$$

The industry average outpatient revenue percentage is 46 percent, so Riverside has a much smaller outpatient program, relative to its size, than the average hospital does. Regardless of relative profitability, a larger percentage of revenue from outpatient services would mean that Riverside's revenue stream would be less dependent on a single source of revenue—inpatient services. Thus, it might be prudent for Riverside's managers to take steps to increase the volume of outpatient services. This might entail increasing capacity, offering more outpatient services (perhaps hiring more hospital-based physicians), or expanding the marketing effort to ensure that prospective patients think about Riverside as more than just a hospital.

Finally, note that because all of Riverside's patients are either outpatients or inpatients, an outpatient revenue percentage of 24.5 percent implies an inpatient revenue percentage of 100.0 − 24.5 = 75.5%.

Payer Mix

Medicare payment percentage
Medicare revenues as a percentage of total revenues.

Medicare payment percentage measures the exposure of a hospital to Medicare patients and hence to payments set by political, rather than economic, processes. For inpatient services, Riverside Memorial Hospital has 7,642 Medicare discharges annually out of a total of 18,281 discharges. Thus, its Medicare payment percentage is 41.8 percent:

$$\text{Medicare payment percentage} = \text{Medicare discharges/Total discharges}$$
$$= 7{,}642/18{,}281 = 41.8\%.$$

With an industry average of 45 percent, Riverside has a somewhat lower percentage of Medicare patients than the average hospital does. To the extent that Medicare payments are lower than payments from other third-party payers, a higher Medicare payment percentage puts pressure on operating revenues. Conversely, if Medicare payments are higher than reimbursements by managed care plans, then in some situations, a higher Medicare payment percentage might be good. Similar metrics could be constructed for Medicaid, managed care plans, and bad debt and charity care patients.

Average Length of Stay

Average length of stay
The average time an inpatient spends in the hospital (per stay).

Average length of stay (ALOS), or just *length of stay (LOS)*, is the number of days that an average inpatient is hospitalized with each admission. Riverside had a total of 95,061 inpatient days in 2008 from 18,281 discharges. Thus, the ALOS is 5.2 days.

$$\text{ALOS} = \text{Inpatient days/Total discharges}$$
$$= 95{,}061/18{,}281 = 5.2 \text{ days.}$$

On average, Riverside keeps its patients in the hospital longer than the average hospital does, with an ALOS of 3.9 days. Still, Riverside has a lower cost structure, and hence lower costs per discharge, than does the average hospital. It would be useful for Riverside's managers to ensure that its ALOS is consistent with the intensity of services provided. It may be possible to lower its ALOS, which would mean even lower costs and greater profitability of inpatient services.

PRICE AND COST METRICS

Although volume is important to a provider's financial success, a high volume coupled with losses on each patient encounter will lead to disaster. To achieve financial soundness, the individual services provided must be profitable. Here are some metrics that focus on prices and costs.

Inpatient Prices

Price per discharge measures the average revenue collected on each inpatient discharge. In 2008, Riverside Memorial Hospital reported $123,740,000 in inpatient service revenue and discharged 18,281 patients, so the net price per discharge is $6,769:

Price per discharge
The average revenue on each inpatient stay.

Net price per discharge = Net inpatient revenue/Total discharges
= $123,740,000/18,281 = $6,769.

With an industry average of $6,905, Riverside collects somewhat less per discharge than the average hospital does. However, if Riverside's cost per discharge is lower than average, perhaps its net price per discharge is appropriate, even though it is below the industry average. Thus, the net price per discharge cannot be completely interpreted without knowing Riverside's cost per discharge.

Inpatient Costs

Cost per discharge measures the dollar amount of resources, on average, expended on each discharge. Because Riverside's inpatient operating expenses for 2008 were $114,865,000, its cost per discharge was $6,283:

Cost per discharge
The average cost of each inpatient stay.

Cost per discharge = Inpatient operating expenses/Total discharges
= $114,865,000/18,281 = $6,283.

Riverside's cost per discharge is well below the industry average of $7,046. Thus, even though Riverside's price per discharge is below average, its cost per discharge is even more so. Thus, the hospital's average profitability on each discharge is more than that for the hospital industry.

Inpatient Profits

We can easily calculate *profit per discharge*, given net price per discharge and cost per discharge, as follows:

Profit per discharge
The average profit made on each inpatient stay.

Profit per discharge = Net price per discharge – Cost per discharge
= $6,769 – $6,283 = $486.

The average hospital is barely making money on each discharge, so Riverside is doing comparatively well on its inpatient services.

(!) **CRITICAL CONCEPT**
Key Performance Indicators and Dashboards

A key performance indicator (KPI) is a metric chosen by a business to routinely monitor one aspect of operational or financial performance. For example, number of visits (or net admissions) might be the KPI that monitors volume. A dashboard is a way to present KPIs in an easily readable format. Here, metrics are presented as dials or with color codes to signify whether benchmarks are being met. Note that some KPIs (e.g., volume) are reviewed daily, while others are reviewed less often (e.g., weekly, monthly, or quarterly).

KEY PERFORMANCE INDICATORS AND DASHBOARDS

We have just scratched the surface of the number of metrics available to help managers control operations. Furthermore, these metrics are usually created on an annual, quarterly, monthly, or even weekly or daily basis. Managers need to monitor operational metrics on a regular basis so that problem areas can be identified and corrective action can be taken in a timely manner. However, tracking a large number of metrics on a daily or weekly basis would overload managers and, as a result, important findings could be missed.

To help solve the data overload and timeliness problems, many healthcare organizations use key performance indicators and dashboards. **Key performance indicators (KPIs)** are a limited number of metrics that measure performance critical to the success of an organization. In essence, KPIs assess the current state of the business, measure progress toward organizational goals, and prompt managerial action to correct deficiencies.

The KPIs chosen by any business depend on the line of business and its mission, objectives, and goals. In addition, KPIs usually differ by timing. For example, a hospital might have a daily KPI of number of net admissions (admissions minus discharges), while the corresponding quarterly and annual KPI might be occupancy rate.

Clearly, the number of KPIs used must be kept to a minimum to allow managers to focus on the most important aspects of operational performance. Yet, managers need a sufficient number to ensure that all critical areas of clinical and financial operations are monitored. This is a tough balancing act to accomplish.

Dashboards are a common way to present an organization's KPIs. The term stems from an automobile's dashboard, which presents key information (for example, speed, engine temperature, and oil pressure) about the car's performance. Often, KPIs are shown as gauges, which allow managers to quickly interpret the indicators. The basic idea here is to allow managers to monitor the business's most important metrics on a regular basis (daily for some metrics) in a form that is easy to read and interpret.

(?) **SELF-TEST QUESTIONS**

1. Why are operational and financial metrics important to good management?

2. Describe three metrics commonly used to track operations.

THEME WRAP-UP   REVENUE CYCLE MANAGEMENT

In 2007, the managers at Big City Medical Center were concerned that collecting receivables from third-party payers took about 60 days, while the average hospital was collecting in roughly 50 days. To help address the problem, Big City hired a consulting firm. How did Big City improve its revenue cycle performance?

For starters, Big City created an executive-level position—chief revenue officer (CRO)—to focus organizational attention on the revenue cycle and achieving best-practice results. The idea here is to recognize that the revenue cycle is not simply a function of the business office but rather requires cooperation from a large number of Big City's clinical employees and physicians (who start the entire billing process with their diagnoses). In addition, revenue cycle improvement requires close and continuous dialogue with Big City's payer partners, primarily City Health Plan, Metropolis Blue Cross and Blue Shield, Medicare, and Medicaid.

To help meet Big City's revenue cycle goals, the CRO assembled a system-level revenue cycle management team that has full responsibility for revenue cycle management, which includes information technology, at all five of Big City's hospitals. Of course, implementation of all directives was accomplished through each hospital's chief financial officer and receivables management staff.

To monitor progress, the CRO established a set of revenue cycle performance metrics. The choice of metrics was driven by a focus on performance reporting and employee accountability. Without the ability to measure progress, to identify areas suitable for improvement, and to hold employees responsible for meeting goals, it would be difficult to make much progress. In total, almost 50 metrics were selected. Such a large number was required because it was essential to monitor hospital-specific and payer-specific performance in addition to aggregate (system) performance.

However, much of the attention was paid to six KPIs, which were called the "Big City 6": (1) days in accounts receivable (average collection period), (2) proportion of receivables over 90 days old, (3) percentage of claim rejections (based on revenues), (4) percentage of final denials (based on revenues), (5) cash as a percentage of revenue, and (6) billed revenues per FTE revenue cycle management employee.

To give Big City's management a quick view of revenue cycle performance, each of the KPIs was compared against a management-established goal (standard) and best-practices benchmark. Then, variances were calculated in both numerical and percentage formats. (For example, if the initial standard was an average collection period of 55 days, and the first quarter's value was 60 days, then the variance was -5 days, or -5/55 = -9%.)

After two years of effort, the end result was a decrease in the average collection period to 48.3 days, which puts Big City below the industry average of 53 days (which is better-than-average performance). The money saved by reducing receivables provided a one-time cash flow of more than $30 million and now saves more than $1.5 million a year in receivables financing costs.

KEY CONCEPTS

This chapter examines some day-to-day financial issues related to revenue cycle and cash, inventory, and receivables management, including operational monitoring. Here are the key concepts:

➤ The *revenue cycle* includes all activities associated with billing and collections for services provided.

➤ The revenue cycle can be broken down into these activity categories, depending on when they occur: (1) *before-service* activities, (2) *at-service* activities, (3) *after-service* activities, and (4) *continuous* activities.

➤ When a healthcare organization does not receive immediate payment for services rendered, an *account receivable* is created. Receivables accumulate until the amounts due are collected.

➤ Businesses can use an *aging schedule* and *average collection period (ACP)* to help keep track of their receivables position and to help avoid the buildup of possible bad debts.

➤ The *primary goal of cash management* is to reduce the amount of cash held to the minimum necessary to conduct business.

➤ *Float* is the difference between the amount of cash in a checking account and the amount shown on the business's checkbook. The larger the float, the better.

➤ Float is increased by *speeding up the collection* of checks received and *slowing down the processing* of checks written.

➤ *Marketable securities* serve both as a substitute for cash and as a temporary investment for funds that are not needed now but will be needed in the near future. Safety is the primary consideration when selecting marketable securities.

➤ Proper *inventory management* requires close coordination among several departments. Because the cost of holding inventories is high, but *stockouts* can be disastrous, inventory management is very important.

➤ Inventories consist of a *base stock* to meet expected usage and a *safety stock* to account for unexpected increases in usage or delays in receiving reorders.

➤ *Just-in-time (JIT), stockless inventory,* and *consigned inventory* systems are used to minimize inventory costs and, simultaneously, to improve operations.

➤ Healthcare managers use *metrics* to monitor performance. Some metrics focus on operational performance, while others (discussed in more detail in Chapter 13) focus on financial performance.

➤ *Key performance indicators (KPIs)* are a limited number of metrics that focus on measures that are most important to an organization's mission success. Often, KPIs are presented in a format that resembles a *dashboard*.

In Part III (beginning with Chapter 8), we begin a new topic: financing and capital investment decisions.

END-OF-CHAPTER QUESTIONS

7.1 What is the revenue cycle? Why is it so important to healthcare organizations?

7.2 What is a receivable? Explain how receivables are built up over time.

7.3 Define average collection period. How is it used to monitor a firm's accounts receivable?

7.4 What is an aging schedule? How is it used to monitor a firm's accounts receivable?

7.5 What is the goal of cash management?

7.6 Briefly describe float and why it is a useful cash management concept.

7.7 a. Give two reasons that businesses hold marketable securities.

b. Which types of securities are most suitable for holding as marketable securities?

c. Suppose Southwest Regional Medical Center has just raised $6 million in new capital that it plans to use to build three freestanding clinics, one each year over the next three years. (For the sake of simplicity, assume that equal payments have to be made at the end of each of the next three years.) What securities should be bought for the firm's marketable securities portfolio, assuming that the firm has no other excess cash? (Hint: Consider both the type and maturity of the securities.)

d. Now, consider the situation faced by the Huntsville Physical Therapy Group. It has accumulated $20,000 in cash above its target cash balance, and it has no immediate needs for this excess cash. However, the firm may at any time need some part or all of the $20,000 to meet unforeseen cash needs. What securities should be bought for the firm's marketable securities portfolio?

7.8 a. What is a just-in-time (JIT) inventory system?

b. What are the advantages and disadvantages of JIT systems?

c. Can JIT inventory systems be used by healthcare providers? Explain your answer.

7.9 What are key performance indicators (KPIs)? What is a dashboard, and how is it used?

END-OF-CHAPTER PROBLEMS

7.1 On a typical day, Park Place Clinic writes $1,000 in checks. Generally, those checks take four days to clear. Each day the clinic typically receives $1,000 in checks, which take three days to clear. What is the clinic's float?

7.2 Drugs 'R Us operates a mail-order pharmaceutical business in San Francisco. The firm receives an average of $325,000 in payments per day. On average, it takes four days from the time customers mail their checks until the firm receives them. The company is considering establishing a lockbox system, in which customers' payments would be sent to nearby (local) banks instead of directly to San Francisco. Banks in the lockbox locations would then wire the daily receipts to a single (concentration) bank.

  The lockbox system, which would consist of ten local depository banks and a concentration bank, would cost Drugs 'R Us $6,500 per month. Under this system, customers' checks would be received at the lockbox locations one day after they are mailed, and the daily total would be wired to the concentration bank at a cost of $9.75 each.

  Assume that the firm could earn 10 percent on short-term investments and that there are 260 working days and hence 260 transfers from each lockbox location per year.
  a. What is the total annual cost of operating the lockbox system?
  b. What is the dollar benefit of the system to Drugs 'R Us?
  c. Should the firm initiate the lockbox system?

7.3 Fargo Memorial Hospital has annual patient service revenues of $14,400,000. It has two major third-party payers, and some of its patients are self-payers. The hospital's patient accounts manager estimates that 10 percent of the hospital's paying patients (its self-payers) pay on Day 30, 60 percent pay on Day 60 (Payer A), and 30 percent pay on Day 90 (Payer B). (Five percent of total billings end up as bad-debt losses, but that is not relevant to this problem.)
  a. What is Fargo's average collection period? (Assume 360 days per year throughout this problem.)
  b. What is the firm's current receivables balance?
  c. What would be the firm's new receivables balance if a newly proposed electronic claims system resulted in collecting from third-party payers in 45 and 75 days, instead of in 60 and 90 days?

d. Suppose the firm's annual cost of carrying receivables is 10 percent. If the electronic claims system costs $30,000 a year to lease and operate, should it be adopted? (Assume that the entire receivables balance has to be financed.)

7.4 Milwaukee Surgical Supplies, Inc. sells on terms of 3/10, net 30. That means customers that pay in ten days get a 3 percent discount on their purchases, while customers that do not take the discount must pay in 30 days. Gross sales (sales before any discounts taken) for the year are $1,200,000 and the collections department estimates that 30 percent of the customers pay on the 10th day and take discounts, 40 percent pay on the 30th day, and the remaining 30 percent pay, on average, on the 40th day after the purchase. (Assume 360 days per year.)

a. What is the firm's average collection period?

b. What is the firm's current receivables balance?

c. What would the firm's new receivables balance be if Milwaukee Surgical toughened up on its collection policy, with the result that all nondiscount customers paid on the 30th day?

d. Suppose that the firm's cost of carrying receivables was 8 percent annually. How much would the toughened credit policy save the firm in annual receivables carrying expense? (Assume that the entire amount of receivables has to be financed.)

7.5 Sacred Heart Hospital has the following receivables amounts, listed by age:

Age of Account (Days)	Value of Account	Percentage of Total Value
0–30	$ 5,450,000	
31–60	3,666,000	
61–90	1,278,000	
91–120	867,000	
Over 120	49,000	
	$11,310,000	

a. Complete the aging schedule by filling in the Percentage of Total Value column.

b. Interpret your results.

c. Using these data, estimate the hospital's average collection period (days in patient accounts receivable). (Hint: Assume that the average age in the first category is 15 days [the midpoint of the range], the average age in the second category is 45 days, and so on. Ignore the receivables over 120 days.)

7.6 Sacramento Memorial Hospital has the following financial data and operational metrics:

Number of beds	250
Total inpatient admissions	12,250
Total outpatient visits	90,754
Total patient revenues	$111,900,050
Outpatient mix	16.2%
Medicare payment percentage (revenues)	28.0%
Average length of stay	5.8 days
Net price per discharge	$7,653
Cost per discharge	$6,292

a. What is the hospital's profit per discharge?

b. What is the hospital's total inpatient and total outpatient revenue? (Hint: Apply patient mix metrics to total revenues.)

c. Verify your Part b answer for total inpatient revenue using volume and profitability metrics. (Hint: Calculate price per discharge.)

d. What are the hospital's total revenues from Medicare patients?

e. What is the total number of inpatient days?

f. What is the hospital's occupancy rate?

7.7 Northeast Medical Group, a family practice, has the following financial data and operational metrics:

Number of physicians	5
Total revenue	$2,748,360
Total operating costs	$1,557,615
Total procedures per physician	12,353
Patients per physician	1,941
Visits per physician	5,333

a. What is the group's revenue per physician?

b. What is the group's operating cost per physician?

c. What is the group's total operating profit?

d. What is the group's profit per physician? Per patient? Per visit? Per procedure?

e. Assume that the group plans to reinvest $50,000 of its profits in the practice. (It plans to buy a new EKG [electrocardiogram] machine.) Also, assume that the remainder of profits will be distributed equally to the group's physicians as salary. What compensation will each physician receive?

FINANCING AND CAPITAL INVESTMENT DECISIONS

Hospitals need buildings and equipment to provide inpatient and outpatient services, while clinics and physician practices require similar assets to provide outpatient services. To obtain these assets, healthcare organizations need capital (money). A large hospital requires a large amount of capital (some hospitals have more than $1 billion of capital), while a small home health care business requires a small amount of capital.

Chapter 8 discusses how healthcare organizations are financed. Two primary types of capital are available to healthcare businesses. Debt capital is borrowed money supplied by lenders, while ownership (equity) capital is obtained from owners of for-profit businesses and from the community at large for not-for-profit businesses. Because debt and ownership capital have different characteristics, managers must learn the impact of these differences on the financial condition of the business.

Chapters 9 and 10 cover capital investment decisions: Once capital is in the healthcare provider's hand, how should it be best spent? In other words, what capital investments (investments in land, buildings, and equipment) should be made? To make the best possible decisions, assessing the financial impact of proposed capital investments is necessary. This requires an understanding of discounted cash flow analysis, financial risk, and other issues related to capital investment decisions.

CHAPTER 8

BUSINESS FINANCING AND THE COST OF CAPITAL

THEME SET-UP STARTING A NEW MEDICAL PRACTICE

A few months ago, six primary care physicians in Seattle met to discuss the feasibility of creating a new group practice. Of the six, four were operating solo practices, while the other two were just completing family practice residencies. Although a solo practice offers some advantages, such as complete control, it presents numerous disadvantages.

Perhaps the largest disadvantage is that the business's administrative and clinical overhead costs must be borne by a single physician, while larger group practices can benefit from economies of scale (the spreading of fixed administrative and clinical costs over more patients). Also, solo practitioners are, in effect, always on call for handling medical emergencies outside of regular working hours. Finally, by forming groups, physicians increase their bargaining power with third-party payers.

The bottom line here is that more and more individual physicians are joining together to form groups. The trend toward multiphysician practices was recognized by the six physicians, who agreed to form a new business, Puget Sound Family Practice.

The start-up of a new group practice is not an easy task. First, legal issues must be settled, such as what type of business organization to establish (the physicians decided on a professional corporation) and who would have the greatest say in running the practice. Next, space has to be rented and equipped. Then, clinical and administrative staffs have to be hired and trained to ensure that the practice runs smoothly and that patients receive quality care in a timely, patient-friendly setting.

All of these start-up tasks require capital. In fact, the initial analysis of capital needs for Puget Sound Family Practice indicated that about $1.8 million was required to get the business up and running. The next steps in the start-up process are to (1) decide how to raise the required capital and (2) estimate how much the financing will cost.

By the end of the chapter, you will see how the physicians at Puget Sound Family Practice decided to fund the new business. Furthermore, you will get a feel for the cost of the capital raised, and how that cost will feed into the practice's decisions regarding equipment purchases and other capital expenditures.

LEARNING OBJECTIVES

After studying this chapter, you will be able to

➤ Describe how interest rates are set on debt financing.

➤ Discuss the various types of long-term and short-term debt instruments and their features.

➤ Define the two types of equity and their features.

➤ Briefly describe the capital structure decision.

➤ Explain the corporate cost of capital and its use.

8.1 INTRODUCTION

If a business is to operate, it must have assets (e.g., land, buildings, and equipment). To acquire these assets, it must raise capital. *Capital* comes in two basic forms: debt and equity. Most healthcare organizations use some debt capital, which is provided by lenders such as banks. Alternatively, equity capital is furnished by the owners of investor-owned businesses and by the community at large for not-for-profit businesses. In this chapter, many facets of business financing are discussed, starting with how interest rates are set on borrowed capital.

> *Capital*
> For finance purposes, the funds used to acquire a business's assets, including land, buildings, equipment, and inventories. Note that in economics, capital generally means the assets owned by a business.

8.2 SETTING INTEREST RATES

The **interest rate** is the price paid to obtain debt capital. Many factors influence the interest rates set on business loans, but the two most important are risk and inflation. To see how these factors operate, note that the owners of Puget Sound Family Practice do not have sufficient personal funds to start the business, so they must supplement their funds with a loan.

RISK

The risk inherent in the prospective group practice, and thus in the ability to repay the loan, would affect the return lenders would require. In effect, lenders would assess the likelihood of the practice earning enough to make the required payments in full and on time. If there is a high probability that this will occur, the loan has minimal risk. Conversely, the higher the probability that the practice will have difficulties making the payments, the higher the risk to the lender.

Lenders would be unwilling to lend to high-risk businesses unless the interest rate on such loans is higher than on loans to low-risk businesses.

CRITICAL CONCEPT
Interest Rate

The interest rate is the price paid by borrowers to obtain debt capital. Put another way, it is the price charged by lenders to provide debt financing. For example, First National Bank might provide a loan to Puget Sound Family Practice with an 8 percent interest rate, which means that the practice must pay the bank 0.08 x $1,000 = $80 per year for each $1,000 borrowed. The interest rate set on a loan is primarily dependent on two factors: the riskiness of the loan and the expected inflation.

In this instance, the bank would likely require personal guarantees from the owner-physicians so that if the practice fails, the owners would be personally liable for repaying the loan.

INFLATION

Inflation has a major impact on interest rates because it erodes the purchasing power of the dollar and lowers the value of investment returns. Think of it this way: Suppose a loaf of bread at the local supermarket cost $1.29 five years ago. Today, that same loaf costs $1.69. Furthermore, assume a lender made a business loan five years ago that pays $1,000 in annual interest. When the loan was made, the interest received would buy $1,000/$1.29 = 775 loaves of bread. Today, the same interest payment would buy only $1,000/$1.69 = 592 loaves. Thus, the interest payments received by a lender who made a loan five years ago will buy less bread today than when the loan was made. In effect, price inflation has reduced the purchasing power of the interest payments received on the loan.

Lenders are well aware of the impact of inflation, and hence the greater the expected rate of inflation, the greater the interest rate required to offset the loss of purchasing power. In the bread example, the price increased 40 cents over five years, which represents an inflation rate of 5.5 percent. Thus, the interest rate on loans over this time has to be at least 5.5 percent just to cover the effects of inflation.

Of course, we just looked at bread. A more meaningful measure of inflation would be the increase in overall prices in the economy. Also, the relevant rate of inflation to a lender is the rate expected in the future, not the rate experienced in the past. Thus, the latest inflation report may indicate an annual rate of 5.5 percent, but that is for a past period. If lenders expect a 4 percent inflation rate in the future, then 4 percent would be the relevant amount used to set current interest rates.

Finally, the inflation rate built into the interest rate on a loan is the average rate expected over the life of the loan. Thus, the inflation rate relevant to a one-year loan is the rate expected for the next year, but the inflation rate relevant to a ten-year loan is the average rate of inflation expected over the next ten years.

⍰ SELF-TEST QUESTIONS

1. What is the "price" of debt capital?

2. What are the two primary factors that affect a loan's interest rate?

8.3 DEBT FINANCING

There are many different types of debt. Some types, such as home mortgages and personal auto loans, are used by individuals, while other types are used primarily by businesses. Some debt is used to meet short-term needs, while other debt is for longer terms.

Principal
The amount of money borrowed in a loan transaction.

When money is borrowed, the borrower (whether a business or an individual) has a contractual obligation to repay the loan, so debt obligations are "fixed by contract." The repayment consists of two parts: (1) the amount borrowed (or *principal*) and (2) the amount of interest stated on the loan.

In this section, we discuss the types of debt most commonly used by healthcare organizations. In subsequent sections, we explore the most important features of debt financing.

LONG-TERM DEBT

Long-term debt is defined as debt that has a *maturity* greater than one year. Thus, the amount borrowed (principal amount) on a long-term loan has to be paid back to the lender at some time in the future longer than one year. Long-term debt typically is used to finance assets that have a long useful life, such as buildings and equipment. The two major types of long-term debt used by healthcare organizations are term loans and bonds.

Term Loans

A **term loan** is long-term debt financing that is arranged directly between the borrowing business and the lender. In essence, the lender provides the capital and the borrower agrees to pay the stated interest rate over the life of the loan and return the amount borrowed.

Typically, the lender is a financial institution such as a commercial bank, mutual fund, or insurance company, but it can also be a wealthy private investor. Most term loans have maturities of three to ten years. Like personal auto loans, term loans usually are paid off in equal installments over the life of the loan, so part of the principal amount is repaid with each loan payment.

The interest rate on a term loan either is fixed for the life of the loan or is variable (*floating rate*). If fixed, the interest rate stays the same over the life of the loan. If variable, the interest rate is usually set at a certain number of percentage points over some index rate. When the index rate goes up or down, so does the interest rate that must be paid on the outstanding balance of the variable-rate loan.

To illustrate a term loan, Apria Healthcare Group, a company with 370 home respiratory and infusion locations across the United States, recently obtained a $125 million five-year term loan from Bank of America. The loan had a floating (variable) interest rate that was set at 175 *basis points* (1.75 percentage points) above the index rate. (The index used on the loan was the London Interbank Offered Rate [LIBOR], which is the interest rate that London banks charge to one another on short-term loans.)

Bonds

A **bond** is a long-term loan under which a borrower agrees to make payments of interest and principal, on specific dates, to the holder of the bond. Although bonds are similar in

> ⓘ **CRITICAL CONCEPT**
> Term Loan
>
> A term loan is a type of long-term debt financing used by businesses. It typically has a maturity of three to ten years and is obtained directly from financial institutions, such as commercial banks. The interest rate on a term loan may be fixed for the life of the loan or variable, which means that the rate changes (floats) as the general level of interest rates in the economy changes. Term loans typically are amortized, which means that the borrower pays back some of the principal amount with each interest payment.

Maturity
The amount of time until a loan matures (must be repaid). Short-term debt has a maturity of one year or less, while long-term debt has a maturity greater than one year.

Floating rate
A loan with an interest rate that changes over time as the designated index value rises and falls.

Basis point
One-hundredth of a percentage point. For example, 50 basis points equals 0.5 percent, or one-half a percentage point.

many ways to term loans, a bond issue generally is offered to the public and sold to many different investors. Indeed, thousands of individual and institutional investors may participate when a business sells a bond issue, while a term loan generally has only one lender.

Additionally, bonds have a terminology of their own. The issuer of a bond is equivalent to the borrower on a term loan, the bondholder is the lender, and the interest rate often is called the coupon rate.

Because bonds are sold to many investors, large amounts of capital can be raised in a bond issue. To illustrate, in late 2006, HCA (Hospital Corporation of America) raised more than $5 billion of debt capital in a single bond issue. Each bond had a principal amount of $1,000, so more than 5 million individual bonds were sold to thousands of investors to complete the issue. To reach so many investors, bonds generally are sold through brokers rather than directly by the borrowing company.

Bonds are categorized as either government (Treasury), corporate, or municipal. Treasury bonds are used to raise money for the federal government. Corporate bonds are issued by investor-owned businesses, while municipal bonds are issued by states, counties, cities, and not-for-profit healthcare organizations.

Although bonds generally have maturities in the range of 10 to 30 years, shorter maturities, as well as longer maturities, are occasionally used. In fact, in 1995, HCA (then Columbia/HCA) issued corporate bonds with a 100-year maturity. Unlike term loans, bonds usually pay only interest over the life of the bond, with the entire amount borrowed returned to lenders at maturity. Most bonds have a fixed interest rate, which locks in the current rate for the entire maturity of the bond and hence minimizes interest payment uncertainty. However, some bonds have floating, or variable, rates so the interest payments move up and down with the general level of interest rates in the economy.

Although municipal, or "muni," bonds typically are issued by states, counties, and cities, not-for-profit healthcare providers are entitled to issue such securities through government-sponsored healthcare financing authorities. Whereas the vast majority of Treasury and corporate bonds are held by institutions, primarily mutual funds, close to half of all outstanding municipal bonds are held by individual investors.

The primary attraction of most municipal bonds is the fact that bond owners (lenders) do not have to pay income taxes on the interest earned. Because such bonds are

> **CRITICAL CONCEPT**
> Bond
>
> A bond is a type of long-term debt used to raise large amounts of capital. Corporate bonds are issued by investor-owned corporations; Treasury bonds are issued by the U.S. government; and municipal bonds are issued by states, counties, cities, and not-for-profit healthcare providers. Bonds typically have maturities in the range of 10–30 years. Because of the high administrative costs involved in selling bonds, as compared to term loans, bonds are not used unless the amount required is greater than $10 million, although smaller-size issues do occasionally occur. To ensure that the entire issue is sold (the full amount of money is raised), bonds typically are issued in small denominations ($1,000 or $5,000) and sold through brokers to institutions and the general public.

tax-exempt, the interest rate set on municipal bonds is less than the rate set on similar corporate bonds. The idea here is that municipal bond buyers are willing to accept a lower interest rate because they do not have to pay income taxes on the interest payments received.

Historically, when an investor (lender) bought a bond, he or she received a very impressive engraved certificate that indicated the principal amount purchased and the terms of repayment. Today, however, bonds typically are issued in registered form, so instead of a certificate, owners receive statements from the issuer (or its agent). However, old bond certificates have become collectibles. For example, a Boston and Maine Railroad $1,000 bond issued in 1940 (which has no financial value) was recently sold for $150, and older certificates signed by well-known industrialists can easily sell for thousands of dollars.

Short-Term Debt

Short-term debt, with a maturity of one year or less, generally is used to finance temporary needs, such as increasing the level of inventories to meet busy-season demand. Short-term debt has several advantages over long-term debt. For example, administrative (i.e., accounting, legal, and selling) costs generally are higher for long-term debt than for short-term debt. Also, long-term loan agreements usually contain more restrictions on the firm's future actions, whereas short-term debt agreements typically are less onerous in this regard. Finally, the interest rate on short-term debt generally is lower than the rate on long-term debt because longer maturities pose more risk to lenders.

In spite of these advantages, short-term debt has one serious disadvantage: It subjects the borrower to more risk than does long-term financing. The increased risk occurs for two reasons.

First, if a business borrows on a long-term basis, its interest costs will be relatively stable over time, but if it uses short-term debt, its interest expense can fluctuate widely, at times possibly going quite high. For example, the short-term rate that banks charge their best business customers (the prime rate) more than tripled over a two-year period in the early 1980s, rising to 21 percent from about 6 percent. Thus, businesses that used large amounts of short-term debt financing during those years saw their interest costs rise to unimaginable levels, forcing many into bankruptcy.

Second, the principal amount on short-term debt comes due on a regular basis (one year or less). If the financial condition of a business temporarily deteriorates, it may find itself unable to repay this debt when it matures. Furthermore, the business may be in such a weak financial position that the lender will not extend the loan. Such a scenario can result in severe problems for the borrower, which, like unexpectedly high interest rates, could force the business into bankruptcy.

Commercial banks are the primary provider of short-term debt financing. Although banks make longer-maturity (term) loans, the bulk of their lending is on a short-term basis

> ### ⓘ CRITICAL CONCEPT
> #### Line of Credit
>
> A line of credit is a common type of short-term debt financing used by businesses. Typically, lines of credit, which are offered by commercial banks, specify a maximum loan size over a specified period—often a year. The borrowing business can borrow up to the maximum amount (and pay it back) at any time while the line is in effect. However, any funds borrowed on the line must be repaid to the bank when the line expires. Lines of credit typically are used to meet a business's short-term capital needs, such as to build up inventories in advance of the busy season. The idea here is that revenues from busy-season patient services will be available to "pay down" the line before it expires.

(about two-thirds of all bank loans mature in a year or less). Bank loans to businesses are frequently written as 90-day notes, so the loan must be repaid or renewed at the end of 90 days.

Alternatively, a business may obtain short-term financing by establishing a **line of credit** with a bank. This is an agreement that specifies the maximum credit the bank will extend to the borrower over a designated period of time, often a year. For example, in December a bank might indicate to managers of Pine Garden Nursing Care that the bank regards the nursing home as being good for up to $100,000 during the forthcoming year. Thus, at any time during the year Pine Garden can borrow up to $100,000, the full amount of the line. Borrowers typically pay an up-front fee to obtain the line, and interest must be paid on any amounts borrowed. Furthermore, the line must be fully repaid by the end of the year.

> ### ⓘ SELF-TEST QUESTIONS
>
> 1. Describe the primary features of a term loan, the features of a bond.
>
> 2. What is a corporate bond? Treasury bond? Municipal bond?
>
> 3. What are the advantages and disadvantages of using short-term versus long-term debt financing?
>
> 4. Describe the features of a line of credit.

Restrictive covenant
A provision in a loan agreement that protects the interests of the lender by restricting the actions of the borrower.

8.4 DEBT CONTRACTS

Debt contracts, which have various names such as loan agreement or bond indenture, spell out the rights and obligations of borrowers and lenders. These contracts vary substantially in length depending on the type of debt. Some contracts, particularly bond indentures, can be several hundred pages in length.

Many debt contracts include provisions, called *restrictive covenants*, which are designed to protect lenders from managerial actions that would be detrimental to lenders' interests. For example, a typical bond indenture may contain several restrictive covenants, such as specifying that the borrower maintains a certain amount of cash on hand. By specifying this minimum, lenders have some assurance that the debt payments coming due in the near future can be met.

When debt is supplied by a single creditor, there is a one-to-one relationship between the lender and borrower. However, bond issues can have thousands of buyers (lenders), so a single voice is needed to represent bondholders. This function is performed by a *trustee*, usually an institution such as a bank, who represents the bondholders and ensures that the terms of the contract (indenture) are being carried out.

What happens if a borrower fails to make a payment required by a debt contract—that is, if the borrower *defaults*? Usually, the debt contract spells out the actions that can be taken by lenders when this occurs. In any event, upon default, lenders have the legal right to force borrowers into bankruptcy, which could result in closure and liquidation. Although lenders have this right, it may not be the prudent action to take. In some default situations, it might be better for lenders to help the borrowing business get through the bad times rather than push the business under.

Finally, many bond contracts have *call provisions*, which give the borrower the right to redeem (call) the bonds prior to maturity. Thus, the issuer can pay off the principal amount and any interest due and retire the issue. The call privilege is valuable to the borrower but potentially detrimental to bondholders, because bonds typically are called when interest rates have fallen. This enables the borrower to replace an old, higher-interest issue with a new, lower-interest issue and hence reduce interest expense. However, the old bondholders are now compelled to reinvest the principal returned in new bonds that have a lower interest rate.

> **Trustee**
> An individual or institution, often a bank, that represents the interests of bondholders.

> **Default**
> Failure by a borrower to make a promised interest or principal repayment.

> **Call provision**
> A provision in a bond contract that gives the issuing company the right to redeem (call) the bonds prior to maturity.

⍰ SELF-TEST QUESTIONS

1. What is a restrictive covenant?

2. What is the purpose of a trustee?

3. What happens when a borrower defaults?

4. What is a call provision, and when are bonds typically called?

8.5 DEBT RATINGS

Major debt issuers, as well as their specific debt issues, are assigned creditworthiness (quality) ratings that reflect the probability of default. The three primary rating agencies are

Investment grade debt

Debt with a BBB or higher rating. Generally considered to be suitable (relatively low risk) investments for conservative individuals and institutions.

Junk debt

Debt with a BB or lower rating. Generally considered to be more speculative than investment-grade debt, and hence inappropriate for conservative investors.

Fitch Ratings, Moody's Investors Service (Moody's), and Standard & Poor's (S&P). All three agencies rate both corporate and municipal debt.

Standard & Poor's rating designations are shown in Table 8.1, but all three have similar rating designations. Debt with a BBB and higher rating is called *investment grade*, while double B and lower debt is called speculative, or *junk*, debt because it has a much higher probability of going into default than do higher-rated issues. Although the rating assignments are subjective, they are based on both qualitative characteristics, such as quality of management, and quantitative factors, such as a business's financial strength.

Debt ratings are important both to borrowers and to lenders for several reasons. First, the rating is an indicator of the issue's default risk, so the rating has a direct influence on the interest rate required by lenders: the lower the rating, the greater the risk and hence the higher the interest rate.

Second, most corporate bonds are purchased by institutional investors rather than by individuals. Many of these institutions are restricted to investment-grade securities. Also, most individual investors who buy municipal bonds are unwilling to take much risk in their bond purchases. Thus, if a new issue is rated below BBB, it will be more difficult to sell because the number of potential purchasers is reduced.

As a result of their higher risk and more restricted market, low-grade bonds typically carry much higher interest rates than do high-grade bonds. To illustrate, in mid-2008, the interest rate on ten-year CCC-rated corporate bonds was about 4.5 percentage points higher than the rate on AAA-rated bonds.

TABLE 8.1
Standard & Poor's
Debt Ratings

Credit Risk	Rating Category
Prime	AAA
Excellent	AA
Upper medium	A
Lower medium	BBB
Speculative	BB
Very speculative	B
	CCC
	CC
Default	D

Note: S&P uses plus and minus modifiers for bond ratings below triple A. Thus, A+ designates the strongest A-rated bond and A– the weakest.

Because of the impact of debt ratings on the cost of financing, healthcare borrowers (particularly not-for-profits) often use *credit enhancement (bond insurance)* to raise the rating on a bond issue. Regardless of the inherent creditworthiness of the issuer, bond insurance guarantees that bondholders will receive the promised interest and principal payments. Thus, bond insurance protects lenders against default by the issuer. Because the insurer gives its guarantee that payments will be made, an insured bond carries the credit rating of the insurance company rather than that of the issuer.

Credit enhancement gives the issuer access to the lowest possible interest rate, but not without a cost. Insurers charge an up-front fee that is related to the underlying rating of the issue: the lower the borrower's inherent credit rating, the higher the cost of insurance.

> ⚠️ **CRITICAL CONCEPT**
> Debt Ratings
>
> Major debt issues are rated by several different rating agencies, such as Standard & Poor's, on their probability of default (creditworthiness). In general, ratings range from AAA, which indicates the safest issues (most creditworthy), through AA, A, BBB, BB, and so on to D (in default). Because debt ratings indicate risk, the lower the rating the higher the interest rate that must be set on the issue to make it attractive to buyers. To assess creditworthiness, rating agencies consider both quantitative factors, such as financial condition, and qualitative factors, such as quality of management and the competitive position of the borrower.

Credit enhancement (bond insurance)
Insurance that guarantees the payment of interest and repayment of principal on a bond if the borrower (issuer) defaults. Insured bonds carry the rating of the insurer rather than the issuer.

> ❓ **SELF-TEST QUESTIONS**
>
> 1. What are debt ratings?
> 2. What are some criteria that the rating agencies use when assigning ratings?
> 3. What impact do ratings have on a borrower's cost of debt?
> 4. Why would healthcare borrowers seek bond insurance?

8.6 EQUITY FINANCING

The second primary source of capital to healthcare businesses is equity financing. Equity financing is provided by owners in for-profit businesses and by religious or governmental entities or by the community at large in not-for-profit businesses. Although there are many similarities between the equity in for-profit and in not-for-profit businesses, there are some key differences. In this section, we describe the most important features of equity financing.

EQUITY IN FOR-PROFIT BUSINESSES

In for-profit businesses, equity financing is supplied by the owners of the business, either directly through the purchase of an equity (ownership) interest in the business or indirectly through earnings retention.

Most large for-profit healthcare businesses are organized as corporations, in which case the owners are stockholders who contribute equity to the company by buying shares of newly issued stock. (The sale of stock from one individual to another that was sold by the company in the past does not create equity financing for the business.) Smaller businesses are organized as proprietorships or partnerships, or as some other hybrid form of business such as a professional corporation. Regardless of type, equity capital is raised when owners provide start-up or additional capital to the business.

Owners of for-profit businesses have certain rights and privileges. Perhaps the most important is a claim on the *residual earnings* of the business. A business's residual earnings, which are the profits that remain after all expenses have been paid, belong to the owners. Some portion of these earnings may be paid out to owners as dividends (in the case of corporations) or bonuses (in the case of proprietorships or partnerships), while the remainder is retained (reinvested) within the business. Such retentions are a major source of equity capital in for-profit businesses.

In addition to the claim on residual earnings, owners of for-profit businesses have the right of control. In small businesses, the owners typically are the managers of the business and hence directly control its operations. In large businesses (corporations), the owners (stockholders) elect the firm's directors, who in turn elect the officers who manage the business.

Businesses need equity capital because it provides a financing base with no maturity date. Thus, businesses can use equity financing for long periods of time without concern that the capital must be repaid. Furthermore, dividends (or bonuses) to equity holders are not guaranteed; they are paid only when the business's managers believe it is prudent to do so. Thus, equity financing does not entail the same mandatory periodic payment to capital suppliers as does debt financing.

Finally, lenders do not make business loans if the business has no equity to share the risk, so equity financing is an important precondition to obtain debt financing.

EQUITY IN NOT-FOR-PROFIT BUSINESSES

Most not-for-profit healthcare organizations received their initial, start-up equity capital from religious, educational, or governmental entities. Today, some organizations continue to receive funding from these sources. However, since the 1970s, these sources have provided a much smaller proportion of hospital funding, forcing not-for-profit hospitals to rely more on profits and outside contributions.

Not-for-profit businesses obtain much of the equity capital from retained earnings. In fact, all profits earned by a not-for-profit organization must be retained within the or-

---

Residual earnings

The earnings (profits) of a business after all expenses, including interest on debt financing, have been paid.

ganization, as there are no owners to receive dividends. In theory, not-for-profit organizations provide "dividends" to the community at large by offering healthcare services to the poor, educational programs, and other charitable endeavors.

In addition to retained earnings, not-for-profit businesses raise equity capital through charitable contributions. Individuals, as well as businesses, are motivated to contribute to not-for-profit healthcare organizations for a variety of reasons, including concern for the well-being of others, the recognition that often accompanies large contributions, and tax deductibility.

Because only contributions to not-for-profit organizations are tax deductible, this source of funding is, for all practical purposes, not available to investor-owned businesses. Although charitable contributions are not a substitute for profit retentions, charitable contributions can be a significant source of equity capital for not-for-profit businesses.

Equity in not-for-profit healthcare organizations serves the same function as in for-profit businesses. It provides a permanent financing base and supports the business's ability to use debt financing. Note that, within not-for-profit businesses, equity financing may be called fund capital or net assets, but for all practical purposes it is equivalent to a for-profit business's equity financing.

---

⑦ SELF-TEST QUESTIONS

1. What are the sources of equity financing for for-profit businesses? For not-for-profit businesses?

2. What is the purpose of equity financing?

3. Do both for-profit and not-for-profit healthcare organizations have access to contribution capital?

8.7 THE CHOICE BETWEEN DEBT AND EQUITY FINANCING

The mix of debt and equity financing used by a business is called its *capital structure*. One of the most perplexing issues for healthcare organizations is how much debt financing, as opposed to equity financing, to use.

Is there an optimal mix of debt and equity (i.e., is there an optimal capital structure)? If optimal capital structures do exist, do hospitals' optimal structures differ from those of home health agencies or medical group practices? Is there an optimal mix of short-term and long-term debt?

Capital structure
The business's mix of debt and equity financing, often expressed as the percentage of debt financing.

These questions, although difficult to answer, are important to the financial well-being of any business and hence are discussed in the following sections.

IMPACT OF DEBT FINANCING ON RISK AND RETURN

To fully understand the consequences of capital structure decisions, it is essential to understand the effects of debt financing on a business's risk and return as reflected in a profit and loss (P&L) statement. Consider the situation that faces Super Health, Inc., a for-profit (investor-owned) business that is just being formed. Its founders have identified two financing alternatives for the business: all equity or 50 percent debt financing.

To begin the analysis, note that the asset requirements for any business depend on the nature and size of the business rather than on how the business will be financed. Assume that Super Health requires $200,000 in assets (e.g., equipment, inventories) to begin operations. If all-equity financed, Super Health's owners will put up the entire $200,000 needed to purchase the assets. However, if 50 percent debt financing is used, the owners will contribute only $100,000, with the remaining $100,000 obtained from a lender—say, a bank loan with a 10 percent interest rate.

Table 8.2 contains the business's projected P&L statements under the two financing alternatives. What is the impact of the two financing alternatives on Super Health's projected first-year profitability?

Revenues are projected to be $150,000 and operating costs are forecasted at $100,000, so the firm's operating income is expected to be $50,000. Because a business's mix of debt and equity financing does not affect revenues and operating costs, the operating income projection is the same under both financing alternatives.

However, interest expense must be paid if debt financing is used. Thus, the 50 percent debt alternative results in a $0.10 \times \$100,000 = \$10,000$ annual interest charge, while

TABLE 8.2
Super Health, Inc.:
Projected P&L
Statements

	All Equity	*50% Debt*
Revenues	$150,000	$150,000
Operating costs	100,000	100,000
Operating income	$ 50,000	$ 50,000
Interest expense	0	10,000
Taxable income	$ 50,000	$ 40,000
Taxes (40%)	20,000	16,000
Profit	$ 30,000	$ 24,000
ROE	15%	24%

no interest expense occurs if the firm is all-equity financed. The result is taxable income of $50,000 under all-equity financing and a lower taxable income of $40,000 under the 50 percent debt alternative.

Because the business anticipates being taxed at a 40 percent rate, the expected tax liability is 0.40 × $50,000 = $20,000 under the all-equity alternative and 0.40 × $40,000 = $16,000 for the 50 percent debt alternative. Finally, when taxes are deducted, the business expects to earn $30,000 in profit if it is all-equity financed but only $24,000 if it is 50 percent debt financed.

At first glance, the use of debt financing appears to be the inferior alternative. After all, if 50 percent debt financing is used, the business's projected profitability will fall by $30,000 – $24,000 = $6,000. But the conclusion that debt financing is bad requires closer examination. What is most important to the owners of Super Health is not the business's dollar profitability but rather the return expected on their equity investment.

The best measure of return to the owners of a business is the rate of *return on equity (ROE)*, which is defined here as projected profit divided by the amount of equity invested. Under all-equity financing, projected ROE is $30,000 / $200,000 = 0.15 = 15%, but with 50 percent debt financing, projected ROE increases to $24,000 / $100,000 = 24%.

The key to the increased ROE is that although profit decreases when debt financing is used, the amount of equity needed also decreases, and this capital requirement decreases more than does profit. The bottom line here is that debt financing can increase owners' expected rate of return. Because the use of debt financing increases, or leverages up, the return to equityholders, such financing often is called *financial leverage*. Hence, the use of financial leverage is merely the use of debt financing.

At this point, it appears that Super Health's financing decision is a no brainer. Given these two financing alternatives, 50 percent debt financing should be used because it promises owners the higher rate of return. Unfortunately, like the proverbial no free lunch, there is a catch. The use of financial leverage increases not only the owners' projected return but also their risk.

To see this, consider what would happen if actual revenues were $25,000 less than expected and actual operating costs were $25,000 higher than expected. In this situation, operating income, and hence ROE, would be zero if all equity financing is used. This would not be a good situation. However, it could be worse: with 50 percent debt financing, $10,000 in interest must be paid to the bank. But with no operating income to pay the interest expense, the owners would either have to put up additional equity capital to pay the interest due or declare the business bankrupt. (The business could theoretically borrow an additional $10,000 to pay the interest, but, based on the first year's results, it is unlikely that any lenders would be interested.) Clearly, the use of 50 percent debt financing has increased the riskiness of the owners' investment.

This simple example illustrates that debt financing can increase both the owners' return and risk. When risk is considered, the ultimate decision on which financing alternative

Return on equity (ROE)
Profit divided by the amount of equity invested Measures the dollars of earnings per dollar of equity investment, or the rate of return to the owners of the business

Financial leverage
The use of debt financing, which typically increases (leverages up) the return to owners.

should be chosen is not so clear-cut. The zero debt alternative has a lower expected ROE but lower risk. The 50 percent debt alternative offers a higher expected ROE but carries more risk.

Thus, the decision is a classic risk–return trade-off: Higher returns can be obtained only by assuming greater risk. What Super Health's founders need to know is whether the higher return is enough to compensate them for the higher risk assumed. To complicate the decision even more, an almost unlimited number of debt-level choices are available, not just the 50/50 mix used in the illustration. This example vividly illustrates that healthcare managers face a difficult decision in setting a business's optimal capital structure.

CAPITAL STRUCTURE THEORY

Trade-off theory
A theory proposing that a business's optimal capital structure balances the costs and benefits associated with debt financing.

At this point, Super Health's founders are left in a quandary because debt financing brings with it both higher returns and higher risk. To help make the decision, academicians have developed several theories of capital structure. The goal of these theories is to determine whether or not businesses have optimal capital structures.

The most widely accepted theory is the *trade-off theory*, which holds that the capital structure decision involves a trade-off between the costs and benefits of debt financing, where the costs are increasing bankruptcy risk and the benefits are increasing return.

The trade-off theory tells managers that every business has an **optimal capital structure** that balances the costs and benefits associated with debt financing. In effect, the optimal capital structure is the mix of debt and equity financing that produces the lowest cost of capital for the business. (Cost of capital is discussed in a later section.) The key implication of the trade-off theory is that some debt financing is good because owners can capture the benefits of increased return, but too much debt is bad because the increased risk of bankruptcy outweighs the higher expected returns.

> (!) **CRITICAL CONCEPT**
> Optimal Capital Structure
>
> When a business uses debt (as opposed to equity) financing, two consequences arise. First, under most conditions, the expected return to owners increases. (For this reason, debt financing is called *financial leverage*.) Second, owners' risk increases. The greater the proportion of debt financing, the greater the impact on return and risk, so the choice as to how much debt financing to use involves a risk–return trade-off. Theory tells us that a business has an optimal capital structure that balances the costs and benefits of debt financing. In essence, some debt financing is good, but too much debt is bad. Unfortunately, theory cannot identify the optimal structure for any given business, so managers must use qualitative factors to make the judgment.

IDENTIFYING THE OPTIMAL CAPITAL STRUCTURE IN PRACTICE

Unfortunately, the trade-off theory cannot identify the optimal capital structure for any given business because the costs and benefits of debt financing to a specific business cannot be estimated at alternative capital structures with any precision. Thus, healthcare managers must apply judgment in making the capital structure decision. Here are some of the more important factors that managers must consider.

◆   *Business risk.* A certain amount of risk, called *business risk*, is inherent in business operations, even when no debt financing is used. This risk is associated with the ability of managers to forecast future profitability. The more uncertainty in the process—say, in forecasting future ROE—the greater the inherent risk of the business. When debt financing is used, owners must bear additional risk above the inherent business risk of the organization. The additional risk to owners (or to the community in the case of not-for-profits) when debt financing is used is called *financial risk*. In general, managers will place some limit on the total amount of risk, including both business and financial, undertaken by a business. Thus, the greater the inherent business risk, the less "room" available for the use of financial leverage and hence the lower the optimal proportion of debt financing.

◆   *Lender and rating agency attitudes.* The attitudes of lenders and rating agencies are important determinants of capital structures. In the majority of situations, managers discuss the business's financial structure with lenders and rating agencies and give a great deal of weight to their advice. In large organizations, managers usually have a target debt rating—say, single A. In small businesses, managers want to restrict debt financing to that readily available from commercial banks. In effect, lenders and rating agencies set a limit on the proportion of debt financing that a business can raise at "reasonable" interest rates.

◆   *Reserve borrowing capacity.* Businesses generally maintain a reserve borrowing capacity that preserves their ability to add additional debt capital. In essence, managers want to maintain financial flexibility, which includes the ability to survive tough times (should they occur) by taking on more debt financing. This can only be accomplished at reasonable interest rates if businesses regularly use less debt than other factors may indicate.

◆   *Industry averages.* Presumably, managers act rationally, so the capital structures of other firms in the industry, particularly the industry leaders, should provide insights about the optimal structure. In general, there is no reason to believe that the managers of one firm are better than the managers of other firms. Thus, if one business has a capital structure that is significantly different from others in its industry, the managers of that firm should identify the unique circumstances that contribute to the anomaly. If unique circumstances cannot be identified, then it is doubtful that the firm has identified the correct capital structure.

Business risk
The risk inherent in the operations of a business, assuming it uses no debt financing.

Financial risk
The additional risk placed on the business's owners (or the community) when debt financing is used.

Debt capacity
The amount of debt in a business's optimal capital structure. A business with excess debt capacity is operating with less than the optimal amount of debt.

♦   *Asset structure.* Firms whose assets are suitable as security (collateral) for loans pay lower interest rates on debt financing than do other firms and hence tend to use more debt. Thus, hospitals tend to use more debt than do biotechnology companies. Both the ability to use assets as collateral and low inherent business risk give a firm more *debt capacity*, and hence a target capital structure that includes a relatively high proportion of debt.

NOT-FOR-PROFIT BUSINESSES

Do not-for-profit businesses have optimal capital structures? The same general concepts we have discussed apply to not-for-profits—namely, some debt financing is good, but too much is bad. In essence, debt financing permits not-for-profits to offer more programs and services than are possible using only equity financing. However, just as with for-profits, using debt financing brings more risk to the owners (in this case the community), and the greater the proportion of debt, the greater the risk.

In spite of the theoretical similarity in capital structure decisions between for-profit and not-for-profit businesses, not-for-profits have a unique problem: They cannot sell equity to raise new capital. If an investor-owned business needs more equity capital than it can obtain through retained earnings, it can always go to the owners (to the equity markets) for the needed funds. Additionally, investor-owned firms can easily adjust their capital structures. If they are financially underleveraged (using too little debt), they can simply issue more debt and use the proceeds to repurchase equity from the owners. On the other hand, if they are financially overleveraged (using too much debt), they can issue additional equity and use the proceeds to reduce the amount of debt outstanding.

Because not-for-profit organizations cannot raise equity by merely asking investors to contribute more capital, they do not have the same degree of flexibility in adjusting their capital structures as do their for-profit counterparts. Thus, it is sometimes necessary for not-for-profits to delay new programs or services, even profitable ones, or to temporarily use more than the optimal amount of debt financing because that is the only way that needed services can be provided.

OPTIMAL CAPITAL STRUCTURE IMPLICATIONS

Target capital structure
The capital structure that a company strives to achieve and maintain over time. Generally the same as the optimal capital structure.

Once a business estimates its optimal capital structure—say, 30 percent debt financing— it will take the financing actions necessary to attain that structure. Then, as the business needs additional capital to finance asset replacement and growth, it will raise capital over time so as to maintain its optimal capital structure. Thus, future financing decisions will be mostly based (targeted) on the optimal capital structure, so the optimal capital structure often is called the *target capital structure.* Other considerations will come into play when raising new capital, but, over the long run, businesses attempt to keep their actual capital structures close to the target.

8.8 THE CHOICE BETWEEN LONG-TERM AND SHORT-TERM DEBT

Once the optimal mix of debt and equity financing has been identified, the next decision arises: What is the optimal mix of debt maturities? In other words, what is the **optimal debt maturity structure**? The answer, like the optimal capital structure, involves a trade-off between risk and return.

In general, the optimal debt maturity structure involves matching the maturities of the debt used with the maturities of the assets being financed. That is, if debt financing is used to increase a business's inventories in preparation for the coming busy season or to pay the salary of a three-month temporary employee, then short-term debt is appropriate. Conversely, if the debt is being used to buy a new scanner or to finance the construction of a new clinic, then long-term debt is appropriate.

The idea here is that the inventory level and payroll will return to their initial, lower levels

> **(!) CRITICAL CONCEPT**
> Optimal Debt Maturity Structure
>
> After a business estimates its optimal mix of debt and equity financing (optimal capital structure), a second decision arises: Should the business's debt financing be all long term, all short term, or some combination of the two? In general, a business's debt maturities should match the maturities of the assets being financed with that debt. Thus, if debt financing is being used to build a new facility, the debt should have a long maturity because the facility has a long life. Conversely, if the debt is taken on to undertake a two-month marketing campaign, it should probably have a short maturity to match the short-term nature of the cash need.

when the busy season is over, so the need for financing is temporary (short term). However, the new diagnostic equipment or clinic will likely be operating for many years, so its financing need is more or less permanent (long term).

In theory, a business could attempt to match exactly the maturity structure of its assets and financing. Inventory expected to be sold in 30 days could be financed with a 30-day bank loan, an x-ray machine expected to last for five years could be financed by a five-year term loan, a 20-year building could be financed by a 20-year bond, and so forth. However, two factors make this approach unpractical: (1) uncertainty about the lives of assets and (2) some equity capital must be used, and this capital has no maturity.

(?) SELF-TEST QUESTION

1. What factor most influences a business's debt maturity structure?

(*) INDUSTRY PRACTICE Capital Structure Decisions in Not-for-Profit Hospitals

Capital structure decisions in not-for-profit healthcare businesses have never been as clear-cut as they are in for-profit businesses. A great deal of theory is available to for-profit businesses to help them make these decisions. Essentially, for-profits have the goal of maximizing their owners' wealth, and this is accomplished by lowering capital costs. However, not-for-profits do not have wealth maximization as a goal, so capital structure theory breaks down in such businesses.

Several studies have been conducted to shed light on how not-for-profit hospitals make capital structure decisions. Although some findings are in conflict, the results are sufficiently consistent to give an idea of what drives the decision. To begin, not-for-profit hospitals do establish a target capital structure and try to stick to it. Most hospitals have target structures in the 35–40 percent debt range, as measured by the debt-to-financing ratio. (The debt-to-financing ratio is defined as long-term debt divided by long-term financing [long-term debt plus equity].)

The most important factor in setting the target capital structure is maintaining a sound bond rating (often A). This is accomplished by using the right amount of debt: too little debt produces a higher rating, while too much debt produces a lower rating.

The focus on bond ratings cannot be overstated. Most not-for-profit hospitals view a high bond rating as an essential element of capital structure policy. The logic here is that not-for-profits are more reliant on debt financing because of their inability to raise capital by selling equity. Note that more reliance on debt does not mean that they use more debt than their for-profit counterparts. In fact, not-for-profit hospitals historically have used less debt than for-profit hospitals. But it is more important for not-for-profits to preserve access to highly rated (low cost) debt financing should a critical need arise.

Not-for-profit hospitals have other reasons to keep debt costs low by using modest amounts and maintaining a high bond rating. For example, the fear of increasing business risk and lower profitability resulting from recent reductions in reimbursement rates makes it less desirable to take on large interest-payment obligations.

Still, the motivation to limit debt usage is somewhat offset by the fact that not-for-profit hospitals can engage in a practice called tax arbitrage, which involves using low-cost municipal (tax-exempt) financing to invest in higher-return Treasury securities, and hence capture a riskless return. (Laws restrict the abilities of not-for-profits to engage in large-scale tax arbitrage, but many hospitals still benefit from the practice by taking on large amounts of debt to fund new facilities that take years to build. Then, before the funds are actually needed to pay for construction and equipment, they are invested in higher-return securities.)

Note: This industry practice is based on information in Wheeler, J. R. C., D. G. Smith, H. L. Rivenson, and K. L. Reiter. 2000. "Capital Structure Strategy in Health Care Systems." *Journal of Health Care Finance* (Summer): 42–52.

8.9 COST OF CAPITAL

Capital suppliers do not provide financing to businesses just for the fun of it. Lenders and owners provide capital with the expectation of earning a return on their investments. Thus, there is a cost when businesses raise capital, and to make good business decisions, managers

---

⚠ CRITICAL CONCEPT
Corporate Cost of Capital

The corporate cost of capital is the weighted average of the costs of a business's debt and equity financing. The weights used in the calculation are the target (optimal) capital structure weights. Once estimated, the corporate cost of capital sets the minimum acceptable (required) rate of return on new capital investments. For example, assume Bayside Memorial Hospital has a corporate cost of capital of 10 percent. If a new open MRI investment, which has been judged to have average risk, is expected to return at least 10 percent, then it is financially attractive to the hospital. If the open MRI is expected to return less than 10 percent, accepting it will have an adverse impact on the hospital's financial condition.

Cost of debt
The return (interest rate) required by lenders to furnish debt capital.

must know this cost. The ultimate goal of the cost of capital estimation process is to estimate a business's **corporate cost of capital**. This cost, in turn, is used as the required rate of return, or hurdle rate, when evaluating the business's capital investment opportunities. (Capital investment decisions are discussed in detail in Chapters 9 and 10.)

The corporate cost of capital is a weighted average of the capital component costs; that is, the costs of debt and equity. After the component costs have been estimated, they are combined to form the corporate cost of capital, with the weights representing the business's target capital structure.

COST OF DEBT

A firm's managers likely will not know at the start of a planning period the exact types and amounts of debt that will be used to finance new asset acquisitions; the type of debt will depend on the specific assets to be financed and on future market conditions. However, a firm's managers do know what types of debt the business usually issues. For example, Puget Sound Family Practice plans to use a bank line of credit to obtain short-term funds to finance temporary needs and a ten-year bank term loan to raise long-term debt capital. Because the practice does not use short-term debt to finance permanent (long-term) assets, its corporate cost of capital estimate will include only long-term debt, which is assumed to be a ten-year loan. (The corporate cost of capital primarily is used to evaluate long-term asset purchases, so it makes sense to base it solely on the cost of long-term financing.)

How should the practice's physicians estimate the component *cost of debt*? For them it is easy; they would call a commercial bank and ask how much a term loan would cost. The answer might be 8 percent. If so, that would be the practice's cost of debt when estimating its corporate cost of capital.

For large businesses that use bonds for long-term debt financing, the process is essentially the same, except the call would be to an investment bank, an institution that helps companies sell stocks and bonds. The bottom line here is that estimating a business's cost of debt financing is relatively easy. Just talk to the people that arrange the financing and find out the going rate.

Note that the appropriate cost of debt for use in estimating the corporate cost of capital is not the interest rate on debt financing that was obtained in the past. Rather, it is the rate today, which is assumed to be the cost of debt financing throughout the planning period.

COST OF EQUITY

The cost of debt is based on the return (interest rate) that lenders require to provide debt financing, and the *cost of equity* to investor-owned businesses can be defined similarly: It is the rate of return that owners require to provide equity to a business. The idea here is that rational investors expect to earn a return on their ownership interest. The return may come in the form of dividends, bonuses, or capital gains (selling the ownership interest for more than its cost). Before the investment is made, equity investors set a minimum required rate of return based on the riskiness of that investment—the higher the risk, the higher the required rate of return. This required rate of return on an ownership investment in a business defines its cost of equity.

> ***Cost of equity***
> The return required by owners to furnish equity capital.

Several methods can be used to estimate a business's cost of equity. We will only discuss one—the **debt cost plus risk premium method**, which relies on the premise that equity investments are riskier than debt investments. Under this assumption, the cost of equity for any business can be thought of as the cost of debt to that business plus a risk premium.

> ⓘ **CRITICAL CONCEPT**
> Debt Cost Plus Risk Premium Method
>
> The debt cost plus risk premium method is used to estimate a business's cost of equity. It is based on the premise that an ownership investment in a business is riskier than a lender's position. Thus, the cost of equity can be estimated by adding a risk premium to the business's cost of debt. The size of the premium varies over time, but generally it is thought to be in the range of 3–5 percentage points for large corporations. To illustrate, assume that the current estimate of the risk premium is 4 percentage points. Then, a large business (such as HCA) with a cost of debt of 7 percent would have a cost of equity estimate of 7 + 4 = 11%.

The assumption that an owners' position in a business is riskier than a lender's is based on the following facts. Lenders have a contractually guaranteed return as specified in the debt agreement. If the borrower fails to make the promised payments, lenders have recourse against the business. In fact, if circumstances dictate, lenders can force a business into bankruptcy with the goal of recovering their investment in a court-ordered liquidation.

Conversely, owners have no contractually guaranteed return. If things work out well, owners' returns can be high. But if things go sour, owners can lose it all. If a company goes bankrupt, lenders typically get some of their principal amount returned, while equityholders typically get nothing back.

Studies suggest that the risk premium for use in the debt cost plus risk premium method has ranged from 3 to 5 percentage points, with an average of 4 percentage points. However, this premium is based on data from large nationwide corporations. Using this premium estimate as a starting point, Puget Sound Family Practice, with a cost of debt of 8 percent, would have a cost of equity estimate of 12.0 percent:

$$\text{Cost of equity} = \text{Cost of debt} + \text{Risk premium}$$
$$= 8.0\% + 4.0\% = 12.0\%.$$

However, we are applying the model to a small business. In such situations, it is typical to add an additional premium to account for the fact that small businesses are, by nature, riskier than large businesses. Furthermore, the ownership position in a small business cannot easily be sold if the owner wants out. (In large businesses with many stockholders, the stock can easily and quickly be sold at a known price through a stockbroker.)

Thus, it is typical to add an additional premium of about 5 percentage points to account for small business ownership risk and lack of marketability. When the practice's physicians added this premium to their initial estimate, they concluded that the cost of equity estimate for Puget Sound Family Practice is 17.0 percent.

Even though the cost of equity estimation process is difficult for investor-owned businesses, the underlying concept is well accepted. However, the basis for a cost of equity for not-for-profit organizations is controversial. Indeed, many different viewpoints exist regarding a not-for-profit's cost of equity. For example, some argue that the cost of equity to a not-for-profit business should be the same as for a similar for-profit business. Others argue that the cost of equity should be the return that is required to maintain the desired debt rating. We will not explore the controversy here—suffice it to say that not-for-profits do have a cost of equity that represents the return required on the community's equity investment in the organization.

COMBINING THE COMPONENT COSTS

The final step in the process is to combine the debt and equity cost estimates to form the **corporate cost of capital**. As discussed in a previous section, each business has a target capital structure in mind. Furthermore, when a firm raises new capital, it generally tries to finance in a way that will keep the actual capital structure reasonably close to its target over time. Here is the general formula for the corporate cost of capital (CCC) for all businesses, regardless of ownership:

$$CCC = [W_d \times \text{Cost of debt} \times (1 - T)] + [W_e \times \text{Cost of equity}].$$

Here W_d and W_e are the target weights for debt and equity, respectively, and T is the business's tax rate.

For Puget Sound, the cost of debt estimate is 8.0 percent and the cost of equity estimate is 17.0 percent. Furthermore, the business's target capital structure is 30 percent debt and 70 percent equity, and its tax rate is 35 percent. Thus, the practice's CCC estimate is 13.5 percent:

$$
\begin{aligned}
CCC &= [W_d \times \text{Cost of debt} \times (1 - T)] + [W_e \times \text{Cost of equity}] \\
&= [0.30 \times 8.0\% \times (1 - 0.35)] + [0.70 \times 17.0\%] \\
&= [0.30 \times 5.2\%] + [0.70 \times 17.0\%] \\
&= 1.6\% + 11.9\% \\
&= 13.5\%.
\end{aligned}
$$

Note that the before-tax cost of debt is reduced by $(1 - T)$ in the formula. This calculation recognizes the fact that the effective cost of debt to a for-profit business is reduced because interest expense is tax deductible. Thus, the effective cost of debt to Puget Sound is not 8.0 percent, but rather $8.0\% \times (1 - 0.35) =$ $8.0\% \times 0.65 = 5.2\%$. The logic here is that every dollar of interest expense reduces the practice's taxes by 35 cents, so the effective interest payment is only 65 cents.

> ### ! CRITICAL EQUATION
> Corporate Cost of Capital
>
> The corporate cost of capital (CCC) is a blend (weighted average) of the costs of a business's debt and equity financing, with the weights being the business's target capital structure. Thus, the CCC estimation can be expressed as:
>
> $$CCC = [W_d \times \text{Cost of debt} \times (1 - T)] + [W_e \times \text{Cost of equity}].$$
>
> Here W_d and W_e are the target weights for debt and equity, respectively, and T is the business's tax rate.

As mentioned briefly in our discussion of optimal capital structure, the optimal structure for any business is the mix of debt and equity financing that produces the lowest corporate cost of capital. Thus, if the capital structure and cost estimates for Puget Sound are correct, 13.5 percent is the lowest corporate cost of capital attainable. By minimizing the practice's capital costs, the physicians have taken the first step in ensuring financial success.

If the business is not-for-profit, the same equation is used, except that the tax rate entered for T would be zero. This might lead to the conclusion that for-profit businesses have a lower corporate cost of capital because their cost of debt is reduced by taxes. However, the starting cost of debt is lower in not-for-profit businesses because their debt is tax exempt. The end result is an effective cost of debt that is roughly the same, whether a provider is for-profit or not-for-profit.

INTERPRETING THE CORPORATE COST OF CAPITAL

The component cost estimates (the costs of debt and equity) that make up a business's corporate cost of capital are based on the returns that investors require to supply capital to the business. Thus, if the business cannot earn at least the corporate cost of capital on its investments, it cannot pay the minimum returns required by its capital suppliers.

From a pure financial perspective, if a business (especially investor owned) cannot earn its corporate cost of capital on new facilities investments, no new investments should be made and no new capital should be raised. If existing investments are not earning the corporate cost of capital, they should be terminated, the assets liquidated, and the proceeds returned to investors for reinvestment elsewhere.

The primary purpose of estimating a business's corporate cost of capital is to help make capital investment decisions; that is, the cost of capital will be used as the minimum return necessary for a new product or service to be attractive financially. However, the corporate cost of capital reflects the aggregate risk of the business. Thus, the corporate cost of capital can be applied without modification only to those projects under consideration that have average risk, where average is defined as that applicable to the firm's current overall operations. If a project under consideration has risk that differs significantly from that of the firm's average, then the corporate cost of capital must be adjusted to account for the differential risk when the project is being evaluated. (We will have much more to say about this in Chapter 10.)

To illustrate the impact of risk, Bayside Memorial Hospital's corporate cost of capital, 10 percent, is appropriate for use in evaluating a new open MRI (magnetic resonance imaging) facility, which has risk similar to the hospital's average project. Clearly, it would *not* be appropriate to apply Bayside's 10 percent corporate cost of capital without adjustment to a new project that involves establishing a managed care subsidiary; this project does not have the same risk as the hospital's average project, which involves patient services.

(?) SELF-TEST QUESTIONS

1. What is the equation for the corporate cost of capital?

2. What weights should be used in the formula? Why?

3. How is the cost of debt estimated? What about the cost of equity?

4. What is the primary difference between the corporate cost of capital for investor-owned firms and that for not-for-profit firms?

5. Explain the interpretation of the corporate cost of capital.

6. Is the corporate cost of capital the appropriate hurdle rate for all projects that a business evaluates?

THEME WRAP-UP   STARTING A NEW MEDICAL PRACTICE

One of the first tasks undertaken by the six physician owners of Puget Sound Family Practice was to figure out the business's optimal capital structure (the appropriate financing mix).

After looking at industry averages for medical practices and discussing the situation with a local banker, the partners decided on an optimal capital structure of 30 percent debt financing and 70 percent equity financing. Thus, their start-up capital of $1.8 million consisted of $1,260,000 in equity put up by the physicians and a $540,000 ten-year term loan from the bank.

Because two of the six physicians were just completing residencies, each of the four practicing physicians put up $315,000 to start the practice. The two new physicians would be paid at a lower rate for the first five years of employment until they funded their equity portion of the practice. The salaries withheld would be distributed to the four physicians who put up the initial capital, so at the end of five years all six physicians would each have an equity stake in the practice of $210,000.

Because Puget Sound's initial financing requirement was primarily used to purchase assets that have relatively long lives, the business's initial debt structure consisted of all long-term debt. However, at the same time, the practice negotiated a $200,000 line of credit with the bank that could be tapped to meet short-term needs as they occur during the first year of operation.

In addition to identifying the target capital structure, the physicians wanted an estimate of their corporate cost of capital. The bank loan interest rate was 8.0 percent, so that set the cost of debt to the business. Furthermore, the cost of equity (the return required on the physician's ownership contributions) was estimated to be 17.0 percent by using the debt cost plus risk premium method and then applying an additional premium to account for the small size of the business. Finally, the component (debt and equity) costs were combined into a weighted average that produced a corporate-cost-of-capital estimate of 13.5 percent.

The 13.5 percent corporate cost of capital represents Puget Sound's overall cost of financing. Furthermore, the practice is being financed at the lowest possible cost, because it is using the optimal mix of debt and equity. Any future financing needed by the practice will be done in such a way as to keep the business at its target capital structure. If the practice's costs of debt and equity stay constant in the future, any new facilities investments should return at least 13.5 percent to maintain a sound financial position.

KEY CONCEPTS

This chapter provides an overview of debt and equity financing. Optimal capital structure and the cost of capital are discussed as well. Here are the key concepts:

➤ To operate, any business must have assets; to acquire assets, the business must raise *capital*. Capital comes in two basic forms: *debt* and *equity*.

➤ Two fundamental factors affect a loan's interest rate: *risk* and *inflation*.

➤ *Term loans* and *bonds* are long-term debt contracts under which a borrower agrees to make a series of interest and principal payments on specific dates to the lender. A term loan generally is provided by a single lender, while a bond typically is offered to the public and sold to many different investors.

➤ In general, bonds are categorized as *Treasury*, which are issued by the federal government; *corporate*, which are issued by taxable businesses; and *municipal*, which are issued by nonfederal governmental entities, including debt issued on behalf of not-for-profit healthcare providers.

➤ A *debt contract* is a legal document that spells out the rights and obligations of both lenders and borrowers.

➤ A *trustee* is assigned to make sure that the terms of a bond contract are carried out.

➤ Bond contracts often include *restrictive covenants*, which are provisions designed to protect bondholders against detrimental managerial actions.

➤ A *call provision* gives the issuer the right to redeem the bonds before maturity under specified terms. A business will call a bond issue and refund it if interest rates fall sufficiently after the bond has been issued.

➤ Bonds and other forms of debt are assigned *ratings* that reflect the probability of default. Ratings range from AAA (the highest) to D (the lowest). The higher the rating, and hence the greater the probability of lenders being paid in full, the lower the interest rate.

➤ The choice between debt and equity financing is a risk–return trade-off. The use of debt financing can *leverage up* the return to owners, but at the same time it *increases owners' risk*.

➤ The *optimal*, or *target*, *capital structure* balances the costs and benefits of debt financing and hence minimizes the business's corporate cost of capital.

➤ The optimal capital structure decision is based on several factors, including business risk, lender and rating agency attitudes, reserve borrowing capacity, industry averages, and asset structure.

➤ Managers of not-for-profit businesses must grapple with the same capital structure decisions faced by managers of investor-owned firms. However, not-for-profit firms do not have the same flexibility in making financing decisions because not-for-profit firms cannot sell equity to owners.

➤ In estimating a firm's corporate cost of capital, the *cost of debt* is the interest rate set on new debt.

➤ The *cost of equity* to investor-owned firms is the return required by its owners. One method for estimating this cost is the *debt cost plus risk premium model,* which adds a premium to the business's cost of debt. The cost of equity to not-for-profit businesses is more problematic.

➤ A business's *corporate cost of capital (CCC)* is estimated as follows:

CCC = [W_d x Cost of debt x (1 – T)] + [W_e x Cost of equity].

Here W_d is the weight of debt, W_e is the weight of equity, and T is the tax rate. Note that the effective cost of debt is reduced in for-profit businesses to recognize the tax deductibility of interest payments. In not-for-profit businesses, the starting cost of debt is lower because the interest on municipal debt is tax exempt.

➤ When making *capital investment decisions*, a business will use the corporate cost of capital as the *hurdle rate* for average-risk projects.

From here, our focus turns to how new project proposals are evaluated. In Chapters 9 and 10, we discuss the role that the corporate cost-of-capital estimate plays in the capital investment evaluation process.

END-OF-CHAPTER QUESTIONS

8.1 The two primary factors that affect interest rates on debt securities are risk and inflation. Explain the role of each of these factors.

8.2 Briefly describe the features of the following types of debt:

a. Term loan

b. Bond

c. Line of credit

d. Municipal bond

8.3 Briefly explain the following debt features:

a. Loan agreement

b. Restrictive covenant

c. Trustee

d. Call provision

8.4 a. What do bond ratings measure?

b. How do investors interpret bond ratings?

c. Why are bond ratings important?

d. What is credit enhancement?

8.5 Critique this statement: The use of debt financing lowers the profits of the firm, and hence debt financing should be used only as a last resort.

8.6 Discuss some factors that healthcare managers must consider when setting a firm's target capital structure.

8.7 How is a business's cost of debt estimated? Its cost of equity?

8.8 Explain the calculation and interpretation of the corporate cost of capital.

END-OF-CHAPTER PROBLEMS

8.1 Seattle Health Plans currently uses zero debt financing. Its operating profit is $1 million, and it pays taxes at a 40 percent rate. It has $5 million in assets and, because it is all-equity financed, $5 million in equity. Suppose the firm is considering replacing half of its equity financing with debt financing that bears an interest rate of 8 percent.

a. What impact would the new capital structure have on the firm's profit, total dollar return to investors, and return on equity?

b. Redo the analysis, but now assume that the debt financing would cost 15 percent.

c. Repeat the analysis required for Part a, but now assume that Seattle Health Plans is a not-for-profit corporation and hence pays no taxes. Compare the results with those obtained in Part a.

8.2 Calculate the effective (after-tax) cost of debt for Wallace Clinic, a for-profit healthcare provider, assuming that the interest rate set on its debt is 11 percent and its tax rate is

a. 0 percent

b. 20 percent

c. 40 percent

8.3 St. Vincent's Hospital has a target capital structure of 35 percent debt and 65 percent equity. Its cost of equity estimate is 13.5 percent and its cost of tax-exempt debt estimate is 7 percent. What is the hospital's corporate cost of capital?

8.4 Richmond Clinic has obtained the following estimates for its costs of debt and equity at various capital structures:

Percent Debt	After-Tax Cost of Debt	Cost of Equity
0%	—	16.0%
20	6.6%	17.0
40	7.8	19.0
60	10.2	22.0
80	14.0	27.0

What is the firm's optimal capital structure? (Hint: Calculate its corporate cost of capital at each structure. Also, note that data on component costs at alternative capital structures are not reliable in real-world situations.)

8.5 Morningside Nursing Home, a not-for-profit corporation, is estimating its corporate cost of capital. Its tax-exempt debt currently requires an interest rate of 6.2 percent and its target capital structure calls for 60 percent debt financing and 40 percent equity (fund capital) financing. Its estimated cost of equity is 16.4 percent. What is Morningside's corporate cost of capital?

CHAPTER 9

CAPITAL INVESTMENT DECISION BASICS

Palm Coast Radiology Associates is a group practice affiliated with Bayside Memorial Hospital. In essence, the hospital provides the equipment and technicians necessary to create radiological images, while the radiologists at the practice perform the required readings and interpretations.

At the last scheduled meeting between hospital and group executives, a new MRI (magnetic resonance imaging) system was proposed by Dr. Fisher, the group's CEO. Although the hospital currently has a conventional MRI system, Dr. Fisher thinks replacing the old one with a new, open system would be beneficial.

MRI technology uses magnets, radio frequencies, and a computer to generate three-dimensional images of organs and structures inside the body. It offers a painless alternative to diagnostic surgeries and can provide early detection and diagnosis of a number of diseases and disabilities, including multiple sclerosis. Bayside's current MRI system requires patients to be surrounded by the scanner, which means that patients must lie in a narrow tube that covers the entire body. The fully enclosed space creates a great amount of patient apprehension and discomfort, and it can be especially uncomfortable for patients who suffer from claustrophobia.

As opposed to a conventional MRI system, the open system does not place the patient in a tube. Rather, the patient is placed in a much less confining imaging space. A receiver coil is placed around the body part that is to be scanned and then that portion of the body is centered in the machine. An open MRI system greatly reduces the feeling of constraint associated with conventional systems yet still produces high-quality images. Additionally, the open system can accommodate pediatric patients who need parental support, as well as patients who are too large to fit in a conventional MRI.

During the meeting, all of the radiologists expressed familiarity with and enthusiasm for the new system, but the hospital's chief financial officer, Jane Adams, voiced her concern about the cost. "Sure, the new system will be great for patients, but it costs $2.5 million. Can we afford it?" she asked. Dr. Fisher thought about the question for a moment, and then replied, "If we can get at least that much in new patient revenue, it should be worth it." On that comment, several meeting attendees became involved in a heated argument about how to assess the financial merits of the potential investment.

By the end of the chapter, you will see how discounted cash flow techniques can be applied to estimate the financial attractiveness of the proposed MRI system. Then, with all the facts at hand, you can make the final decision!

LEARNING OBJECTIVES

After studying this chapter, you will be able to

➤ Explain how managers use project classifications and post-audits in the capital investment decision process.

➤ Describe the role of financial analysis in healthcare capital investment decisions.

➤ Discuss the key elements of breakeven analysis.

➤ Answer why discounted cash flow (DCF) analysis is such an important concept in healthcare finance.

➤ Perform basic DCF calculations.

➤ Define the opportunity cost principle.

➤ Measure the financial return on an investment in both dollar and percentage terms.

9.1 INTRODUCTION

This chapter focuses on *capital investment decisions*, which involve the acquisition of land, buildings, and equipment. Capital investment decisions are among the most critical decisions healthcare managers must make, because the results of such decisions generally affect the business's operations and financial status for an extended period.

Good capital investment decisions are essential to good financial management. In this chapter, and the next, we discuss many of the concepts necessary for building an effective capital investment analysis system.

9.2 PROJECT CLASSIFICATIONS

Although benefits can be gained from the careful analysis of capital investment proposals, such efforts can be costly. For certain projects, a relatively detailed analysis may be warranted, along with senior management involvement; for others, simpler procedures should be used. Accordingly, large healthcare providers generally classify projects into categories, and by cost within each category, and then analyze each project on the basis of its category and cost.

For example, Bayside Memorial Hospital uses the following classifications:

◆ *Category 1: Mandatory replacement.* Category 1 consists of expenditures related to replacing worn-out or damaged equipment necessary to the operations of the hospital. In general, these expenditures are mandatory, so they are usually made with limited analyses.

◆ *Category 2: Discretionary replacement.* This category contains expenditures to replace serviceable but technologically obsolete equipment. The purpose of these projects is to lower costs or to provide more clinically effective services. Because Category 2 projects are not mandatory, a detailed decision process is generally required to support these expenditures.

◆ *Category 3: Expansion of existing services or markets.* Expenditures to increase capacity, or to expand within markets currently served by the hospital, are included here. These decisions are more complex, so detailed analysis is required, and the final decision is made at a high level within the organization.

◆ *Category 4: Expansion into new services or markets.* These are projects necessary to provide new services or to expand into geographic areas not currently served. Such projects involve strategic decisions that could change the fundamental nature of the hospital, and they normally require the expenditure of large sums of money over

Capital investment decision
The decision whether or not to invest in long-term assets such as land, buildings, and equipment. Such decisions often are referred to as capital budgeting decisions.

long periods. Invariably, a particularly detailed analysis is required, and the board of trustees generally makes the final decision as part of the hospital's strategic plan.

◆ *Category 5: Environmental projects.* This category consists of expenditures for complying with government orders, labor agreements, accreditation requirements, and the like. Unless the expenditures are large, Category 5 expenditures are treated like Category 1 expenditures.

◆ *Category 6: Other.* This category is a catchall for projects that do not fit neatly into another category. The primary determinant of how Category 6 projects are evaluated is the amount of funds required.

In general, relatively simple analyses and only a few supporting documents are required for replacement decisions and safety/environmental projects, especially those that are mandatory. A detailed analysis is necessary for expansion and other projects.

Note that, within each category, projects are classified by size: larger projects need more detailed analyses and approval at higher organizational levels. Thus, for example, at Bayside Memorial Hospital, department heads can authorize spending up to $50,000 on discretionary replacement projects, while the full board of directors must approve expansion projects that cost more than $5 million.

(?) SELF-TEST QUESTIONS

1. What is the primary advantage of classifying capital projects?

2. What are some typical project classifications?

3. What role does project size (cost) play in the classifications?

4. Into what category would the open MRI project be placed?

9.3 THE ROLE OF FINANCIAL ANALYSIS IN CAPITAL INVESTMENT DECISIONS

For investor-owned businesses, the role of financial analysis in capital investment decision making is clear: Projects that contribute to owners' wealth should be undertaken, while those that do not should be ignored.

However, what about not-for-profit businesses, which do not have wealth maximization as a goal? In such businesses, the appropriate goal typically is providing quality, cost-effective services to their communities. (A strong argument could be made that this should also be the goal of investor-owned businesses in the healthcare industry.) In this situation, capital investment decisions must consider many factors besides a project's financial implications.

Still, good decision making, and hence the future viability of the business, requires that the financial impact of capital investments be recognized. If a business takes on a series of highly unprofitable projects that meet nonfinancial goals, and such projects are not offset by profitable ones, the firm's financial condition will deteriorate. If this situation persists over time, the business will eventually lose its financial viability and could even be forced into bankruptcy.

Because bankrupt businesses cannot meet a community's needs, even managers of not-for-profit healthcare businesses must consider a capital investment's potential impact on the organization's financial condition. Managers may make a conscious decision to accept a project with a poor financial prognosis because of its nonfinancial virtues, but managers must know the financial impact up front so that they are not surprised when the project drains the business's financial resources.

Financial analysis provides managers with the relevant information about a capital investment's financial impact and hence helps managers make better decisions, including decisions based primarily on nonfinancial factors. (Later in the chapter we discuss how nonfinancial factors can be formally considered in the capital investment decision process.)

(?) SELF-TEST QUESTIONS

1. What is the role of financial analysis in capital investment decisions within for-profit firms?

2. Why are such analyses important in not-for-profit businesses?

9.4 OVERVIEW OF CAPITAL INVESTMENT FINANCIAL ANALYSIS

The financial analysis of capital investment proposals typically involves the following four steps:

1. *Cash flow estimation.* First, estimate the project's cash flows. Usually, this estimation consists of the initial cost, the cash flows that arise from operating the project, and the cash flows associated with closing down the project at the end of its useful life. (Cash flow estimation is discussed in Chapter 10.)

2. *Project risk assessment.* Second, assess the riskiness of the cash flows. (Risk assessment is addressed in Chapter 10.)

3. *Cost of capital estimation.* Third, estimate the project cost of capital. As discussed in Chapter 8, a business's corporate cost of capital reflects the aggregate risk of the business's assets—that is, the riskiness inherent in the average project. If the project being evaluated does not have average risk, the corporate cost of capital must be adjusted to obtain the project cost of capital.

4. *Financial impact assessment.* Fourth, assess the project's financial merit. Several measures can be used for this purpose; we will discuss three in this chapter.

(?) SELF-TEST QUESTION

1. Explain the four steps in capital investment financial analysis.

9.5 CREATING THE TIME LINE

Consider the situation facing Bayside Memorial Hospital (see the Theme Set-Up). The CEO of the hospital-affiliated radiology group proposed an open MRI project. The system costs $2 million, and Bayside would have to spend another $500,000 for site preparation and installation, for a total initial cost of $2.5 million.

The open MRI system is expected to be in operation for five years, at which time the hospital's strategic plan calls for a new imaging facility. As discussed earlier, the first step in the financial analysis of a proposed capital investment is to estimate the project's cash flows. Cash flows, basically, are the amounts of money expected to flow into and out of the hospital as a result of acquiring the open MRI system.

We will leave the details of this step for Chapter 10, but here is a rough idea of what was done. Bayside's managers, with help from the radiology group physicians, estimated the volume of procedures (scans), the reimbursement amounts expected on each scan, the costs to operate the MRI, and any other cash flows that would result from operating the system.

Time line
A graphical representation of time and cash flows. It may be an actual horizontal line with dates and cash flows or cells on a spreadsheet.

These flows were then combined with the cost of the system and the flows expected when the system is shut down after five years of operation. The end result is the following set of cash flows, placed on a *time line*:

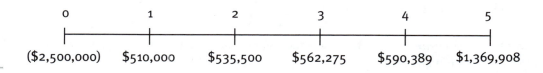

0	1	2	3	4	5
($2,500,000)	$510,000	$535,500	$562,275	$590,389	$1,369,908

⊤

Time lines make it easier to visualize when the cash flows in a particular analysis occur. Time 0 is any starting point (typically the time of the first cash flow in an analysis). In our situation,

◆   Time 0 is when the MRI would be purchased;

◆   Time 1 is one period from the starting point, or the end of Period 1; and

◆   Time 2 is two periods from the starting point, or the end of Period 2.

The time line goes on until Period 5. Thus, the numbers (0, 1, 2, etc.) represent end-of-period values.

Often, as in this case, the periods are years, but other time intervals such as quarters or months can be used when needed to fit the timing of the cash flows being evaluated. Because, in this example, the time periods are years, the interval from 0 to 1 is Year 1, and 1 represents both the end of Year 1 and the beginning of Year 2. (Years are often used in project analyses because the flows are too difficult to forecast with confidence on a more frequent basis.)

Cash flows are shown on a time line directly below the points in time in which the flows are expected to occur. The $2,500,000 under Year 0 is a cost (outflow), so it is set in parentheses. (Outflows are sometimes designated by minus signs rather than by parentheses.) The $510,000 shown under Year 1 is an estimate of the net cash inflow resulting from the first year's operation of the open MRI, considering both the system's expected operating revenues and costs. The Year 5 net cash flow includes both the net operating cash flow and the cash flow expected from selling the MRI at the end of the project's five-year life.

Time lines play an essential role in capital investment financial analyses because they depict the amount and timing of a project's expected cash flows. The time line may be an actual line, as illustrated earlier, or it may be a series of columns (or rows) on a spreadsheet. Time lines are used extensively in investment analyses, so get into the habit of using them as you work on the problems in Chapters 9 and 10.

⑦ SELF-TEST QUESTIONS

1. Why are time lines so important in capital investment financial analyses?

2. Draw a three-year time line that illustrates the following situation: An investment of $10,000 at Time 0 and inflows of $5,000 at the end of Years 1, 2, and 3.

9.6 BREAKEVEN ANALYSIS

Breakeven analysis was introduced in Chapter 5 in conjunction with profit analysis. There, we estimated the volume required for both accounting and economic breakeven.

CRITICAL CONCEPT
Payback

Payback is the number of years that it takes to recover the cost of an investment. For example, assume that an EKG (electrocardiogram) machine that costs $2,500 is expected to net $1,000 in cash flow in each of the next five years. If things go as expected, the $2,500 investment will be recovered in three years (with $500 left over), so the payback is 3 years, or more precisely, 2.5 years. The shorter the payback, the better, as the business will more quickly recover its investment in the project.

Here, we apply the breakeven concept in a capital investment setting. In such analyses, many types of breakeven can be calculated. Rather than discuss all the possible types here, let's focus on time breakeven, which is measured by **payback**.

The best way to calculate the open MRI's expected payback is to examine the project's cumulative cash flows. At any point in time, the cumulative cash flow is merely the sum of all the cash flows (with a proper sign indicating an inflow or outflow) that have occurred up to that point. Payback occurs when the cumulative cash flow turns positive.

Here are the open MRI's annual cash flows and cumulative cash flows:

Year	Annual Cash Flow	Cumulative Cash Flow
0	($2,500,000)	($2,500,000)
1	$510,000	(1,990,000)
2	535,500	(1,454,500)
3	562,275	(892,225)
4	590,389	(301,836)
5	1,369,908	1,068,072

We see that the cumulative cash flow at Year 0 is -$2,500,000; at Year 1 it is -$2,500,000 + $510,000 = -$1,990,000; at Year 2 it is -$1,990,000 + $535,500 = -$1,454,500; and so on.

As shown in the far-right column, the $2,500,000 cost of the open MRI project will be recovered at the end of Year 5 *if the cash flow forecasts are correct*, because Year 5 is the year that the cumulative flow turns positive. Furthermore, if the cash flows are assumed to come in evenly during the year, breakeven will occur $301,836 / $1,369,908 = 0.22 years (or about .2 years) into Year 5, so the open MRI project's payback is 4.2 years. (At the end of Year 4, $301,836 remains to be recovered, while the cash flow expected in Year 5 is $1,369,908.)

At one time, payback was used by managers as the sole measure of a project's financial attractiveness: A business might accept all projects with paybacks of five years or less. However, payback has two serious deficiencies when it is used in this way.

First, payback ignores all cash flows that occur after the payback period. To illustrate, Bayside might be evaluating a competing project that has the same cash flows as the open MRI project in Years 0 through 5. However, the alternative project might have a cash inflow of $2 million in Year 6. Both projects would have the same payback—4.2 years—and hence be ranked the same, even though the alternative project clearly is better from a financial perspective.

Second, payback ignores the time value of money. (Time value is discussed in the next section.) For these two reasons, payback generally is no longer used as the primary evaluation tool.

In spite of its deficiencies, payback is useful in capital investment analysis. The shorter the payback, the more quickly the funds invested in a project will become available for other purposes. Also, cash flows expected in the distant future generally are regarded as riskier than near-term cash flows because they are harder to estimate, so projects with long paybacks are considered to be more risky than projects with short paybacks. Considering both these factors, shorter payback projects usually are more financially attractive than longer payback projects.

? SELF-TEST QUESTIONS

1. What is payback?

2. What are the benefits of payback?

3. What are its deficiencies?

9.7 DISCOUNTED CASH FLOW ANALYSIS

Up to this point, our financial analysis of the open MRI investment has been limited to breakeven analysis. We have laid out the expected cash flows from the project on a time line and estimated that it would take 4.2 years for Bayside to recover its investment, assuming that everything occurs as expected. If we were whizzes at processing information, we might be able to merely look at the cash flows and the payback and make a complete judgment about the project's financial attractiveness. But most people cannot do this, so summarizing the information contained in the project's cash flows would be useful.

The process of assigning appropriate values to cash flows that occur at different points in time and then summarizing this information in a single value is called *discounted cash flow (DCF) analysis*. DCF analysis is an important part of healthcare finance because most financial analyses involve future cash flows. In fact, of all the investment analysis techniques, none is more important than DCF analysis. The concepts presented

Discounted cash flow (DCF) analysis
The use of time value of money techniques to estimate the value of an investment's expected cash flows.

The time value of money principle is based on the fact that money in hand is worth more than funds expected to be received in the future. For example, consider $100 in hand today versus $100 to be received in one year. If the $100 in hand today is invested in a bank account that pays 5 percent interest, it will earn $5 in interest and be worth $105 at the end of one year. However, the $100 to be obtained at the end of the year is only worth $100 when received. Discounted cash flow (DCF) analysis is used to account for the time value of money.

here are the cornerstones of all investment analyses, so an understanding of DCF concepts is essential to good capital investment decision making.

The economic principle that underlies DCF analysis is **time value of money**. This principle is based on the fact that a dollar to be received in the future is worth less than a current dollar because a dollar in hand today can be invested in an interest-bearing account and hence can be worth more than one dollar in the future. Because current dollars are worth more than future dollars, capital investment decisions must account for both the magnitude and the timing of the forecasted cash flows.

FUTURE VALUE (COMPOUNDING)

Compounding
The process of finding the future value of a current (starting) amount or series of cash flows.

We start our discussion of DCF analysis by examining how money invested today grows over time. The process of moving from today's value to a future value is called *compounding* because the value increases, or compounds, over time.

Although compounding is not used a great deal in capital investment analyses, it is the best starting point for learning DCF concepts. To illustrate compounding, suppose you deposit $100 in a bank account that pays 5 percent annual interest (interest is credited to the account at the end of each year). How much would be in the account at the end of one year?

To put the analysis on a time line, note that the account is opened with a deposit of $100 at Year 0. This is shown as an outflow, because you will be turning the money over to the bank. The question mark at Year 1 signifies that you want to know the value of the account at that time, after being on deposit for one year.

During one year's time, you will earn 5 percent interest on the initial $100, so the interest earned is $100 × 0.05 = $5. Thus, at the end of one year the amount in the account is $100 + $5 = $105. Note that the balance in the account at Year 1 can be calculated directly by multiplying the starting amount, $100, by 1 + Interest rate (expresses as a decimal). Thus, the ending amount after one year is $100 × (1 + 0.05) = $100 × 1.05 = $105.

What would be the value of the $100 if you left the money in the account for two years? At the start of the second year, the account balance is $105. Interest of $105 × 0.05 = $5.25 is earned on the now larger beginning amount during the second year, so the account balance at the end of Year 2 is $105 + $5.25 = $110.25.

The Year 2 interest, $5.25, is higher than the first year's interest, $5, because $5 × 0.05 = $0.25 in interest was earned on the first year's interest. Again, we could calculate the balance after two years as $105 × 1.05 = $110.25. In addition, we could calculate the balance at the end of Year 2 directly from the initial starting amount, $100, as follows: $100 × 1.05 × 1.05 = $100 × (1.05)^2 = $110.25. By multiplying by 1.05 two times, we recognize that the initial deposit is compounded at a 5 percent rate over two years.

What about the balance after five years? The compounding process continues, and because the beginning balance is higher in each succeeding year, the annual interest earned increases in each year. At the end of Year 5, the balance would be $100 × (1.05)^5 = $127.63. Thus, after five years, you would earn $27.63 in total interest on your initial $100 investment.

These calculations demonstrate that a pattern exists in future value calculations. In general, the future value of a single starting amount at the end of N years can be found by applying this equation:

$$FV_N = PV \times (1 + I)^N.$$

Here,

◆ FV_N is the future value at the end of N years.

◆   PV is the initial starting amount (present value).

◆   I is the interest rate (expressed in decimal form).

Future values, as well as most other DCF calculations, can be performed in three ways: regular calculator, financial calculator, or spreadsheet. We include the regular calculator solution in our discussions (when applicable). Financial calculator and spreadsheet solutions are presented in boxes.

To use a regular calculator to solve compounding problems, multiply the PV by (1 + I) for N times or use the exponential function to raise (1 + I) to the Nth power and then multiply the result by the PV. Perhaps the easiest way to find the future value of $100 after five years when compounded at 5 percent is to enter $100, then multiply this amount by 1.05 for five times. If the calculator is set to display two decimal places, the answer would be $127.63:

```
         0            1            2            3            4            5
         |------------|------------|------------|------------|------------|
   $100 × 1.05     × 1.05       × 1.05       × 1.05       × 1.05 = $127.63
         ----->       ----->       ----->       ----->       ----->
```

As denoted by the arrows, compounding involves moving to the right along the time line.

SOLUTION TECHNIQUE Financial Calculator

Financial calculators have been preprogrammed to solve many types of time value analyses, including future value of a single starting amount. In effect, the future value equation is programmed directly into the calculator. With a financial calculator, the future value is found using three of the following five time value input keys:

To find the future value of $100 after five years at 5 percent interest using a financial calculator, just enter PV = 100, I = 5, and N = 5, and then press the FV key. The answer, 127.63 (rounded to two decimal places), will appear.

Some financial calculators require that cash flows be designated as either inflows or outflows (entered as either positive or negative values). Applying this logic to the illustration, you deposit the initial amount, which is an outflow to you, and take out, or receive, the ending amount, which is an inflow to you. If the calculator requires a sign convention, the PV would be entered as −100. (If the PV was entered as 100, a positive value, the calculator would display −127.63 as the answer.) The calculator solution can be shown pictorially as follows:

Inputs   5   5   −100

Output   =127.63

Different financial calculators require slight changes to the procedures given here. For example, sometimes the time value buttons are keys on the calculator, whereas on other calculators the time value variables appear on a screen. Also, some calculators require that the compute (CPT) button be pressed before pressing FV. Thus, if you are using a financial calculator to perform DCF calculations, be sure to read the user's manual.

Spreadsheet programs are ideally suited for time value analyses. For simple time value calculations, it is easy to enter the appropriate formula directly into the

SOLUTION TECHNIQUE Spreadsheet

	A	B	C	D
1				
2	5	Nper	Number of periods	
3	$ 100.00	Pv	Present value	
4	5.0%	Rate	Interest rate	
5				
6	$ 127.63	=100*(1.05)^5 (entered into Cell A6)		
7				
8	$ 127.63	=A3*(1+A4)^A2 (entered into Cell A8)		
9				
10	$ 127.63	=FV(A4,A2,,−A3) (entered into Cell A10)		

spreadsheet. For example, you could enter the spreadsheet version of the future value equation into Cell A6: =100*(1.05)^5. Here, = tells the spreadsheet that a formula is being entered into the cell; * is the spreadsheet multiplication sign; and ^ is the spreadsheet exponential, or power, sign.

When this formula is entered into Cell A6, the value $127.63 appears in the cell (when formatted with a dollar sign to two decimal places). Note that different spreadsheet programs use slightly different syntax in their time value analyses. The examples presented here use Excel syntax.

In most situations, it is more useful to enter a formula that can accommodate changing input values than to embed these values directly in the formula, so it would be better to solve this future value problem with this formula: =A3*(1+A4)^A2, as done in Cell A8. Here, the present value ($100) is contained in Cell A3, the interest rate (0.05, which is displayed as 5%) in Cell A4, and the number of periods (5) in Cell A2. With this formula, future values can be easily calculated with different starting amounts, interest rates, or number of years by changing the values in the input cells.

In addition to entering the appropriate formula, many DCF calculations are preprogrammed by the spreadsheet software. The preprogrammed formulas are called functions. Like any formula, a function consists of a number of arithmetic calculations combined into one statement. By using functions, spreadsheet users can save the time and tedium of building formulas from scratch.

(Continued)

SOLUTION TECHNIQUE Spreadsheet

Each function begins with a unique name that identifies the calculation to be performed, along with one or more arguments (the input values for the calculation) enclosed in parentheses. The best way to access the time value functions is to use the spreadsheet's function wizard (also called the paste function).

For this future value problem, first move the cursor to Cell A10 (the cell where you want the answer to appear). Then, click on the function wizard; select Financial for the function category and FV (future value) for the function name; and enter A4 for Rate, A2 for Nper (number of periods), and –A3 for PV. (Note that the Pmt and Type entries are left blank for this problem. These entries are used for solving different types of problems. Also, note that the cell address entered for PV has a minus sign. This is necessary for the answer to be displayed as a positive number.) Finally, press OK and the result, $127.63, appears in Cell A10.

PRESENT VALUE (DISCOUNTING)

Suppose you have been offered the opportunity to purchase a low-risk security that will pay $127.63 at the end of five years. How much would you be willing to pay for that security? In other words, what is the security worth today? To answer that question, you need another piece of information: the interest rate you could earn on other investments of similar risk to the security being offered. If similar investments offer a 5 percent annual rate of return (interest rate), then 5 percent should be used to value the offer.

The compounding example presented in the previous section shows that an initial amount of $100 invested at 5 percent per year would be worth $127.63 at the end of five years. Thus, you should be indifferent to the choice between $100 today and $127.63 at the end of five years. Today's $100 is defined as the present value of $127.63 due in five years when 5 percent is the comparison rate of return. If the price of the security being offered is exactly $100, you could buy it or turn it down because that is the security's fair value. If the price is less than $100, you should buy it. But, if the price is greater than $100, you should decline the offer.

Conceptually, the present value of a cash flow due N years in the future is the amount that, if it were on hand today, would grow to equal the future amount when compounded at the appropriate comparison rate. In effect, the present value tells us what amount would have to be invested to earn the return available on similar alternative investments. If the investment can be obtained for a lesser amount, a higher rate will be earned. If the investment costs more than the present value, the rate earned will be less than that available on similar alternatives.

Finding present values is called *discounting*, because the amount you are calculating (the present value) is smaller than the starting amount (the future value). Discounting is simply the reverse of compounding: If the PV is known, compound to find the FV; if the FV is known, discount to find the PV.

Discounting
The process of finding the present value of an amount or series of cash flows expected to be received in the future.

Here is the time line for calculating the security's present (current) value:

To develop the discounting equation for a single ending amount, solve the compounding equation for PV:

Compounding: $FV_N = PV \times (1 + I)^N$.
Discounting: $PV = FV_N/(1 + I)^N$.

The equations show us that compounding problems are solved by multiplication, while discounting problems are solved by division.

To solve this problem using a regular calculator, enter $127.63 and divide it five times by 1.05:

As shown by the arrows, discounting is moving left along the time line.

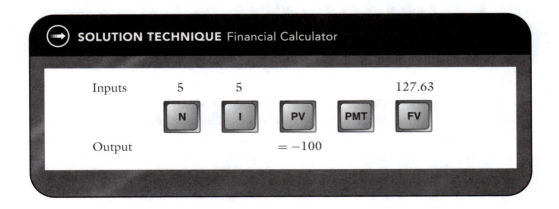

SOLUTION TECHNIQUE Spreadsheet

	A	B	C	D
1				
2	5	Nper	Number of periods	
3	$ 127.63	Fv	Future value	
4	5.0%	Rate	Interest rate	
5				
6	$ 100.00	=A3/(1+A4)^A2 (entered into Cell A6)		
7				
8	$ 100.00	=PV(A4,A2,,–A3) (entered into Cell A8)		
9				
10				

One solution would be to enter the applicable formula, as shown to the right of Cell A6: =A3/(1+A4)^A2. Here, the future value ($127.63) is contained in Cell A3, the interest rate (0.05, which is displayed as 5%) in Cell A4, and the number of periods (5) in Cell A2. With this formula, present values easily can be calculated with different starting future amounts, interest rates, or number of years.

The function approach is illustrated in Cell A8. First, move the cursor to that cell (the cell where you want the answer to appear). Then, click on the function wizard; select Financial for the function category and PV (present value) for the function name; and enter A4 for Rate, A2 for Nper (number of periods), and –A3 for Fv. (Note that the Pmt and Type entries are left blank for this problem. Also, note that the cell address entered for Fv has a minus sign. This is necessary for the answer to be displayed as a positive number.) Finally, press OK and the result, $100.00, appears in Cell A8.

OPPORTUNITY COST OF CAPITAL

In the last section, we chose an interest (discount) rate to value the proposed security investment. We used 5 percent, the interest rate offered on alternative investments of similar risk. In doing this, we implemented a concept called the **opportunity cost of capital**.

The opportunity cost of capital plays a crucial role in DCF analysis. To illustrate, suppose you found the winning ticket for the Florida lottery and now have $1 million to invest. Should you assign some cost to these funds? At first blush it might appear that this money has zero cost because its acquisition was purely a matter of luck. However, as soon you think about what to do with the $1 million, you must think in terms of the opportunity costs involved.

By using the money to invest in one alternative (for example, in the stock of Health Management Associates), you forgo the opportunity to make some other investment with the same funds (for example, buying U.S. Treasury securities). Thus, there is an opportunity cost associated with any investment planned for the $1 million, even though the lottery winnings were "free."

Because one investment decision automatically negates all other possible investments with the same funds, the cash flows expected to be earned from any investment must be discounted at

> **⚠ CRITICAL CONCEPT**
> Opportunity Cost of Capital
>
> The opportunity cost of capital (money) is a tried-and-true economic principle. If you invest $100 in Investment A, those funds will not be available for any other purpose. Thus, you should require that the return on Investment A be at least as good as the return on similar alternative investments. If Investment A is not as good as similar Investment B, then the $100 should be invested in B rather than in A. In other words, Investment A has an opportunity cost, and that cost is the return that one would expect to earn on alternative investments with similar risk.

a rate that reflects the return that could be earned on forgone investment opportunities. The problem is that the number of forgone investment opportunities is virtually infinite, so which one should be chosen to establish the opportunity cost discount rate?

The opportunity cost rate to be applied in DCF analyses is the rate that could be earned on alternative investments of similar risk. It is not logical to assign a low opportunity cost rate to a series of risky cash flows, or vice versa. This concept is important, so it is worth repeating: *The opportunity cost rate (i.e., the discount rate) applied to investment cash flows is the rate that could be earned on alternative investments with similar risk.*

Also, it is essential to recognize that the discounting process itself accounts for the opportunity cost of capital (i.e., the loss of use of the funds for other purposes). In effect, discounting a potential investment at, say, 10 percent, produces a present value that provides a 10 percent return. Thus, if the investment can be obtained for less than its present value, it will earn more than its opportunity cost of capital and hence is a good investment.

Alternatively, if the cost of the investment is greater than its present value, it will earn less than its opportunity cost of capital and hence is a bad investment.

Finally, note that the opportunity cost rate does not depend on the source of the funds to be invested. Rather, *the primary determinant of this rate is the riskiness of the cash flows being discounted.* Thus, the same opportunity cost rate would be applied to a potential investment, regardless of whether the funds to be used for the investment were won in a lottery, taken out of petty cash, or obtained by selling securities.

At this point, you may question the ability of analysts to assess the riskiness of a set of cash flows or to choose an opportunity cost rate with any confidence. Fortunately, the process is not as difficult as it may appear here. We discuss risk assessment in more detail in Chapter 10. Furthermore, businesses have a benchmark that can be used as a starting point—the corporate cost of capital, which is covered in Chapter 8.

(?) SELF-TEST QUESTIONS

1. What is compounding? Interest on interest?

2. What is discounting? How is it related to compounding?

3. What are three techniques used to perform DCF calculations?

4. Why does an investment have an opportunity cost of capital even when the funds employed have no explicit cost?

5. How are opportunity cost rates established?

Return on investment (ROI)

The profitability of an investment. Can be measured in either dollars or percentage (rate of) return.

9.8 RETURN ON INVESTMENT

Now that you have a basic understanding of DCF analysis, we can continue with Bayside's open MRI analysis. The most important measure of a project's financial attractiveness is its expected profitability, or *return on investment (ROI)*. With any investment, the most important question is this: Do you expect to make any money? In this section, we discuss two ROI measures that will answer that question.

(!) CRITICAL CONCEPT
Net Present Value

Net present value (NPV) measures the dollar value of an investment on the basis of its opportunity cost of capital. To illustrate, assume a $100 investment is expected to return $120 after one year. Furthermore, the return available on alternative investments of similar risk (opportunity cost of capital) is 5 percent. The NPV of this investment is $120/(1.05)^1 - $100 = $114.29 - $100 = $14.29. Thus, the investment is expected to (1) return the $100 initial investment, (2) provide a 5 percent return on those funds, and (3) create $14.29 of additional value (on a present value basis). An NPV of zero means that the investment just breaks even in the sense that it earns its opportunity cost of capital but no more.

NET PRESENT VALUE

Net present value (NPV), is a dollar ROI measure that uses DCF analysis, so it is often referred to as a DCF profitability measure. NPV is calculated and interpreted as follows:

◆   *Find the present values.* Find the present (Time 0) value of each cash flow, including both inflows and outflows, when discounted at the opportunity cost of capital.

◆   *Sum the present values.* The resulting sum is defined as the project's NPV. (The term NPV is used because it is the sum, or net, of the present values of an investment's expected cash flows.)

◆ *Interpret the NPV.* If the NPV is positive, the project is expected to be profitable; and the higher the NPV, the more profitable the project. If the NPV is zero, the project just breaks even in an economic sense. If the NPV is negative, the project is expected to be unprofitable.

To calculate the NPV of Bayside's open MRI project, we first need a discount rate (opportunity cost of capital). Bayside's corporate cost of capital is 10 percent, so if we assume that the project has average risk, then 10 percent can be used to calculate the project's NPV. (In Chapter 10, we assess the riskiness of the project. If the riskiness of the project is more than or less than the average risk for Bayside, the discount rate will have to be adjusted.)

Using a 10 percent discount rate, the NPV of Bayside's open MRI project is calculated as follows:

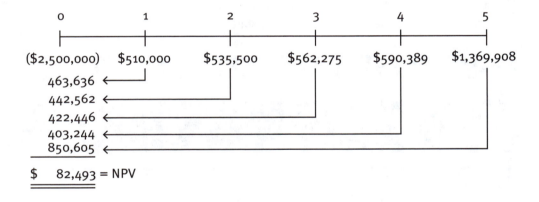

Financial calculators and spreadsheets have NPV functions that easily perform the mathematics, given the cash flows and opportunity cost of capital.

⟹ SOLUTION TECHNIQUE Financial Calculator

The present value of an uneven cash flow stream can be solved with most financial calculators by using the following steps:

- *Enter the cash flows.* Input the individual cash flows, in chronological order, into the cash flow register, where they usually are designated as CF_0 and CF_j (CF_1, CF_2, CF_3, and so on). For the open MRI project, enter

(Continued)

SOLUTION TECHNIQUE Financial Calculator

−2500000, 510000, 535500, 562275, 590389, and 1369908 in that order into the cash flow register.

• *Enter the discount rate.* In this case, enter I = 10.

• *Push the NPV key.* The answer, 82,493, will appear.

Note that amounts entered into the cash flow register remain there until the register is cleared. Thus, if a problem with eight cash flows had been previously worked, and the new problem with only four cash flows is entered, the calculator assumes that the final four cash flows from the first calculation belong to the second calculation. Be sure to clear the register before starting a new time value analysis.

 SOLUTION TECHNIQUE Spreadsheet

	A	B	C	D
1				
2	10.0%		Project cost of capital	
3	$ (2,500,000)		Cash flow 0	
4	510,000		Cash flow 1	
5	535,500		Cash flow 2	
6	562,275		Cash flow 3	
7	590,389		Cash flow 4	
8	1,369,908		Cash flow 5	
9				
10	$ 82,493	=NPV(A2,A4:A8)+A3 (entered into Cell A10)		

In this example, we have merely entered the net cash flows into the spreadsheet. In a typical capital investment analysis, the spreadsheet would be used to calculate the net cash flows. (Chapter 10 discusses cash flow analysis.)

> ⊶ **SOLUTION TECHNIQUE** Spreadsheet
>
> The project's NPV is calculated in Cell A10 using the NPV function. The first entry in the function (A2) is the discount rate (opportunity cost of capital), while the second entry (A4:A8) designates the range of cash inflows from Years 1 through 5. Because the NPV function calculates NPV one period before the first cash flow entered in the range, it is necessary to start the range with Year 1 rather than Year 0. Finally, to complete the calculation in Cell A10, A3 (the initial outlay) is added to the NPV function. The end result, $82,493, is displayed in Cell A10.

The rationale behind the NPV method is straightforward. An NPV of zero signifies that the project's cash inflows are just sufficient to (1) return the capital invested in the project and (2) provide the required rate of return on that capital (meet the opportunity cost of capital). If a project has a positive NPV, it is generating excess cash flows, and these excess cash flows are available to management to reinvest in the business and, for investor-owned firms, to pay bonuses (if a proprietorship or partnership) or dividends.

If a project has a negative NPV, its cash inflows are insufficient to compensate the firm for the capital invested or perhaps even insufficient to recover the initial investment, so the project is unprofitable and acceptance would cause the financial condition of the firm to deteriorate. For investor-owned businesses, NPV is a direct measure of the contribution of the project to owners' wealth, so NPV is considered by many people to be the best measure of project profitability.

The NPV of Bayside's open MRI project is $82,493, so on a present value basis, the project is expected to generate a value of more than $80,000 after all costs, including the opportunity cost of capital, have been considered. Thus, the project is profitable and its acceptance would have a positive impact on Bayside's financial condition. Note that NPV is, in reality, an expected value, although it typically is not called "expected NPV." Thus, the actual (realized) profitability of the MRI project may be greater than or less than the (expected) NPV of $82,493, depending on whether the realized cash flows are greater than or less than those expected when the project is analyzed.

INTERNAL RATE OF RETURN

Like NPV, **internal rate of return (IRR)** is a DCF ROI measure. However, whereas NPV measures a project's dollar profitability, IRR measures a project's percentage profitability (i.e., its expected rate of return).

Mathematically, IRR is defined as the discount rate that equates the present value of the project's expected cash inflows to the investment outlay. (Another way of saying the same thing is that IRR is the discount rate that forces the NPV of the project to be zero.)

For Bayside's open MRI project, the rate that causes the sum of the present values of the cash inflows to equal the $2,500,000 cost of the project is about 11.1 percent:

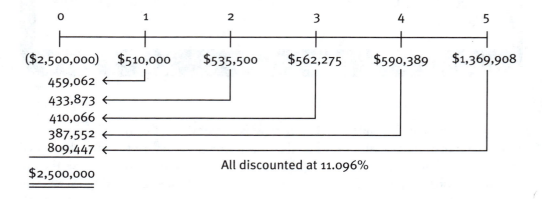

0	1	2	3	4	5
($2,500,000)	$510,000	$535,500	$562,275	$590,389	$1,369,908

459,062 ←
433,873 ←
410,066 ←
387,552 ←
809,447 ←

$2,500,000

All discounted at 11.096%

⊘ CRITICAL CONCEPT
Internal Rate of Return

Internal rate of return (IRR) measures the expected rate of (percentage) return of an investment. Assume that a $100 investment is expected to return $120 after one year. The discount rate that equates the present value of the expected $120 cash inflow to the $100 cost is 20 percent: $120/1.20 = $100. Thus, the IRR of this investment is 20 percent. In other words, the $100 investment is expected to earn a 20 percent return: $100 x 1.20 = $120. If the opportunity cost of capital (the return available on alternative investments of similar risk) is 10 percent, this investment is expected to provide a return above those available on comparable alternatives, and hence the investment is financially attractive.

Thus, the MRI project's IRR is 11.1 percent. Put another way, the project is expected to generate an 11.1 percent rate of return on its $2,500,000 investment. The IRR is the rate of return expected on the investment, assuming all the cash flows anticipated actually occur.

If the IRR exceeds the project cost of capital (opportunity cost rate), a surplus is expected to remain after recovering the invested capital and earning its opportunity cost. If the IRR is less than the project cost of capital, however, taking on the project imposes an expected financial cost on the firm's stockholders or stakeholders.

The open MRI project's 11.1 percent IRR exceeds its 10 percent project cost of capital. Thus, as measured by IRR, the MRI project is profitable, and its acceptance would enhance

SOLUTION TECHNIQUE Financial Calculator

Use the same cash flows that were entered to solve for NPV. However, now push the IRR button to obtain the answer: 11.1 percent.

SOLUTION TECHNIQUE Spreadsheet

	A	B	C	D
1				
2	10.0%		Project cost of capital	
3	$ (2,500,000)		Cash flow 0	
4	510,000		Cash flow 1	
5	535,500		Cash flow 2	
6	562,275		Cash flow 3	
7	590,389		Cash flow 4	
8	1,369,908		Cash flow 5	
9				
10	11.1%	=IRR(A2,A3:A8) (entered into Cell A10)		

Note that we have placed the IRR function in Cell A10. The first entry in the function (A2) gives a starting value for the spreadsheet calculation, while the next entry (A3:A8) specifies the range of cash flows to be used in the calculation. The answer, 11.1%, is displayed in Cell A10.

Bayside's financial condition. As with NPV, a project's IRR actually represents its expected rate of return. After the project is completed, the actual (realized) rate of return may be higher than or lower than that expected.

COMPARISON OF THE NPV AND IRR METHODS

Consider a project with a zero NPV. In this situation, the project's IRR must equal its opportunity cost of capital. The project only earns its opportunity cost of capital, so acceptance would neither enhance nor diminish the firm's financial condition. To have a positive NPV, the project's IRR must be greater than its cost of capital, and a negative NPV signifies a project with an IRR that is less than its cost of capital. Thus, projects that are deemed profitable by the NPV method will also be deemed profitable by the IRR method.

In our open MRI analysis, the project would have a positive NPV for all costs of capital less than 11.1 percent. If the cost of capital were greater than 11.1 percent, the project would have a negative NPV. In effect, the NPV and IRR are perfect substitutes for each other in measuring whether or not a project is profitable.

(?) SELF-TEST QUESTIONS

1. What is the difference between return on investment and profitability?

2. Briefly describe how to calculate net present value (NPV) and internal rate of return (IRR).

3. How are NPV and IRR interpreted?

4. Can NPV and IRR lead to different conclusions about a project's financial attractiveness?

5. Evaluate the following statement: "NPV and IRR are expected values."

(✱) INDUSTRY PRACTICE Capital Investment Analysis in Healthcare Organizations

Over the last 20 years, several surveys have been conducted to assess how healthcare organizations analyze and make capital investment decisions. In the 1980s, approximately half of surveyed hospitals used ROI measures (NPV and IRR) to assess financial attractiveness, while about 40 percent used the payback method.

Fast forward to today. Now, virtually all large healthcare organizations use ROI to assess financial impact. NPV is the most common measure, but many systems use multiple financial measures rather than just one. The most frequently used are NPV, IRR, and payback. It appears that large businesses do not place complete faith in one measure but prefer to paint a complete picture of the expected financial consequences of a proposed capital investment.

(✳) INDUSTRY PRACTICE Capital Investment Analysis in Healthcare Organizations

For example, NPV provides information about the expected dollar contribution to an organization's financial value. IRR gives some information about the "safety margin" inherent in the project, because an IRR much higher than the cost of capital means that the project's cash flows can fall short of predictions yet the project would still be profitable. Finally, payback is useful in screening capital investments in changing technologies, where continuous innovation can make the investment obsolete in a short time.

Interestingly, there appears to be little difference in the financial analysis techniques used by for-profit and not-for-profit businesses. Both types realize that financial soundness is important in meeting organizational goals.

In addition to financial factors, most large healthcare organizations recognize that nonfinancial factors play an important role in the decision process. For example, contribution to the mission and fit with the organization's long-term strategic vision are commonly mentioned as important decision factors.

Furthermore, many healthcare organizations have a formal system for incorporating physician input into the decision process. All organizations reported undertaking projects with poor financial prospects (negative NPVs) because of "mission virtues." Such projects were viewed as paying healthcare dividends to the community as opposed to paying financial dividends to the business.

Although little information is available regarding the capital investment policies of small healthcare businesses (such as small medical practices), evidence from other industries suggests that such businesses are less sophisticated than their larger counterparts. Indeed, most capital investment decisions at small businesses appear to be based solely on need as opposed to financial attractiveness. If some type of financial analysis is done, it is more likely to be a "back of the envelope" calculation as opposed to a spreadsheet analysis. That said, as reimbursement rates tighten and as sophisticated business practices filter down to smaller businesses, the use of ROI measures is expected to become as widespread in small businesses as it is in large businesses.

Note: This industry practice is based on information in Reiter, K. L., D. G. Smith, J. R. C. Wheeler, and H. L. Rivenson. 2000. "Capital Investment Strategies in Health Care Systems." *Journal of Health Care Finance* (Summer): 31–41.

9.9 PROJECT SCORING

Many other factors, beside financial, clearly must be considered in a complete capital investment analysis. To incorporate multiple factors into the decision, many businesses use a quasi-subjective **project scoring** approach that attempts to capture both financial and nonfinancial factors. Table 9.1, which is used by Bayside Memorial Hospital, illustrates one such approach.

Bayside ranks projects on three dimensions: stakeholder, operational, and financial. Within each dimension, multiple factors are examined and assigned scores that range from two points for very favorable impact to minus one point for negative impact. The scores within each dimension are added to obtain scores for each of the three dimensions, and then the dimension scores are summed to obtain a total score for the project. The total score gives Bayside's managers a feel for the relative values of projects under consideration when all factors, including financial, are taken into account.

Table 9.2 contains the scores assigned by Bayside's managers for the open MRI project. By their judgment, the project has a score of 6, which can be compared with scores of

TABLE 9.1
Bayside Memorial Hospital: Project Scoring Table

	Relative Score			
Criteria	*2*	*1*	*0*	*−1*
Stakeholder Factors				
Physicians	Strongly support	Support	Neutral	Opposed
Employees	Greatly helps morale	Helps morale	No effect	Hurts morale
Visitors	Greatly enhances visit	Enhances visit	No effect	Hurts image
Patients	High	Moderate	None	Negative
Operational Factors				
Outcomes	Greatly improves	Improves	No effect	Hurts outcomes
Length of stay	Documented decrease	Anecdotal decrease	No effect	Increases
Technology	Breakthrough	Improves current	Adds to current	Lowers
Productivity	Large decrease in FTEs*	Decrease in FTEs	No change in FTEs	Adds FTEs
Financial Factors				
Payback	Less than 2 years	2–4 years	4–6 years	Over 6 years
IRR	Over 20%	15–20%	10–15%	Less than 10%

Stakeholder factor score   _____

Operational factor score   _____

Financial factor score   _____

  Total score   ＝＝＝＝＝

*Full-time equivalent

other current projects or with the average score of past projects.

Note that the scoring system is completely arbitrary, so the open MRI project with a score of 6, for example, is not necessarily twice as good as a project with a score of 3 or half as good as a project with a score of 12. Nevertheless, Bayside's project scoring system forces its managers to address multiple issues when making capital investment decisions, and the system does provide a relative ranking of projects under consideration.

CRITICAL CONCEPT
Project Scoring

Project scoring is a technique for incorporating both financial and nonfinancial factors in capital investment decisions. The various factors, such as IRR (a financial factor) and social value (a nonfinancial factor), are graded on a numerical scale. These grades are then added, and the total score reflects the overall attractiveness of the project. The higher the score, the more attractive the project, considering both financial and nonfinancial factors.

? SELF-TEST QUESTION

1. Describe the concept and use of a project scoring system.

TABLE 9.2

Bayside Memorial Hospital: Project Score for the Open MRI

Stakeholder Factors	
Physicians	2
Employees	0
Visitors	0
Patients	2
Total stakeholder	4
Operational Factors	
Outcomes	1
Length of stay	0
Technology	1
Productivity	0
Total operational	2
Financial Factors	
Payback	0
IRR	0
Total financial	0
Total score	6

9.10 THE POST-AUDIT

Capital budgeting is not a static process. If there is a long lag between a project's acceptance and its implementation, any new information concerning either capital costs or the project's cash flows should be analyzed before the final start-up occurs. Furthermore, the performance of each project should be monitored throughout the project's life.

The process of formally monitoring project performance over time is called the *post-audit*. It involves comparing actual results with those projected; explaining why differences occur; and analyzing potential changes to the project's operations, including replacement or termination.

The post-audit has several purposes:

Post-audit
The feedback process in which the performance of projects previously accepted is reviewed and necessary changes are made.

- *Improve forecasts.* When managers systematically compare forecasts to actual outcomes, estimates tend to improve. Conscious or unconscious biases that occur can be identified and, one hopes, eliminated; new forecasting methods are sought as the need for them becomes apparent; and managers tend to do everything better, including forecasting, if they know that their actions are being monitored.

- *Develop historical risk data.* Post-audits permit managers to develop historical risk and expected-rates-of-return data on new project proposals. These data can then be used to make judgments about the relative risk and profitability of future projects as they are evaluated.

- *Improve operations.* Managers run businesses, and they can perform at higher or lower levels of efficiency. When a forecast is made, for example, by the surgery department, the department director and medical staff are, in a sense, putting their reputations on the line. If costs are above predicted levels and volume is below expectations, the managers involved will strive, within ethical bounds, to improve the situation and to bring results into line with forecasts. As one hospital CEO put it: "You academics worry only about making good decisions. In the healthcare industry, we also have to worry about making decisions good."

- *Reduce losses.* Post-audits monitor the performance of projects over time, so the first indication that termination or replacement should be considered often arises when the post-audit indicates that a project is performing poorly.

? SELF-TEST QUESTIONS

1. What is a post-audit?

2. Why are post-audits important to the financial effectiveness of a business?

THEME WRAP-UP   EVALUATING A CAPITAL INVESTMENT

Bayside's managers began their capital investment analysis of the proposed open MRI project by performing three steps.

First, they laid out the net cash flows expected from the project, which include both costs and revenues, on a time line. This enabled them to see the amounts and timing of the flows expected if the open MRI is purchased. Then, they used those cash flows to estimate the payback, 4.2 years, which is the expected time required to recover the initial $2.5 million investment.

Second, they applied DCF analysis, which accounts for the time value of money, to assess the profitability, or ROI, of the proposal. To perform ROI analyses, it is necessary to apply an opportunity cost of capital. This is the return that could be earned on alternative investments of similar risk to the project being analyzed. Bayside's managers used the corporate cost of capital, 10 percent, as the opportunity cost of capital.

The ROI analysis determined that the NPV of the project was $82,493 and the internal rate of return was 11.1 percent. NPV measures dollar profitability, and the positive amount signifies that the project is expected to add financial value to the hospital. IRR measures the expected rate of return on the project, and because the 11.1 percent IRR was greater than the 10 percent opportunity cost of capital, IRR confirmed that the project was financially attractive.

Third, Bayside's managers used a project scoring system to incorporate nonfinancial factors into the decision process.

At this point, the open MRI proposal appears financially attractive. However, the analysis is not yet complete. In Chapter 10, we find out how Bayside's managers estimated the project's net cash flows and, more importantly, how they assessed the project's riskiness. If the open MRI project turns out to have either more or less risk than Bayside's average project, the ROI analysis has to be revised, which could change the conclusions about the project's financial attractiveness.

KEY CONCEPTS

This chapter covers the basics of capital investment analysis. Here are the key concepts:

➤ *Capital investment analysis* involves analyzing potential expenditures on land, buildings, and equipment and deciding whether or not the business should undertake those investments.

➤ A capital investment analysis consists of four steps: (1) estimate the expected cash flows, (2) assess the riskiness of those flows, (3) estimate the appropriate opportunity cost of capital, and (4) determine the project's profitability and breakeven characteristics.

➤ Time breakeven, which is measured by *payback,* provides managers with insights into a project's liquidity and risk.

➤ *Compounding* is the process of determining the future value of a current cash flow or series of flows.

➤ *Discounting* is the process of finding the present value of a future cash flow or series of flows.

➤ Project profitability is assessed by *return on investment (ROI)* measures. The two most commonly used ROI measures are net present value and internal rate of return.

➤ *Net present value (NPV),* which is simply the sum of the present values of all the project's cash flows when discounted at the project's opportunity cost of capital, measures a project's expected dollar profitability. An NPV greater than zero indicates that the project is expected to be profitable after all costs, including the opportunity cost of capital, have been considered. Furthermore, the higher the NPV, the more profitable the project.

➤ *Internal rate of return (IRR),* which is the discount rate that forces a project's NPV to equal zero, measures a project's expected rate of return. If a project's IRR is greater than its opportunity cost of capital, the project is expected to be profitable, and the higher the IRR, the more profitable the project.

➤ Firms often use *project scoring* to subjectively incorporate a large number of factors, including financial and nonfinancial, into the capital investment decision process.

➤ The *post-audit* is a key element in capital budgeting. By comparing actual results with predicted results, managers can improve both operations and the cash flow estimation process.

Our discussion of capital investment decisions continues in Chapter 10, which focuses on cash flow estimation and risk assessment.

END-OF-CHAPTER QUESTIONS

9.1 a. What is capital investment analysis? Why are capital investment decisions so important to businesses?

b. What is the purpose of placing capital investments into categories, such as mandatory replacement, or expansion of existing products, services, or markets?

c. Should financial analysis play the dominant role in capital investment decisions? Explain your answer.

d. What are the four steps of capital investment financial analysis?

9.2 a. What is the opportunity cost of capital?

b. How is this rate used in discounted cash flow (DCF) analysis?

c. Is this rate a single number that is used in all situations?

9.3 Describe the following project breakeven and profitability measures. Be sure to include each measure's economic interpretation.

a. Payback

b. Net present value (NPV)

c. Internal rate of return (IRR)

9.4 Describe a project scoring system.

9.5 What is a post-audit? Why is the post-audit critical to good investment decision making?

END-OF-CHAPTER PROBLEMS

9.1 Find the following values for a single cash flow:

a. The future value of $500 invested at 8 percent for one year

b. The future value of $500 invested at 8 percent for five years

c. The present value of $500 to be received in one year when the opportunity cost rate is 8 percent

d. The present value of $500 to be received in five years when the opportunity cost rate is 8 percent

9.2 Consider the following net cash flows:

Year	Cash Flow
0	$ 0
1	250
2	400
3	500
4	600
5	600

a. What is the net present value if the opportunity cost of capital (discount rate) is 10 percent?

b. Add an outflow (or cost) of $1,000 at Year 0. Now, what is the net present value?

9.3 Consider another set of net cash flows:

Year	Cash Flow
0	$2,000
1	2,000
2	0
3	1,500
4	2,500
5	4,000

a. What is the net present value of the stream if the opportunity cost of capital is 10 percent?

b. What is the value of the stream at the end of Year 5 if the cash flows are invested in an account that pays 10 percent annually?

c. What cash flow today (Year 0), in lieu of the $2,000 cash flow, would be needed to accumulate $20,000 at the end of Year 5? (Assume that the cash flows for Years 1 through 5 remain the same.)

9.4 Better Health, Inc., is evaluating two capital investments, each of which requires an up-front (Year 0) expenditure of $1.5 million. The projects are expected to produce the following net cash inflows:

Year	Project A	Project B
1	$ 500,000	$2,000,000
2	1,000,000	1,000,000
3	2,000,000	600,000

a. What is each project's IRR?

b. What is each project's NPV if the opportunity cost of capital is 10 percent? 5 percent? 15 percent?

9.5 Capital Healthplans, Inc. is evaluating two different methods for providing home health services to its members. Both methods involve contracting out for services, and the health outcomes and revenues are not affected by the method chosen. Therefore, the net cash flows for the decision are all outflows. Here are the projected flows:

Year	Method A	Method B
0	($300,000)	($120,000)
1	(66,000)	(96,000)
2	(66,000)	(96,000)
3	(66,000)	(96,000)
4	(66,000)	(96,000)
5	(66,000)	(96,000)

a. What is each alternative's IRR?

b. If the opportunity cost of capital for both methods is 9 percent, which method should be chosen? Why?

9.6 Assume that you are the chief financial officer at Porter Memorial Hospital. The CEO has asked you to analyze two proposed capital investments—Project X and Project Y. Each project requires a net investment outlay of $10,000, and the opportunity cost of capital for each project is 12 percent. The projects' expected net cash flows are as follows:

Year	Project X	Project Y
0	($10,000)	($10,000)
1	6,500	3,000
2	3,000	3,000
3	3,000	3,000
4	1,000	3,000

a. Calculate each project's payback, NPV, and IRR.

b. Which project (or projects) is financially acceptable? Explain your answer.

9.7 The director of capital budgeting for Big Sky Health Systems, Inc., has estimated the following cash flows (in thousands of dollars) for a proposed new service:

Year	Expected Net Cash Flow
0	($100)
1	70
2	50
3	20

The project's opportunity cost of capital is 10 percent.

a. What is the project's payback period?

b. What is the project's NPV?

c. What is the project's IRR?

CHAPTER 10

PROJECT CASH FLOW ESTIMATION AND RISK ANALYSIS

THEME SET-UP   ESTIMATING A PROJECT'S CASH FLOWS AND ASSESSING RISK

In Chapter 9, we explored the financial implications of Bayside Memorial Hospital's potential purchase of an open MRI (magnetic resonance imaging) system. The new MRI system greatly reduces the feeling of constraint associated with conventional MRI technology and produces high-quality images. Additionally, the open MRI system can accommodate pediatric patients who need parental support and patients who are too large to fit in a conventional MRI machine.

Bayside's initial analysis used discounted cash flow (DCF) techniques to assess the payback and profitability of the project. However, in their DCF analysis, Bayside's managers assumed that the project had average risk, so they used the corporate cost of capital, 10 percent, as the opportunity cost of capital. The results so far indicate a payback of 4.2 years, a net present value (NPV) of $82,493, and an internal rate of return (IRR) of 11.1 percent. Additionally, Bayside's managers used a project scoring system to incorporate nonfinancial factors into the decision process. At this point, the open MRI project seems attractive. However, the managers have not finished their analysis.

Now, the managers must assess the project's riskiness. If the proposal was found to have either more or less risk than Bayside's average project, the managers would have to modify the financial analysis. In addition, Dr. Fisher, the radiology group CEO who proposed the project, was not sure of the process that Bayside's managers used to estimate the project's net cash flows. Thus, he asked the managers to explain how the cash flows were developed.

By the end of the chapter, you will learn how project cash flows are estimated. Furthermore, you will understand what investment risk is, how it is assessed, and what impact it has on capital investment decisions.

LEARNING OBJECTIVES

After studying this chapter, you will be able to

➤ Define the key elements of cash flow estimation.

➤ Conduct a basic project cash flow analysis.

➤ Explain the concept of investment risk.

➤ Discuss the techniques used in project risk assessment.

➤ Conduct a project risk assessment.

➤ Incorporate risk into the capital investment decision process.

10.1 INTRODUCTION

Chapter 9 covers the basics of capital investment decisions, including discounted cash flow analysis, breakeven analysis, and return on investment (profitability) measures. This chapter extends this discussion to include cash flow estimation and risk analysis.

Both cash flow estimation and risk analysis are critical to good capital investment decisions. If the cash flow estimates are wrong, the entire financial analysis is of little, or no, value. Furthermore, if risk is ignored, the financial analysis could lead to improper capital investment decisions.

10.2 CASH FLOW ESTIMATION

The most difficult, yet most important, step in evaluating capital investment proposals is cash flow estimation. This step involves estimating the investment outlays, annual net operating flows, and cash flows associated with project termination. Many separate (component) cash flows are involved, and many individuals typically participate in the process.

Often, historical data can be used to help make the cash flow estimates. But, for projects that involve new services, scant data are available. Thus, often, forecasts are not much better than rough estimates. Making accurate forecasts of the costs and revenues associated with many projects is difficult, so forecast errors can be quite large. For this reason, risk analyses must be performed on prospective projects.

Neither the difficulty nor the importance of cash flow estimation can be overstated. However, the following guiding principles can help healthcare managers eliminate most of the common errors that arise.

FOCUS ON INCREMENTAL CASH FLOWS

The relevant cash flows to consider when evaluating a new capital investment are the project's **incremental cash flows**, which are formally defined as the firm's cash flows in each period if the project is undertaken minus the firm's cash flows if the project is not undertaken. In capital investment decisions, the decision must be based on the actual dollars that flow into and out of the business rather than on revenues and expenses defined by accountants for other purposes. After all, it is cash flow that creates value. The focus on cash flow actually makes the estimation process easier, because applying a set of arbitrary accounting rules is not necessary when analyzing capital investments.

In theory, project cash flows should be analyzed exactly as they are expected to occur. Of course, there must be a compromise between accuracy and simplicity. A time line with daily cash flows would, in theory, provide the most accuracy, but daily cash flow estimates would be costly to construct, unwieldy to use, and probably no more accurate than annual cash flow estimates. Thus, in most situations, analysts simply assume that all cash flows occur at the end of each year, so the typical time line for a capital investment analysis uses years as periods.

CRITICAL CONCEPT
Incremental Cash Flow

Incremental cash flows are flows that are properly included in a capital investment analysis. The term *incremental* means that the flows arise solely because of project acceptance—if the project is accepted, and only if the project is accepted, these cash flows will result. The term *cash flow* means that these are the amounts of cash that actually flow into or out of the business. Some flows might appear to be incremental flows, but they occur whether or not the project is undertaken and hence are nonincremental to the decision and should not be included in the analysis. Conversely, the loss of revenues on an existing project that results if a new project is undertaken is incremental to the decision and should be included in the analysis.

Perhaps the first decision that must be made in forecasting a project's cash flows is the life of the project. Does the cash flow forecast need to be for 20 years, or is 5 years sufficient? Many projects, such as a new hospital wing or an ambulatory surgery center, have long productive lives. In theory, the cash flow forecast should extend for the full life of the project, yet most managers would have little confidence in forecasting beyond the near term.

Thus, healthcare organizations often set an arbitrary limit on project life—say, five or ten years. If the forecasted life is less than the arbitrary limit, the forecasted life is used to develop the cash flows. If the forecasted life exceeds the limit, project life is truncated and the cash flows beyond the limit do not appear on the time line.

Terminal value

The cash flow assigned in the last year of a long-life project to account for the value lost because the cash flows were truncated.

Salvage value

The expected market value of an asset (project) at the end of its useful life.

Sunk cost

A cost that has already occurred or is irrevocably committed. Sunk costs are nonincremental to capital investment analyses and hence should not be included.

If truncation occurs, it is important to recognize that some of the project's value is being ignored, because the cash flows omitted from the analysis typically consist of inflows. The recognition of lost value can be quantitative (by assigning a *terminal value* to the project) or qualitative (by merely noting that the NPV of the project understates its true value).

Conversely, many projects have short lives, and hence the analysis will extend over the project's entire life. In such situations, the assets associated with the project may still have some value remaining when the project is terminated. The cash flow expected to be realized from selling the project's assets at termination is called *salvage value*. Even if a project is being terminated for old age, any cash flows that will arise by virtue of scrap value must be included in the analysis. Note that the net cash flow at termination can be negative if the cost of dismantling the project is greater than the market value of the assets to be sold.

IGNORE SUNK COSTS

A *sunk cost* refers to an outlay that has already occurred or has been irrevocably committed, so it is unaffected by the current decision to accept or reject a project. To illustrate, suppose that in 2009 Gold Coast Surgery Center is evaluating the purchase of a robotic surgery system. To help in the decision, in 2008 the center hired and paid $10,000 to a consultant to conduct a feasibility study.

This cash flow is *not* relevant, and hence nonincremental to the capital investment decision, because it is not contingent on the equipment purchase; it has already occurred.

Sometimes a project will appear to be unprofitable when *all* of its associated costs, including sunk costs, are considered. However, on an incremental basis, the project may be profitable and should be undertaken. Thus, the correct treatment of sunk costs can be critical to the decision.

INCLUDE OPPORTUNITY COSTS

All relevant *opportunity costs* must be included in a capital investment analysis. To illustrate, one opportunity cost involves the use of the capital required to finance the project. If a business uses its money to invest in Project A, it cannot use the capital to invest in Project B, or for any other purpose.

> ***Opportunity cost***
> The cost associated with alternative uses of the same asset. For example, if land is used for one project, it is no longer available for other uses, and hence an opportunity cost arises.

The opportunity cost associated with the use of capital is accounted for in the discount rate, which represents the return that the business could earn by investing the funds in alternative investments of similar risk. Thus, the discounting process used to calculate NPV forces the opportunity cost of capital to be considered in the analysis. (Similarly, the opportunity cost of capital is considered when a project's IRR is compared to its cost of capital.)

In addition to the opportunity cost of capital, other types of opportunity costs arise in capital investment analyses. For example, assume that Gold Coast's robotic surgery system would be installed in a separate freestanding facility and that Gold Coast currently owns the land on which the facility would be built.

When analyzing this project, the value of the land cannot be disregarded merely because no cash outlay is required. There is an opportunity cost inherent in the use of the land because using it for the robotic surgery facility deprives Gold Coast of its use for other purposes. The property might be used for conventional surgical suites or a parking garage rather than sold. But the best measure of the land's value, and hence the opportunity cost inherent in its use, is the cash flow that could be realized from selling the property.

Gold Coast purchased the land ten years ago at a cost of $50,000, but the current market value of the property is $130,000, after subtracting all legal, real estate, and other fees required to sell the land. Thus, the robotic surgery system project should have a $130,000 opportunity cost charged against it. After all, if not used for the project, the land could be sold, resulting in a $130,000 net cash inflow to the center.

INCLUDE EFFECTS ON EXISTING BUSINESS LINES

Capital investment analyses must consider the effects of the project under consideration on the organization's existing business lines. Such effects can be either positive or negative. To illustrate, assume that some of the patients who are expected to undergo robotic surgery would have been treated by conventional surgery at the center, so these conventional revenues will be lost if the robotic facility goes into operation. Thus, the incremental cash flows to Gold Coast are the flows attributable to the robotic surgery facility, minus those flows lost from forgone conventional surgery services.

On the other hand, new patients that come to Gold Coast because of the new robotic surgery capability may use other services provided by the center. In this situation, the incremental cash flows generated by the robotic surgery patients' utilization of other services should be credited to the robotic project. If possible, both positive and negative effects on other projects should be quantified, but at a minimum they should be noted so that these effects are subjectively considered when the final decision regarding the project is made.

INCLUDE INFLATION EFFECTS

Because inflation can have a considerable influence on a project's profitability, it must be considered in all capital budgeting analyses. As we discuss in Chapter 8, a business's corporate cost of capital is a weighted average of its costs of debt and equity. These costs are estimated on the basis of investors' required rates of return, and investors incorporate an inflation premium into such estimates.

For example, a lender might require a 3 percent return on a ten-year loan in the absence of inflation. However, if inflation is expected to average 4 percent over the coming ten years, the investor would require a 7 percent return. Thus, investors add an inflation premium to their required rates of return to help protect against the loss of purchasing power that stems from inflation.

Because inflation effects are already embedded in the corporate cost of capital, and because this cost will be used to set the opportunity cost (discount) rate used in the analysis, inflation effects must also be built into the project's cash flow estimates. If the cash flow estimates do not include inflation effects, but a discount rate is used that does include inflation, the profitability of the project will be understated. (The NPV will be too low.)

The best way to deal with inflation is to apply inflation effects to each component cash flow using the best available information about how each component will be affected. For example, labor costs would be increased by the wage inflation rate, inventory costs would be adjusted by the supplies inflation rate, revenues would be adjusted by price inflation, and so on. Because it is impossible to estimate future inflation rates with much precision, errors are bound to occur.

Sometimes inflation is assumed to be neutral—that is, it is assumed to affect all revenue and cost components equally. However, in most years it is unlikely that both revenues and costs would inflate at the same rate. Inflation adds to the uncertainty, and hence risk, of a project under consideration as well as to the complexity of capital investment cash flow estimation.

INCLUDE ANY STRATEGIC VALUE

Sometimes a project will have value, called *strategic value*, that stems from future investment opportunities that can be undertaken only if the project currently under consideration is accepted. Typically, such value is not captured by a project's cash flow estimates. To illustrate, consider University Hospital's decision to start a kidney transplant program. The financial analysis of this project showed the program to be unprofitable, but the hospital's managers considered kidney transplants to be the first step in an aggressive transplant program. Not only would the entire transplant program be profitable, but it would also enhance the hospital's reputation for technological and clinical excellence and hence increase the hospital's ability to attract new patients.

In theory, the best approach to dealing with strategic value is to forecast the cash flows from the follow-on projects, estimate their probabilities of occurrence, and then add the expected cash flows from the follow-on projects to the cash flows of the project under consideration.

In practice, this is usually impossible to do, because either the follow-on cash flows are too nebulous to forecast or the potential follow-on projects are too numerous to quantify. At a minimum, decision makers must recognize that some projects have strategic value, and this value should be qualitatively considered when making capital investment decisions.

> **Strategic value**
> The value inherent in a capital investment that is not captured in its cash flow estimates. For example, a project may provide a foot in the door in a new service area that could lead to other profitable investments.

? SELF-TEST QUESTIONS

1. Briefly discuss the following concepts associated with cash flow estimation:

   · Incremental cash flow

   · Cash flow timing

   · Project life

   · Terminal value

   · Salvage value

   · Sunk costs

   · Opportunity costs

   · Effects on current projects

   · Inflation effects

   · Strategic value

2. Evaluate the following statement: Ignoring inflation effects and strategic value can result in *overstating* a project's financial attractiveness.

10.3 ESTIMATING THE CASH FLOWS FOR THE OPEN MRI PROJECT

In this section, we discuss how Bayside's managers estimated the cash flows for the open MRI project. This illustration reviews some of the concepts we just covered as well as introduces several others that are important to good cash flow estimation.

THE BASIC DATA

Managers at Bayside Memorial Hospital, in collaboration with physicians from the radiology group, developed the required component cash flows (basic input data). The system costs $2 million, and the hospital would have to spend another $500,000 for site preparation, delivery, and installation. Because the system would be installed in the hospital, the space to be used has a very low, or zero, market value to outsiders. Furthermore, its value to Bayside for alternative uses is very difficult to estimate, so no opportunity cost was assigned to account for the value of the site.

Bayside's managers developed the project's forecasted revenues by conducting the analysis contained in Table 10.1. The estimated average charge per scan is $500, but 25 percent of this amount is expected to be lost on discounts to payers, charity care, and bad debt losses. Thus, the actual reimbursement expected, on average, is $375 per scan.

The open MRI system is estimated to have weekly utilization (volume) of 40 scans, and each scan will cost the hospital $15 in supplies. The system is expected to operate 50 weeks a year, with the remaining two weeks devoted to maintenance. The MRI system would require 1.5 FTE (full-time equivalent) technicians, resulting in an incremental increase in annual labor costs of $60,000, including fringe benefits.

TABLE 10.1
Bayside Memorial
Hospital: Open
MRI System
Revenue Analysis

Payer	Number of Scans per Week	Charge per Scan	Total Charges	Basis of Payment	Net Payment per Scan	Total Payments
Medicare	10	$500	$ 5,000	Fixed fee	$370	$ 3,700
Medicaid	5	500	2,500	Fixed fee	350	1,750
Private insurance	9	500	4,500	Full charge	500	4,500
Blue Cross	5	500	2,500	Percent of charge	420	2,100
Managed care	7	500	3,500	Percent of charge	390	2,730
Self-pay	4	500	2,000	Full charge	55	220
Total	40		$20,000			$15,000
Average			$ 500			$ 375

No increase in overhead costs is associated with the new open MRI. (Additional existing overhead may be allocated to the new system, but such a reallocation is not an incremental cash flow—that is, it is not a new cash cost to Bayside.) The open MRI would require maintenance, which would be furnished by the manufacturer for an annual fee of $150,000, payable at the end of each year of operation.

The MRI system is expected to be in operation for five years, at which time the hospital's master plan calls for a new imaging facility. The hospital plans to sell the MRI at that time for an estimated $750,000 salvage value, net of removal costs. The inflation rate is estimated to average 5 percent over the period, and this rate is expected to affect all revenues and costs equally.

CASH FLOW ANALYSIS

The next step in the analysis is to convert the component cash flow data into the project's net cash flows. This analysis is presented in Table 10.2. Here are the key points of the analysis by line number:

TABLE 10.2

Bayside Memorial Hospital: Open MRI System Cash Flow Analysis

	0	Cash Revenues and Costs				
		1	2	3	4	5
1. System cost	($2,000,000)					
2. Installation expenses	(500,000)					
3. Total cost	($2,500,000)					
4. Net revenues		$750,000	$787,500	$826,875	$868,219	$ 911,630
5. Labor costs		(60,000)	(63,000)	(66,150)	(69,457)	(72,930)
6. Maintenance cost		(150,000)	(157,500)	(165,375)	(173,644)	(182,326)
7. Supplies		(30,000)	(31,500)	(33,075)	(34,729)	(36,465)
8. Net operating income		$510,000	$535,500	$562,275	$590,389	$ 619,908
9. Salvage value						750,000
10. Net cash flow	($2,500,000)	$510,000	$535,500	$562,275	$590,389	$1,369,908

Profitability measures (from Chapter 9):
  Net present value = $82,493.
  Internal rate of return = 11.1%.

Note: Some rounding occurs in this table.

◆ *Line 1.* Line 1 contains the estimated cost (price) of the open MRI system—$2,000,000. In general, capital budgeting analyses assume that the first cash flow, normally an outflow, occurs at the end of Year 0, the starting point of the analysis. Note that cash outflows are shown in parentheses.

◆ *Line 2.* The related site-preparation expense, including shipping and installation costs—$500,000—is also assumed to occur at Year 0.

◆ *Line 3.* Line 3 adds the two initial cost components to obtain the project's total cost—$2,500,000.

◆ *Line 4.* Annual net revenues = Weekly volume × Weeks of operation per year × Average reimbursement per scan = 40 × 50 × $375 = $750,000 in Year 1. The 5 percent inflation rate is applied to all revenues and costs that would likely be affected by inflation, so the net revenue amounts shown on Line 4 increase by 5 percent over time.

   Although most of the operating revenues and costs would occur more or less evenly over the year, it is difficult to forecast exactly when the flows would occur. Furthermore, the potential for large errors in cash flow estimation is significant. For these reasons, operating cash flows are assumed to occur at the end of each year. Also, the assumption is that the open MRI system could be placed in operation quickly. If this were not the case, then Year 1's operating flows would be reduced. In some situations, it might take several years from the first cash outflow to the point when the project is operational and begins to generate revenues and hence cash inflows.

◆ *Line 5.* Labor costs are forecasted to be $60,000 during the first year, and these costs are assumed to increase over time at the 5 percent inflation rate.

◆ *Line 6.* Maintenance fees—$150,000 for Year 1—must be paid to the manufacturer at the end of each year of operation. These fees are assumed to increase at the 5 percent inflation rate.

◆ *Line 7.* Each scan uses $15 of supplies, so supply costs in Year 1 total 40 × 50 × $15 = $30,000, and they are expected to increase each year by the inflation rate.

◆ *Line 8.* Line 8 shows the project's net operating income in each year, which is merely net revenues minus all operating expenses. For Year 1, the value is $510,000.

◆ *Line 9.* The project is expected to be terminated after five years, at which time the MRI system would be sold for an estimated $750,000, net of removal and other project shutdown costs. This salvage value cash flow is shown as an inflow at the end of Year 5.

◆ *Line 10.* The project's net cash flows are shown on Line 10. The project requires a $2,500,000 investment at Year 0 but then generates cash inflows over its five-year operating life.

The bottom of the table contains the results of the profitability (return on investment [ROI]) analysis performed in Chapter 9. In Chapter 9, we estimated the project's NPV to be $82,493, when the opportunity cost of capital was assumed to be Bayside's corporate cost of capital, 10 percent. In addition, the project's IRR was found to be 11.1 percent.

Note that the cash flows in Table 10.2 do not include any allowance for interest expense on any debt capital used to acquire the MRI system. On average, Bayside will finance new projects in accordance with its target capital structure, which consists of 35 percent debt financing and 65 percent equity financing. The costs associated with this financing mix, including both interest costs and the cost of equity capital, are incorporated into the firm's 10 percent corporate cost of capital. Because the cost of debt financing is included in the discount rate that is applied to the net cash flows to obtain ROI, recognition of interest expense in the cash flows would be double counting.

If the project were being analyzed by a for-profit provider, some adjustments would have to be made to the cash flows to account for tax effects. Although these adjustments are not complicated, a thorough discussion at this point is not warranted.

Finally, note that this project is a replacement project in the sense that the open MRI system will be replacing the current conventional MRI system. Replacement projects typically have a somewhat more complicated cash flow structure than do entirely new projects. For example, the current revenues and costs are lost to the business. Additionally, the old MRI could be sold if it is replaced.

Bayside's managers believed that these cash flows were either not material or not relevant to the analysis because (1) the current system is leased and hence will merely be returned to the owner, and (2) a competing outpatient imaging center may soon have its own open MRI system, so Bayside patients seeking an open system would be lost whether or not the hospital buys one. Thus, the cash flows were treated as if the project were a new, as opposed to a replacement, project.

(?) SELF-TEST QUESTIONS

1. Briefly, how is a project cash flow analysis constructed?

2. What are the key differences in cash flow analyses performed by investor-owned and not-for-profit businesses?

3. What is the difference between a new and a replacement project?

10.4 RISK ANALYSIS

The higher the risk associated with any investment, the higher its required rate of return. Thus, the ultimate goal in project risk analysis is to ensure that the cost of capital used as the discount rate in a project's ROI analysis properly reflects the riskiness of that project.

Generically, risk is defined as "a hazard; a peril; exposure to loss or injury." Thus, risk refers to the chance that an unfavorable event will occur. If a person engages in skydiving, he or she is taking a chance with injury or death; skydiving is risky. If a person gambles at roulette, he or she is not risking injury or death but is taking a financial risk. Even when a person invests in stocks or bonds, he or she is taking a risk in the hope of earning a positive rate of return. Similarly, when Bayside invests in new assets, such as an open MRI system, it is taking a financial risk.

To illustrate financial risk, consider two potential personal investments. The first investment consists of a one-year, $1,000 investment in a bank certificate of deposit (CD). The interest rate on the CD is 5.0 percent, so the expected interest earned at the end of one year is $1,000 × 0.050 = $50. The return on the CD is fixed by contract and, furthermore, is insured by a governmental agency. Thus, there is virtually a 100 percent probability that the investment will actually earn the 5.0 percent rate of return that is expected. In this situation, the investment is described as *risk-free*.

Now, assume that the $1,000 is invested in a biotechnology partnership that will be terminated in one year. If the partnership develops a new commercially valuable product, its rights will be sold for $2,000, producing a rate of return of 100 percent. But if nothing worthwhile is developed, the partnership will be worthless and no money will be received. The investor may expect to earn $2,000 from the partnership, but there also is a chance of losing the entire $1,000 investment. Because there is some possibility of earning a return that is far less than expected, the partnership investment is described as risky.

Thus, financial risk is related to the probability of earning a return less than expected. The greater the chance of earning a return far below that expected, the greater the amount of financial risk.

Now let's apply the concept of **financial risk** to Bayside's open MRI system project. Table 10.2 contains the project's cash flow analysis. If all of the project's component cash flows (e.g., reimbursement, volume, operating costs) were known with certainty, the project's projected profitability would be known with certainty, and hence the project would be risk-free.

However, in virtually all project analyses, future cash flows, and hence profitability, are uncertain, and in many cases highly uncertain, so risk is present. For example, forecasting patient volume for the open MRI system is not easy. If the forecasts are too high, and hence the actual (realized) volume is lower than that assumed in Table 10.1, then the

Risk-free investment

An investment that has a guaranteed (sure) return. In other words, the probability of earning the return expected is 100 percent.

realized NPV of the project would be less than the forecasted $82,493.

The nature of the component cash flow distributions and their correlations with one another determine the nature of the project's profitability distribution and hence the project's risk. In the following sections, two quantitative techniques for assessing project risk are discussed: sensitivity analysis and scenario analysis. Then, we explore a qualitative approach to risk assessment.

SENSITIVITY ANALYSIS

Historically, **sensitivity analysis** has been classified as a risk assessment tool, although it has many limitations in this regard. However, it does have significant value in project analyses, so we will discuss it in some detail here.

Many of the input variables that determine a project's cash flows are subject to uncertainty. Let's face it, some of the inputs—say, volume—may be nothing more than educated guesses. If the realized (actual) value of such a variable is different from its expected value, the project's realized profitability will differ from that expected.

> ### ! CRITICAL CONCEPT
> Financial Risk
>
> Capital investments are risky because a project's cash flows are not known with certainty when the project is being analyzed. For example, the estimate for the number of scans conducted by Bayside's new open MRI is based on historical volumes for the old system plus estimates of new volume created by the easier-to-use new system. If purchased and put into operation, the actual (realized) number of scans will likely be higher or lower than the initial estimate. The same reasoning applies to the average net reimbursement estimate, labor cost estimate, and the like. The bottom line is that the net cash flows in Table 10.2 are merely estimates of what is expected to happen financially rather than a sure bet. Because of the uncertainty in the cash flow forecasts, the $82,493 NPV (as well as the IRR) is also uncertain. After the project is completed, and hence looking back on realized results, the actual NPV of the project could be much less than expected. In fact, the project could end up being a big loser. It is this fact that makes projects risky.

Sensitivity analysis shows how much a project's profitability (NPV or IRR) will change in response to a given change in a single component cash flow (input variable), with other inputs held constant. In other words, sensitivity analysis tells us how sensitive a project's profitability is to changes in input variable values.

To illustrate sensitivity analysis, assume that Bayside's managers believe that all of the open MRI project's component cash flows (except for weekly volume and salvage value) are known with relative certainty. (For ease of illustration, we are limiting the sensitivity analysis to two variables.) The expected (most likely, or best guess) values for these variables (volume = 40 and salvage value = $750,000) were used in Table 10.2 to obtain the *base case* NPV of $82,493.

Sensitivity analysis is designed to provide managers with the answers to questions such as these: What happens to profitability if volume is more or less than the expected level? What if salvage value is more or less than expected?

Base case
In a capital investment analysis, the situation that is expected (most likely) to occur.

Sensitivity analysis is the process of assessing how changes in one variable affect another variable. In capital investment decisions, sensitivity analysis is used to determine how much a project's profitability—say, as measured by NPV—is affected when the value of an input cash flow component, such as volume, changes. The idea here is that many of the component cash flow estimates are uncertain, so the realized values for these flows may be quite different from those used in the initial analysis. The greater the sensitivity of the project's profitability to changes in the component cash flow estimates, the greater the likelihood that the project's actual profitability will be far less than expected. Sensitivity analysis is most useful in identifying cash flow components that are critical to the analysis—that is, those components that when changed have the greatest effect on profitability.

In a typical sensitivity analysis, each uncertain component cash flow is changed by a fixed percentage amount above and below its expected value, while all other component cash flows are held constant at their expected values. Thus, all input variables, except one, are held at their base case values. The resulting NPVs (or IRRs) are recorded and plotted. Table 10.3 contains the NPV sensitivity analysis for the open MRI project, assuming only two uncertain variables: volume and salvage value.

Note that the NPV is a constant $82,493 when there is no change in either of the component cash flow values. This situation occurs because a 0 percent change recreates the base case. Managers can examine values in Table 10.3 to get a feel for which component cash flow has the greatest impact on the MRI project's NPV—the larger the NPV change for a given percentage input change, the greater the impact. Such an examination shows that the MRI project's NPV is more affected by changes in volume than by changes in salvage value. This result should be somewhat intuitive because salvage value is a single cash flow in the analysis, occurring only at Year 5, whereas volume influences the net cash flow in each year of operation.

TABLE 10.3 Open MRI Project Sensitivity Analysis	Change from Base Case Level	Net Present Value	
		Volume	Salvage Value
	−30%	($814,053)	($ 57,215)
	−20	(515,193)	(10,646)
	−10	216,350	35,923
	0	82,493	82,493
	+10	381,335	129,062
	+20	680,178	175,631
	+30	979,020	222,200

Often, the results of sensitivity analyses are shown in graphical form. For example, the sensitivity analysis presented in tabular form in Table 10.3 is graphed in Figure 10.1. Here, the slopes of the lines show how sensitive the open MRI project's NPV is to changes in each of the two uncertain component inputs—the steeper the slope, the more sensitive NPV is to a change in the variable.

Figure 10.1 vividly illustrates that the open MRI project's NPV is very sensitive to the volume forecast but only mildly sensitive to the salvage value forecast. If a sensitivity plot has a negative slope, it indicates that increases in the value of that input variable decrease the project's NPV.

If two projects are being compared, the one with the steeper sensitivity lines would be regarded as riskier because a relatively small error in estimating a component cash flow—for example, volume—would produce a large error in the project's forecasted NPV. If information were available on the sensitivity of NPV to input changes for Bayside's average project, we could make similar judgments regarding the riskiness of the open MRI project relative to the hospital's average project.

Although sensitivity analysis typically is considered to be a risk assessment tool, it does have severe limitations in this role. For example, suppose Bayside had a contract with an HMO that guaranteed a minimum MRI usage at a fixed reimbursement rate. In that

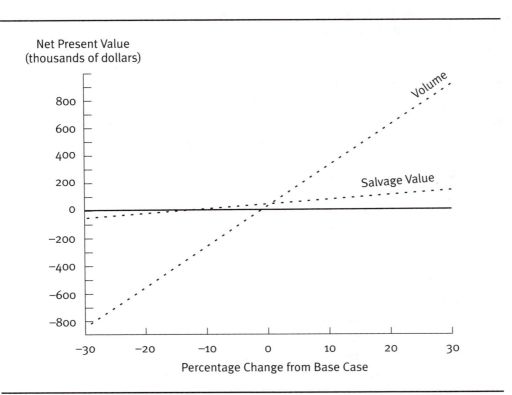

FIGURE 10.1
Open MRI Project Sensitivity Analysis Graphs

situation, the project probably would have very little risk, in spite of the fact that the sensitivity analysis showed NPV to be highly sensitive to forecasted volume.

In general, a project's risk depends on both the sensitivity of its profitability to changes in key input variables and the ranges of likely values of these variables. Because sensitivity analysis considers only the first factor, it can give misleading results. Furthermore, sensitivity analysis does not consider any interactions among the uncertain cash flow components; it considers each component independently of the others.

In spite of the shortcomings of sensitivity analysis as a risk assessment tool, it does present managers with valuable information. First, it provides breakeven information for the project's uncertain variables. For example, Table 10.3 and Figure 10.1 show that just a few percent decrease in expected volume makes the project unprofitable (a negative NPV), whereas the project remains profitable even if salvage value falls by more than 10 percent. Although somewhat rough, this breakeven information is clearly of value to Bayside's managers.

Second, and perhaps more important, sensitivity analysis identifies those cash flow components that are most critical to the analysis. By most critical, we mean those components that have the largest impact on profitability when their realized values differ from their forecasted values. For the open MRI project, volume is clearly the most critical input variable of the two being examined, so Bayside's managers should ensure that the volume estimate is the best possible.

A small overestimate in volume could make the project seem financially attractive when evaluated, yet the actual results could easily be disappointing. The concept here is that Bayside's managers have a limited amount of time to spend on analyzing the open MRI project, so they should spend their resources as productively as possible by focusing on those cash flow components that make the most difference.

In addition, sensitivity analysis can be useful after a project has been initiated. For example, assume Bayside's open MRI project was accepted and the first year's post-audit indicates that the project is not meeting financial expectations. Bayside's managers must take actions to improve the project's financial results.

But what actions should they take? Sensitivity analysis identifies the variables that have the greatest impact on profitability. Thus, managers can try to influence those variables that have the greatest potential for improving financial performance, such as volume, rather than those variables that have little impact on profitability.

SCENARIO ANALYSIS

Scenario analysis is a project risk analysis technique that considers the sensitivity of NPV to changes in uncertain cash flow components, the likely range of component values, and the interactions among components.

To conduct a scenario analysis, managers start with the base case and then pick a bad set of circumstances (e.g., low volume, low salvage value, high labor costs) and a good set (e.g., high volume, high salvage value, low labor costs). Next, managers use the component cash flow values from the bad and good circumstances (scenarios) to forecast profitability under assumptions other than those used in the base case.

To illustrate scenario analysis, again consider Bayside's open MRI project. Assume that Bayside's managers regard a drop in weekly volume below 30 scans as unlikely, and a volume above 50 is also improbable. On the other hand, salvage value could be as low as $500,000 or as high as $1 million. The most likely values for these cash flow components are 40 scans per week for volume and $750,000 for salvage value. Thus, a volume of 30 and a $500,000 salvage value define the lower bound (worst case scenario), while a volume of 50 and a salvage value of $1 million define the upper bound (best case scenario).

Bayside can now use the worst, most likely, and best case values for these cash flow components to obtain the NPV that corresponds to each scenario. Bayside's managers use a spreadsheet model to conduct the analysis, and Table 10.4 summarizes the results. The most likely (base) case results in a positive NPV; the worst case produces a negative NPV; and the best case results in a large, positive NPV.

Typically, the scenario analysis would be interpreted by Bayside's financial staff as described in the Optional Discussion box. However, scenario analysis can also be interpreted in a less mathematical way. The difference between the most likely NPV ($82,493) and the worst case NPV (-$819,844) is $902,337. The larger this difference, the greater the chance that the project will have a return far below that expected, and hence the greater the risk.

> **⚠ CRITICAL CONCEPT**
> *Scenario Analysis*
>
> Scenario analysis is a risk assessment technique that overcomes the problems associated with sensitivity analysis. In essence, scenario analysis examines the impact of several (often three) economic scenarios on a project's profitability. For example, assume a group practice is considering the purchase of an electrocardiogram (EKG) machine. The most likely (base case) estimate for volume is 200 procedures in the first year at an average reimbursement of $40 per procedure. These values result in a base case estimate of $8,000 in annual revenue. In a scenario analysis, the best case estimate may be 250 procedures at $45 and the worst case may be 150 procedures at $35. Thus, the revenue estimate is 250 x $45 = $11,250 for the best case and 150 x $35 = $5,250 for the worst case. By combining these revenue values with the best and worst case estimates for the other uncertain component cash flows, we obtain the net cash flows for all three scenarios. Once the net cash flows are forecasted, the profitability (NPV and IRR) of each scenario can be estimated. The difference between the most likely (base) case and worst case NPV (or IRR) gives managers a feel for the riskiness of the project—the greater the difference in these values, the higher the risk.

Scenario	Volume	Salvage Value	NPV
Worst case	30	$ 500,000	($819,844)
Most likely case	40	750,000	82,493
Best case	50	1,000,000	984,829

TABLE 10.4
Open MRI Project Scenario Analysis

OPTIONAL DISCUSSION Applying Statistical Concepts to Scenario Analysis

The statistical concepts of expected value and standard deviation can be applied to the data in Table 10.4 to determine the expected NPV and standard deviation of NPV. To do this, an estimate is needed of the probabilities of occurrence of the three scenarios. Suppose that Bayside's managers estimate that the following will occur: a 20 percent chance of the worst case, a 60 percent chance of the most likely (base) case, and a 20 percent chance of the best case. (Of course, it is difficult to estimate scenario probabilities with any confidence.)

Using these probabilities, the expected NPV can be found as follows:

$$\text{Expected NPV} = (0.20 \times [-\$819,844]) + (0.60 \times \$82,493) + (0.20 \times \$984,829)$$
$$= \$82,493.$$

The expected NPV in the scenario analysis is the same as the base case NPV, $82,493. The consistency of results occurs because, when coupled with the scenario probabilities, the values of the uncertain variables used in the scenario analysis—30, 40, and 50 scans for volume, and $500,000, $750,000, and $1,000,000 for salvage value—produce the same most likely values used in the base case analysis in Table 10.2.

Using the distribution of NPVs, we can calculate the standard deviation:

$$\sigma_{NPV} = [0.20 \times (-\$819,844 - \$82,49^3)2 + 0.60 \times (\$82,493 - \$82,493)^2$$
$$+ 0.20 \times (\$984,829 - \$82,493)^2]^{\frac{1}{2}}$$
$$= \$570,688.$$

The standard deviation of NPV measures the open MRI project's stand-alone risk. Bayside's managers can compare the standard deviation of NPV of this project with the uncertainty inherent in Bayside's aggregate cash flows, or average project.

Often, the coefficient of variation (CV) is used to measure the stand-alone risk of a project: $CV = \sigma_{NPV} / \text{Expected NPV} = \$570,688 / \$82,493 = 6.9$ for the

OPTIONAL DISCUSSION Applying Statistical Concepts to Scenario Analysis

open MRI project. The CV measures the risk per unit of return and hence is a better measure of comparative risk than the standard deviation, especially when projects have widely differing NPVs.

Bayside's average project has a CV in the range of 8.0 to 10.0, so the open MRI project would be judged to have below-average risk relative to the hospital's average project.

Note that the potential loss of almost $820,000 represents an estimate of the worst possible financial consequences of the MRI project. Bayside is a large hospital in sound financial condition, so it can absorb such a loss in value without much impact. Thus, the project does not represent a significant financial threat to the hospital.

Conversely, if such a loss would mean financial ruin for the hospital, its managers might be unwilling to undertake the project, regardless of its profitability under the base and best case scenarios. Note that the risk of the project is not changing in these two situations—the risk being the spread between the most likely and worst case NPVs.

The focus here is in the ability of the organization to bear the risk inherent in the project. Thus, large businesses in excellent financial condition can afford to take on more capital investment risk than can smaller businesses in poor financial condition.

While scenario analysis provides useful information about a project's risk, it is limited in two ways. First, it considers only a few possible outcomes, whereas, in reality, an almost infinite number of possibilities exist.

Second, scenario analysis implies a definite relationship among the uncertain variables. That is, the scenario analysis assumes that the worst value for volume (30 scans per week) would occur at the same time as the worst value for salvage value ($500,000) because the worst case scenario is defined by combining the worst possible value of each uncertain variable. Although this relationship (all worst values occurring together) may hold in some situations, it may not hold in others. For example, if volume is low, maybe the open MRI will have less wear and tear and hence be worth more after five years of use. The worst value for volume, then, should be coupled with the best salvage value. Conversely, poor volume may be symptomatic of poor medical effectiveness of the open MRI and hence lead to limited demand for used equipment and a low salvage value. Scenario analysis tends to create extreme profitability values for the worst and best cases because it automatically combines all worst and best input values, even if these values actually have only a remote chance of occurring together.

Qualitative risk assessment
A process for assessing project risk that focuses on qualitative factors as opposed to profit variability.

QUALITATIVE RISK ASSESSMENT

In some situations, perhaps in many, conducting a quantitative risk assessment is difficult, because predicting the scenario numbers is simply hard to do. In such situations, rather than ignore project risk, some healthcare businesses use a *qualitative risk assessment* approach. For example, Bayside uses the following questions to subjectively assess project risk:

◆ *Market share.* Does the project require additional market share or represent a new service initiative?

◆ *Scope of expertise.* Is the project outside the scope of current management expertise?

◆ *Recruitment.* Does the project require difficult-to-recruit technical specialists?

◆ *Competition.* Will the project place us in competition with a strong competitor?

◆ *Technology.* Does the project require the use of new, unproven technology?

To assess project risk, each "yes" answer is assigned one point. If the project has zero or one point, it is judged to have low risk. If it has two or three points, it is judged to have average risk, while a score of four or five points indicates high risk.

When Bayside's managers applied the qualitative risk assessment tool to the open MRI project, they assigned "no" as the answer to all questions except this one: Will the project place us in competition with a strong competitor? This question was answered "yes," under the assumption that a competing outpatient imaging center would also purchase an open MRI. Thus, with a total of one point, the project was judged to have low risk when assessed qualitatively.

Although such a subjective approach initially appears to have little theoretical foundation, a closer examination reveals that each question in the above list is tied to cash flow uncertainty. Thus, the greater the number of "yes" answers, the greater the cash flow uncertainty and hence the greater the risk of the project.

Even when a quantitative risk assessment is feasible, a separate qualitative assessment is a good idea. The value of using the qualitative risk assessment approach in conjunction with a quantitative risk assessment is that it forces managers to think about project risk in an alternative framework. If the quantitative and qualitative assessments do not agree, then clearly the project's risk assessment requires more consideration.

? SELF-TEST QUESTIONS

1. Define the concept of financial risk.

2. What makes one project riskier than another?

? SELF-TEST QUESTIONS

3. Briefly describe sensitivity analysis. Is sensitivity analysis a good risk assessment tool? If not, what is its value in the capital budgeting process?

4. Briefly describe scenario analysis. What are its strengths and weaknesses?

5. Describe qualitative risk assessment. Why does it work?

6. Assume a quantitative risk assessment has been conducted on a project. Is a qualitative risk assessment necessary?

10.5 INCORPORATING RISK INTO THE DECISION PROCESS

It may be possible to reach the general conclusion that one project is more or less risky than another or to compare the riskiness of a project with the business as a whole. But it is difficult to develop a really good measure of project risk. This lack of confidence in measuring project risk adds to the difficulties in incorporating differential risk into the capital budgeting decision.

THE RISK-ADJUSTED DISCOUNT RATE METHOD

The method used most often to incorporate risk into the capital investment decision process is the *risk-adjusted discount rate (RADR)* method. Here, the project's most likely (base case) cash flows are discounted using a rate based on the project's risk assessment.

> **Risk-adjusted discount rate**
> A risk adjustment method that changes the discount rate to reflect the unique riskiness of the project being analyzed.

The starting point for the risk adjustment is the corporate cost of capital, which is covered in detail in Chapter 8. Remember that this rate reflects the organization's aggregate risk—that is, the riskiness of the business's average project. In project risk analysis, a project's risk is assessed relative to the firm's average project. The corporate cost of capital is then adjusted to reflect any differential risk, resulting in a **project cost of capital**.

In general, above-average-risk projects are assigned a project cost of capital that is higher than the corporate cost of capital, average-risk projects are evaluated at the corporate cost of capital, and below-average-risk projects are assigned a discount rate that is less than the corporate cost of capital.

Although widely used, the RADR method does have some disadvantages. First, there is no theoretical basis for the size of the adjustment, so the amount remains a matter of judgment. Second, the RADR method combines time value and the adjustment for risk into a single discount rate applied to all cash flows. By lumping together risk and time value, the risk premium is compounded over time; just as interest compounds over time, so does the risk premium. Thus, use of the RADR method implies that risk increases with time, which imposes a greater burden on long-term projects. The end result is that, all else the same, short-term projects will tend to look better financially than long-term projects. In general, this is not a problem, because long-term projects typically will be riskier than

CRITICAL CONCEPT
Project Cost of Capital

The project cost of capital is the discount rate that reflects the unique riskiness of the project being analyzed. Usually, the project cost of capital is estimated by adding or subtracting a specified number of percentage points from the corporate cost of capital. If the project is assessed to be riskier than average, the project cost of capital is greater than the corporate cost of capital. If the project is less risky, the project cost of capital is less than the corporate cost of capital.

short-term projects because of the difficulties in forecasting cash flows well into the future.

MAKING THE FINAL DECISION ON THE OPEN MRI PROJECT

The business's corporate cost of capital provides the basis for estimating the project cost of capital (discount rate). Unfortunately, there is no good way of specifying exactly how much the corporate cost of capital should be adjusted to account for project risk. Given the present state of the art, risk adjustments are necessarily judgmental and somewhat arbitrary.

Bayside's standard procedure is to add 4 percentage points to its 10 percent corporate cost of capital when evaluating higher-risk projects and to subtract 2 percentage points when evaluating lower-risk projects. Because Bayside's open MRI project was judged to have below-average risk, the project cost of capital is reduced to 10% – 2% = 8%. Thus, the final NPV estimate, which incorporates the risk analysis, is $243,969. Because the NPV, after adjusting for risk, is larger than before ($82,493), the risk analysis makes the open MRI project even more attractive financially than indicated in Chapter 9.

But what if the project had been judged to have above-average risk? In this situation, the project cost of capital would be 10% + 4% = 14%, and the project's expected (base case) net cash flows shown in Table 10.2 would be discounted at that project cost of capital. The resultant NPV is -$200,017, so the project becomes unprofitable if the analysis were to judge the project as having above-average risk.

Bayside's managers might still decide to go ahead with the open MRI project for other reasons, but at least they would know that its expected profitability is not sufficient to make up for its riskiness.

? SELF-TEST QUESTIONS

1. Explain the risk-adjusted discount rate (RADR) method for incorporating risk in the capital investment decision process.

2. What assumptions about time and risk are inherent in the RADR method?

3. What is the difference between the corporate cost of capital and a project cost of capital?

4. Is the risk adjustment objective or subjective?

⊛ INDUSTRY PRACTICE Risk Analysis in Healthcare Organizations

Several surveys have been conducted over the last 20 years to assess how businesses, including healthcare organizations, assess and incorporate risk into capital investment decisions.

Most organizations consider a variety of factors when assessing project risk, including market characteristics, uncertainty of cash flow estimates, and strategic fit. When examining cash flow uncertainty, most attention is paid to the estimates for cost, volume, and reimbursement.

Although there is general agreement that the discount rate used in capital investment analyses should be adjusted for project risk, there is less agreement on the method used. However, many organizations set a range of discount rates (for example, one used a range of 10.5 to 21.5 percent) and then applied these rates to projects on the basis of relative risk. Higher-risk projects are assigned higher rates, and vice versa.

Still, the entire capital investment process brings out many concerns. For example, one chief financial officer stated: "I do not believe in NPV. You can make any project look good or bad by selecting the right discount rate. Or, you can spend all of your time arguing about which discount rate is correct." Although this statement has merit, we should not denigrate the entire process because of the difficulties involved. Clearly, some projects are suitable for a quantitative risk analysis, as described in this chapter, and other projects are not. One of the keys to making good analyses is to be able to make such distinctions.

Note: This industry practice is based on information in Reiter, K. L., D. G. Smith, J. R. C. Wheeler, and H. L. Rivenson. 2000. "Capital Investment Strategies in Health Care Systems." *Journal of Health Care Finance* (Summer): 31–41.

10.6 AN OVERVIEW OF THE CAPITAL INVESTMENT DECISION PROCESS

For capital planning purposes, healthcare managers need to forecast the total number of projects that will be undertaken and the dollar amount of capital needed to fund these projects. The list of projects to be undertaken is called the *capital budget*.

While every healthcare provider estimates its optimal capital budget in its unique way, some procedures are common to all firms. This process is illustrated by the procedures followed by the Dallas Medical Group:

Capital budget
A plan (budget) that outlines a business's expected future expenditures on new capital assets, such as land, buildings, and equipment.

◆ *Estimate the corporate cost of capital.* The practice manager estimates the group's corporate cost of capital. As discussed in Chapter 8, this estimate depends on market conditions, the business's inherent risk, and its optimal capital structure.

◆ *Assign project costs of capital.* Each project is assigned a project cost of capital that reflects its risk relative to the overall business.

◆ *Calculate NPVs.* The project costs of capital are used to discount each project's base case net cash flows. From a purely financial standpoint, all projects with positive NPVs are acceptable, while those with negative NPVs should be rejected.

◆ *Consider the relevant subjective factors.* Subjective factors are considered, and these factors may result in a capital budget that differs from a budget based solely on financial considerations. For example, could the project significantly increase the group's liability exposure? Conversely, does the project have any strategic or social value or other attributes that could affect its acceptability? Typically, if the project involves new services and is large (in capital requirements) when compared to the group's average project, then the additional subjective factors will be important to the final decision.

Ultimately, capital budgeting decisions require an analysis of a mix of objective and subjective factors, such as risk, profitability, medical staff and patient needs, and social value. The process is not precise, and often there is a temptation to ignore one or more important factors because they are so nebulous and difficult to measure. Despite the imprecision and subjectivity, a project's risk, as well as its other attributes, should be assessed and incorporated into the capital investment decision process.

(?) SELF-TEST QUESTIONS

1. Describe a typical capital investment decision process.

2. Are decisions made solely on the basis of quantitative factors? Explain your answer.

10.7 CAPITAL RATIONING

Standard capital investment decision processes assume that businesses can raise virtually unlimited amounts of capital to meet investment needs. Presumably, as long as a business is investing the funds in profitable (positive NPV) projects, it should be able to raise the debt and equity needed to fund all worthwhile projects.

This picture of the capital financing/capital investment process is probably appropriate for most large investor-owned businesses. However, not-for-profit businesses do not have unlimited access to capital. Their equity capital is limited primarily to retentions and contributions, and their debt capital is limited to the amount supported by the equity capital base. In addition, small businesses typically do not have unlimited supplies of capital. Thus, many businesses face periods in which the capital needed for investment in new projects exceeds the amount available. This situation is called *capital rationing*.

If capital rationing exists, from a purely financial perspective it is best to accept the set of projects that maximizes aggregate NPV and still meets the capital constraint. This approach could be called "getting the most bang for the buck" because it picks projects that have the most positive impact on the organization's financial condition. Of course, priority may be assigned to some low or even negative NPV projects because of mission considerations, which is fine as long as these projects are offset by the selection of profitable projects to sustain the business's financial strength.

Capital rationing
The condition of having more acceptable projects than funds (capital) to undertake those projects.

(?) SELF-TEST QUESTIONS

1. What is capital rationing?

2. From a financial perspective, how are projects chosen when capital rationing exists?

THEME WRAP-UP ESTIMATING A PROJECT'S CASH FLOWS AND ASSESSING RISK

At the beginning of Chapter 9, we introduced a proposal by Palm Coast Radiology Associates that Bayside Memorial Hospital purchase a new, $2.5 million open MRI system. Although the medical benefits of the new system are clear, there were concerns expressed about the financial implications of the purchase.

To begin, Bayside's managers conducted a base case analysis assuming that the project had average risk. Among the results was an NPV of $82,493. Then, they performed a project risk analysis, first using sensitivity analysis to identify the key cash flow components. (For ease of illustration, we only examined two components of sensitivity analysis here: volume and salvage value.) After conducting scenario and qualitative analyses, the managers concluded that the project has below-average risk. Thus, the 10 percent corporate cost of capital was adjusted downward to obtain an 8 percent project cost of capital, resulting in a final NPV estimate of $243,969.

After all factors (including recommendations from the physicians of Palm Coast Radiology Associates) were considered, and after the estimation and analysis processes were explained to Dr. Fisher, Bayside decided to go ahead with the open MRI project. Bayside's new MRI system went into service one full year before the competition (the outpatient imaging center) brought its own system to the marketplace.

Today, the open MRI system is still going strong. Clearly, Bayside's managers made the right decision.

KEY CONCEPTS

This chapter discusses project cash flow estimation and risk analysis. Here are the key concepts:

➤ The most critical and most difficult step in analyzing a capital investment proposal is estimating the *incremental cash flows* for the project.

➤ In determining incremental cash flows, *opportunity costs* (cash flows forgone by using an asset) must be considered, but *sunk costs* (cash outlays that cannot be recouped) are not included. Furthermore, any impact of the project on the firm's *other projects* must be included in the analysis.

➤ A project may have some *strategic value* that is not accounted for in the estimated cash flows. At a minimum, strategic value should be noted and considered qualitatively in the analysis.

➤ The *effects of inflation* must be considered in project analyses. The best procedure is to build inflation effects directly into the component cash flow estimates.

➤ Project risk is associated with the chance of earning a return less than that expected. The greater the probability of a return far below expected, the higher the risk. Two techniques are commonly used to *assess* a project's risk: (1) sensitivity analysis and (2) scenario analysis.

➤ *Sensitivity analysis* shows how much a project's profitability (for example, as measured by NPV) changes in response to a given change in an input variable such as volume, with other things held constant. Although its use in risk assessment is limited, it is a valuable tool for identifying a project's critical component cash flows.

➤ *Scenario analysis* defines a project's best, most likely, and worst cases and then uses these data to assess risk.

➤ In many situations, conducting a quantitative project risk assessment is impractical. In these cases, many healthcare businesses use a *qualitative approach* to risk assessment.

➤ Projects generally are classified as high risk, average risk, or low risk relative to the business's average project. Higher-risk projects are evaluated at a *project cost of capital* that is greater than the firm's corporate cost of capital. Average-risk projects are evaluated at the firm's corporate cost of capital, while lower-risk projects are evaluated at a rate less than the corporate cost of capital.

➤ The *capital budget* is the list of all projects expected to be undertaken during the next planning period.

➤ *Capital rationing* occurs when a business does not have access to sufficient capital to fund all profitable projects. Under these conditions, the best financial outcome results from accepting the set of projects that has the highest aggregate NPV.

➤ Ultimately, capital budgeting decisions require an analysis of a mix of objective and subjective factors such as risk, profitability, medical staff and patient needs, and service to the community. The process is not precise, but good managers do their best to ensure that none of the relevant factors is ignored.

This chapter concludes our discussion of financing and capital investment decisions. In Chapter 11, we address how businesses report financial results.

END-OF-CHAPTER QUESTIONS

10.1 Briefly define the following cash flow estimation concepts:
- a. Incremental cash flow
- b. Sunk cost
- c. Opportunity cost
- d. Strategic value
- e. Inflation effects

10.2 Define financial risk. Why is risk analysis so important to capital investment decisions?

10.3 a. Briefly describe sensitivity analysis.
- b. What are its strengths and weaknesses?

10.4 a. Briefly describe scenario analysis.
- b. What are its strengths and weaknesses?

10.5 Describe the qualitative approach to risk assessment. Why does this approach, which does not rely on numerical data, work?

10.6 How is project risk incorporated into the capital investment decision?

10.7 What is the difference between the corporate cost of capital and a project cost of capital?

10.8 What is meant by the term capital rationing? From a purely financial standpoint, what is the best capital budget under capital rationing?

10.9 Santa Roberta Clinic has estimated its corporate cost of capital to be 11 percent. What are reasonable values for the project costs of capital for lower-risk, average-risk, and higher-risk projects?

END-OF-CHAPTER PROBLEMS

10.1 Great Lakes Clinic has been asked to provide exclusive healthcare services for next year's World Exposition. Although flattered by the request, the clinic's managers want to conduct a financial analysis of the project. An up-front cost of $160,000 is needed to get the clinic in operation. Then, a net cash inflow of $1 million is expected from operations in each of the two years of the exposition. However, the clinic has to pay the organizers of the exposition a fee for the marketing value of the opportunity. This fee, which must be paid at the end of the second year, is $2 million.

a. What are the net cash flows associated with the project?

b. What is the project's IRR?

c. Assuming a project cost of capital of 10 percent, what is the project's NPV?

10.2 California Imaging Center, a not-for-profit business, is evaluating the purchase of new diagnostic equipment. The equipment, which costs $600,000, has an expected life of five years and an estimated salvage value of $200,000 at that time. The equipment is expected to be used 15 times a day for 250 days a year for each year of the project's life. On average, each procedure is expected to generate $80 in cash collections during the first year of use. Thus, net revenues for Year 1 are estimated at 15 x 250 x $80 = $300,000.

Labor and maintenance costs are expected to be $100,000 during the first year of operation, while utilities will cost another $10,000 and cash overhead will increase by $5,000 in Year 1. The cost for expendable supplies is expected to average $5 per procedure during the first year. All costs and revenues are expected to increase at a 5 percent inflation rate after the first year.

The center's corporate cost of capital is 10 percent.

a. Estimate the project's net cash flows over its five-year estimated life. (Hint: Use the following format as a guide.)

	Year					
	0	1	2	3	4	5
Equipment cost						
Net revenues						
Less: Labor/maintenance costs						
Utilities costs						
Supplies						
Incremental overhead						
Operating income						
Equipment salvage value	___	___	___	___	___	___
Net cash flow	═══	═══	═══	═══	═══	═══

b. What are the project's NPV and IRR? (Assume for now that the project has average risk.)

c. Assume the project is assessed to have high risk and California Imaging Center adds or subtracts 3 percentage points to adjust for project risk. Now, what is the project's NPV? Does the risk assessment change how the project's IRR is interpreted?

10.3 You have been asked to evaluate the proposed acquisition of a new clinical laboratory test system. The system's price is $50,000, and it will cost another $10,000 for transportation and installation. The system is expected to be sold after three years because the laboratory is being moved at that time. The best estimate of the system's salvage value after three years of use is $20,000. The system will have no effect on volume or reimbursement (and hence revenues), but it is expected to save $20,000 per year in operating costs. The not-for-profit business's corporate cost of capital is 10 percent, and the standard risk adjustment is 4 percentage points.

a. What is the project's net investment outlay at Year 0?

b. What are the project's operating cash flows in Years 1, 2, and 3?

c. What is the terminal cash flow at the end of Year 3?

d. If the project has average risk, is it expected to be profitable?

e. What if the project is judged to have lower-than-average risk? Higher-than-average risk?

10.4 The staff of Jefferson Medical Services has estimated the following net cash flows for a food services operation that it may open in its outpatient clinic:

Year	Expected Net Cash Flow
0	($100,000)
1	30,000
2	30,000
3	30,000
4	30,000
5	30,000
5 (salvage value)	20,000

The Year 0 cash flow is the net investment outlay, while the final amount is the terminal cash flow. (The clinic is expected to move to a new building in five years.) All other flows represent net operating cash flows. Jefferson's corporate cost of capital is 10 percent.

a. What is the project's IRR?

b. Assuming the project has average risk, what is its NPV?

c. Now, assume that the operating cash flows in Years 1 through 5 could be as low as $20,000 or as high as $40,000. Furthermore, the salvage value cash flow at the end of Year 5 could be as low as $0 or as high as $30,000. What is the worst case and best case IRR? The worst case and best case NPV?

10.5 (This optional problem requires statistics know-how.) Heywood Home Healthcare is evaluating a project with the following net cash flows and probabilities:

Year	Prob = 0.2	Prob = 0.6	Prob = 0.2
0	($100,000)	($100,000)	($100,000)
1	20,000	30,000	40,000
2	20,000	30,000	40,000
3	20,000	30,000	40,000
4	20,000	30,000	40,000
5	30,000	40,000	50,000

The Year 5 values include salvage value. Heywood's corporate cost of capital is 10 percent.

a. What is the project's most likely (base case) NPV assuming average risk?

b. What are the project's most likely, worst, and best case NPVs?

c. What is the project's expected NPV on the basis of the scenario analysis?

d. What is the project's standard deviation of NPV?

e. Assume that Heywood's managers judge the project to have lower-than-average risk. Furthermore, the company's policy is to adjust the corporate cost of capital up or down by 3 percentage points to account for differential risk. Is the project financially attractive?

10.6 The managers of United Medtronics are evaluating the following four projects for the coming budget period. The firm's corporate cost of capital is 14 percent.

Project	Cost	IRR
A	$15,000	17%
B	15,000	16
C	12,000	15
D	20,000	13

a. What is the firm's capital budget?

b. Now, suppose Medtronics's managers want to consider differential risk in the capital budgeting process. Project A has average risk, B has below-average risk, C has above-average risk, and D has average risk. What is the firm's optimal capital budget when differential risk is considered? (Hint: The firm's managers lower the IRR of high-risk projects by 3 percentage points and raise the IRR of low-risk projects by the same amount.)

PART IV

REPORTING RESULTS

In Part IV, our focus is on how businesses report overall financial results and how those results are analyzed to assess financial condition. A business's financial status is reported in its financial statements—the three most important are the income statement, the balance sheet, and the statement of cash flows.

Chapter 11 provides an introduction to financial statements as a whole and to the income statement (which reports profitability) specifically.

Chapter 12 covers the balance sheet (which reports a business's assets and the way those assets are financed) and the statement of cash flows (which concerns the cash flowing into and out of a business). Together, Chapters 11 and 12 offer a comprehensive treatment of the format and content of a business's financial statements.

Chapter 13 illustrates various techniques that are frequently used to gain better insights into a business's financial condition. Financial statements contain a great deal of information about a business's financial condition, but much of this information is masked by the vast amount of data reported.

CHAPTER 11

REPORTING PROFITS

CONSTRUCTING AN INCOME STATEMENT

Five years ago, Lori Gibbs, a nurse practitioner, opened Park Ridge Homecare, a not-for-profit home health agency located in a suburb of Chicago. After working for almost 15 years at a gerontology group practice, she felt ready to embark on a new career that would combine her nursing knowledge with a desire to run her own business.

In the beginning, the business provided basic healthcare services—such as wound and dressing care, catheter care, IV (intravenous) therapy, and colostomy care—to patients that are homebound. To support these services, the business sold medical supplies and equipment such as bandages, IV solutions, wheelchairs, and walkers. After the first year, the business expanded to offer additional services, including physical, occupational, and speech therapy.

The first several years of the business were hectic. In fact, Lori devoted most of her time to the work, often putting in 12 or more hours per day. Much of her effort involved fundraising, and she realized that running a start-up business was no piece of cake. Her time off was limited to emergencies and a few days here and there. However, all of her work eventually paid off—the business prospered, and she was able to hire an administrator to handle day-to-day operations.

Now, Lori is considering opening a second location in Barrington, a relatively affluent suburb about 20 miles from Park Ridge. The success of Park Ridge Homecare made her feel confident that she can start a second business. However, rather than struggle with fundraising, as she did for the first location, she wants to use the financial resources of the Park Ridge business to open the Barrington site.

This is the question Lori faces: What is the current financial condition of Park Ridge Homecare, and can it be used to support the opening of a second location?

By the end of the chapter, you will learn how Park Ridge Homecare reports its profitability and get an idea of how to convert profit to cash flow. By the end of Part IV, you will be able to assess the financial condition of a business on the basis of the data reported in its financial statements.

LEARNING OBJECTIVES

After studying this chapter, you will be able to

➤ Explain why financial statements are important to managers and to outside parties.

➤ Discuss the basic concepts behind the creation of financial statements.

➤ Describe the components of the income statement (revenues, expenses, and profitability) and the relationships among these components.

➤ Differentiate among operating income, net income, and cash flow.

11.1 INTRODUCTION

When you think about a healthcare business, what do you visualize? Most people see buildings, equipment, and people. What we often do not readily consider are the costs involved—for example, salaries, medical supplies, and interest on debt financing. To be successful, these costs must be covered by revenues from patients and third-party payers (private and public insurance). The bottom line here is that a large number of economic (financial) events support the physical elements (facilities and people) of the business.

In this chapter, we begin our discussion of how an organization reports its financial status. By the time you finish Chapter 13, you will have a good feel for financial reporting and how these reports can be used to assess a business's financial condition.

Financial accounting
The field of accounting that focuses on the measurement and communication of the economic events and status of an entire organization.

11.2 FINANCIAL ACCOUNTING

Financial accounting involves identifying, measuring, recording, and communicating the economic events and status of an organization. This information is summarized and presented in a set of **financial statements**, the three most important of which are the income statement, the balance sheet, and the statement of cash flows. Because these statements communicate financial information, financial accounting is often called "the language of business."

Most people consider only the actual statements, such as the income statement shown in Table 11.1, when looking for financial data.

> ### ⓘ CRITICAL CONCEPT
> #### Financial Statements
>
> Using tables and footnotes, financial statements report the financial status of an organization. The three most important financial statements are the income statement, the balance sheet, and the statement of cash flows. Financial statements provide information about the profitability, cash flows, assets, and liabilities of a business that is useful to a wide range of users, including investors and managers.

However, the notes that follow the statements contain a wealth of information as well. These notes, commonly called *footnotes*, provide details that are left out of the primary documents. The footnote system ensures that important information is provided to financial statement users without clogging up the actual statements with excessive detail.

The predominant users of financial statements are *stakeholders*—parties who have a financial interest in the organization and hence are concerned with its economic welfare. In a not-for-profit organization, such as a community hospital, stakeholders include managers, staff physicians, employees, suppliers, creditors, patients, and even the community at large. Investor-owned organizations, such as a medical practice, have essentially the same set of stakeholders, plus the owners.

Although financial statements were developed primarily to meet the information needs of outside parties, the owners and managers of an organization, including its board of directors (trustees), also are important users of these statements. After all, managers are charged with ensuring that the organization has the financial strength to accomplish its mission. Managers are involved not only in creating financial statements but also in assessing

Footnotes
The notes that accompany the financial statements to explain and amplify the information presented in the statements.

Stakeholder
An individual (or business) that has an interest in an organization. For example, owners (in for-profit businesses), managers, suppliers, and patients.

Annual report
A report issued annually by a business that contains descriptive information about operations over the past year and several years of historical financial statements.

current financial condition and formulating plans to ensure that the organization will be able to support its mission in the future.

Financial statements usually are distributed to the public as part of a business's *annual report*. Many large businesses, both for-profit and not-for-profit, make their annual reports available on their websites. In addition, for-profit corporations with publicly traded stock must submit financial information, including financial statements, to the Securities and Exchange Commission, which in turn makes the information available to the public.

? SELF-TEST QUESTIONS

1. What is the purpose of a business's financial statements?

2. Who are the primary users of financial statements?

11.3 HISTORICAL FOUNDATION

Financial statements can be easily regarded as mere pieces of paper with numbers. However, if you know how and why financial statements were developed and used, you can better understand what happens within a business and why financial statements play an important role.

Thousands of years ago, individuals or families were self-contained in the sense that they gathered their own food, made their own clothes, and built their own shelters. When specialization began, some individuals became good at hunting, others at making arrowheads, others at making clothing, and so on. With specialization came trade, initially by bartering one type of goods for another.

At first, each producer worked alone, and trade was strictly local. Over time, some people set up production shops that employed workers, simple forms of money were developed, and trade expanded beyond the local area. As these simple economies expanded, more formal forms of money developed and a primitive form of banking began, with wealthy merchants lending profits from past dealings to enterprising shop owners and traders who needed money to expand their operations.

When the first loans were made, lenders could physically inspect borrowers' assets and judge the likelihood of repayment. Eventually, though, lending became much more complex. Industrial borrowers were developing large factories, merchants were acquiring fleets of ships and wagons, and loans were being made to finance business activities at distant locations. At that point, lenders could no longer easily inspect the assets that backed their loans, and they needed a practical way of summarizing the value of those assets.

Also, certain loans were made on the basis of a share of the profits of the business, so a uniform, widely accepted method for expressing income was necessary. In addition, owners required reports to see how effectively their own enterprises were being operated, and governments needed information for use in assessing taxes. For all these reasons, a need arose for financial statements, for accountants to prepare the statements, and for auditors to verify the accuracy of the accountants' work.

The economic systems of the industrialized countries have grown enormously since the early days, and financial statements have become much more complex. However, the original reasons for these statements still apply: Bankers and other investors need the information to make intelligent investment decisions, managers rely on it to operate their organizations efficiently, and taxing authorities use it to assess taxes in an equitable manner.

Unfortunately, many problems can arise when translating physical assets and economic events into accounting numbers. Nevertheless, that is what healthcare businesses must do when they construct financial statements. To illustrate the translation problem, the numbers used to reflect a business's assets and liabilities generally reflect historical costs and prices. However, inventories may be spoiled, obsolete, or even missing; land, buildings, and equipment may have current values that are much higher or lower than their historical costs; and money owed to the business may be uncollectible.

Also, some liabilities—such as obligations to make lease payments—may not even show up in the numbers. Similarly, costs that are reported may be understated or overstated, and some costs, such as depreciation, do not even represent current cash expenses. When examining a set of financial statements, you should keep in mind the physical reality that underlies the numbers and recognize that many problems can occur in the translation process.

(?) SELF-TEST QUESTIONS

1. What are the historical foundations of financial statements?

2. Do any problems arise when translating physical assets and economic events into monetary units? Give one or two illustrations to support your answer.

11.4 FINANCIAL STATEMENT REGULATION AND STANDARDS

As a consequence of the Great Depression of the 1930s, which caused many businesses to fail with subsequent large losses to investors, the federal government began regulating the form and content of financial information reported by businesses. This regulation is based on the theory that financial information constructed and presented according to standardized rules allows investors and other stakeholders to make the best informed decisions.

Securities and Exchange Commission (SEC)
The government agency that regulates the sale of securities and the content and format of financial statements.

Generally accepted accounting principles (GAAP)
The set of guidelines that have evolved over time that prescribe the content and format of financial statements.

External audit
An examination of a business's financial statements by an outside party to ensure that the statements follow GAAP principles and are a fair representation of the economic status of the business.

The *Securities and Exchange Commission (SEC)*, an independent regulatory agency of the U.S. government, was given the authority to establish and enforce the form and content of financial statements for large, stockholder-owned corporations. In addition, not-for-profit corporations must file financial statements with state authorities that conform to SEC standards. Most for-profit small businesses that are not technically bound by SEC-established guidelines still follow these standards to ensure uniformity of presentation of financial data. The end result is that most businesses create SEC-conforming financial statements.

Rather than directly manage the process, the SEC relies on other organizations, such as the Financial Accounting Standards Board (FASB) and the American Institute of Certified Public Accountants (AICPA) to develop and implement the rules and regulations. Over time, the regulating organizations developed guidelines called *generally accepted accounting principles (GAAP)*. GAAP can be thought of as a set of objectives, conventions, and principles that have evolved through the years to guide the preparation and presentation of financial statements. In essence, GAAP set the rules for preparing financial statements.

For large organizations, the final step in the financial statement quality-assurance process is the *external audit*, which is performed by an independent (outside) accounting firm. The results of the external audit are reported in a letter attached to the financial statements stating whether or not the statements are judged to be a fair presentation of the business's financial status as specified by GAAP.

The preparation of financial statements is as much art as it is science. Furthermore, the GAAP in force today represent years of negotiation, compromise, and interpretation, and the organizations involved are continuously reviewing and revising the standards to ensure that they stay relevant as business operations and financing evolve over time.

(?) SELF-TEST QUESTIONS

1. Why are widely accepted principles important for measuring and recording economic events?

2. What does GAAP stand for, and what is its primary purpose?

3. What is the purpose of the auditor's opinion?

11.5 REPORTING METHODS

Two different methods can be used to prepare financial statements: cash accounting and accrual accounting. Although each method has its own set of advantages and disadvantages, GAAP require the accrual method, so it dominates the preparation of financial statements. Still, many small businesses use the cash method, and knowledge of the cash method helps our understanding of the accrual method, so we will discuss both methods here.

CASH ACCOUNTING

Under **cash accounting**, economic events are recognized when a financial transaction occurs. For example, suppose Sunnyvale Clinic, a large multispecialty group practice, provided services to a patient in December 2008. At that time, the clinic billed the insurer, Blue Cross/Blue Shield of Florida, $700, which represents the full amount that the insurer is obligated to pay. However, Sunnyvale did not receive payment from the insurer until February 2009.

If it used cash accounting, the $700 payment obligation on the part of the insurer would not appear in Sunnyvale's 2008 financial statements. The books would be closed on December 31, and the $700 payment expected from Blue Cross/Blue Shield of Florida would be nowhere in sight! Rather, the revenue would be recognized (included in the financial statements) when the cash was actually received in February 2009.

The core argument in favor of cash accounting is that the most important financial event is the receipt of cash, not the provision of the service and the resulting obligation to pay.

Similarly, Sunnyvale's costs of providing services would be reported when the cash is physically paid out: Inventory costs would be recognized as supplies are purchased, labor costs would be recognized when employees are paid, new equipment purchases would be recognized when the invoices are paid, and so on. To put it simply, cash accounting records the actual flow of money into and out of a business.

There are two advantages to cash accounting:

◆ It is simple and easy to understand. No complex rules are required for the preparation of financial statements.

◆ It is closely aligned to accounting for tax purposes, and hence cash accounting statements are easy to translate into income tax filing data.

Because of these advantages, a large number of medical practices—typically smaller ones—use cash accounting. However, cash accounting has one big disadvantage: It does not present information on a business's revenue or cost obligations, which clearly affect financial condition.

CRITICAL CONCEPT
Cash Accounting Versus Accrual Accounting

Reporting financial transactions can be done in two ways. Under cash accounting, economic events are defined by the transfer of cash. Thus, revenues are reported when the payments for services are actually received and costs are reported when the payments are made. Under accrual accounting, economic events are defined by the creation of payment obligations. Revenues are reported when the service is rendered (payment obligation is created), and costs are reported when the obligation to pay is created. Cash accounting is simpler and closely mimics the data needed for income tax filing, but accrual accounting creates statements that better represent the financial status of the business. Because GAAP require accrual accounting, most businesses, including both for-profit and not-for-profit, use this method. However, many small businesses, which do not have to provide financial statements to the public, use cash accounting.

ACCRUAL ACCOUNTING

Under **accrual accounting**, the economic event that creates the financial transaction, rather than the transaction itself, is the basis for reporting. When applied to revenues, the accrual concept implies that revenue earned does not necessarily correspond to the receipt of cash. Why? Earned revenue is recognized in financial statements when a service has been provided that creates an expectation of payment, rather than when payment is actually received.

For healthcare providers, the payment obligation typically falls on the patient, a third-party payer, or both. If the obligation is satisfied immediately, such as when a patient makes full payment at the time the service is rendered, the revenue is in the form of cash. Thus, the revenue is reported whether cash accounting or accrual accounting is used. However, in most situations, the bulk of the payment for services is not received until later—perhaps several months after the service is provided. In this situation, the revenue created by the service does not create an immediate cash payment.

Consider the Sunnyvale example presented in the last section. Although the services were provided in December 2008, the clinic did not receive its $700 payment until February 2009. Sunnyvale's accounting (fiscal) year ended on December 31, so the clinic's books were closed after the revenue obligation was created but before the cash was received. But, because Sunnyvale uses accrual accounting, it reported this $700 of revenue on its 2008 financial statements even though no cash was collected. Under cash accounting, the $700 in revenues would not be reported until 2009, when the cash was actually received. (Note that when accrual accounting is used, the fact that the $700 was not actually received in 2008 will be disclosed elsewhere in the financial statements.)

The accrual accounting concept also applies to expenses. To illustrate, assume that Sunnyvale had payroll obligations of $50,000 for employees' work during the last week of 2008 that would not be paid until the first payday in 2009. Because the employees actually performed the work, the obligation to pay the salaries was created in 2008. Thus, the $50,000 expense would be reported in 2008 even though no cash payment will be made until 2009 (the next accounting period). (The fact that the cash has not actually been paid out will also be disclosed elsewhere in the financial statements.)

As we discuss the specific financial statements in detail, remember the difference between cash and accrual accounting. This knowledge will make it much easier for you to understand and interpret the statements.

? SELF-TEST QUESTIONS

1. Briefly explain the difference between cash and accrual accounting.

2. Why do GAAP favor accrual over cash accounting?

11.6 INCOME STATEMENT BASICS

In this section, we begin our discussion on the content and interpretation of a business's financial statements. Unfortunately, the financial statements of large organizations can be long and complex, and there is significant leeway regarding the format used, even within healthcare organizations. Thus, to keep our discussion manageable, we provide simplified illustrations of the key issues.

The most frequently asked, and perhaps the most important, question about an organization's financial status is, Is it making money? The **income statement** summarizes the operations of an organization with a focus on its revenues, expenses, and profitability. Thus, the income statement is also called the **statement of operations** or statement of revenues and expenses.

To illustrate, consider the income statements of Park Ridge Homecare in Table 11.1. Most financial statements contain two years of data, with the most recent year presented first. The idea here is that newer data are more important than older data, so the statements are listed in descending order of age.

The title tells us that these are annual income statements, ending on December 31, for the years 2008 and 2007. Whereas the balance sheet, which is covered in Chapter 12, reports a business's financial position at a single point in time, the income statement contains operational results over a specified period of time. Because these income statements are part of Park Ridge Homecare's annual report, the time period is one year. (Most businesses also prepare quarterly income statements, and many prepare monthly statements.)

! CRITICAL CONCEPT
Income Statement (Statement of Operations)

The income statement (statement of operations or statement of revenues and expenses) reports the results of operations of a business over some period of time—often one year. The three major sections are revenues, expenses, and profitability (which is the difference between revenues and expenses). Many healthcare businesses create income statements that report two different types of profitability: (1) profits that stem solely from patient service activities, and (2) profits from all activities. Other businesses report only total profits. Because the income statement itself only summarizes the financial results of business operations, a great deal of explanatory and supplementary information is contained in the statement's footnotes.

TABLE 11.1
Park Ridge Home-
care Statements of
Operations for
Years Ended
December 31,
2008 and 2007 (in
thousands)

	2008	2007
Revenues:		
Net patient service revenue	$4,042	$2,687
Other operating revenue	27	32
Total revenues	$4,069	$2,719
Expenses:		
Salaries and benefits	$2,714	$1,835
Supplies and drugs	1,042	675
Insurance	90	83
Provision for bad debts	46	21
Depreciation	21	15
Interest	16	19
Total expenses	$3,929	$2,648
Operating income	$ 140	$ 71
Nonoperating income:		
Contributions	$ 10	$ 22
Investment income	13	6
Total nonoperating income	$ 23	$ 28
Net income (excess of revenues over expenses)	$ 163	$ 99

Also, note that the dollar amounts reported are listed in thousands of dollars, so the $4,042 reported as net patient service revenue for 2008 is actually $4,042,000.

The core components of the income statement are straightforward: revenues, expenses, and profitability. In this illustration, there are two profitability measures—one based solely on operating revenues, called operating income, and the other based on total revenues, called net income (by for-profits) and excess of revenues over expenses (by not-for-profits).

Note that profitability, as measured either by operating income or net income, may be positive or negative. When expenses exceed revenues, the result is an operating loss or net loss. Operating income and net income are important measures of a business's profitability.

(Several other measures of profitability are discussed in Chapter 13.) In general, the greater the profitability of a business, the better its financial position.

The income statement, then, summarizes the ability of an organization to generate profits. Basically, it lists the organization's income (revenues), the costs that must be incurred to produce the income (expenses), and the differences between the two (profitability). In the following sections, the major components of the income statement are discussed in detail.

Before we close this section, note that the footnotes to the income statement usually run many pages, while the statement itself typically takes up only a single page. The explanatory and supplemental information contained in the footnotes is as important to read and understand as the actual income statement.

? SELF-TEST QUESTIONS

1. What is the primary purpose of the income statement?

2. In regards to time, how do the income statement and balance sheet differ?

3. What are the major components of the income statement?

4. Are the footnotes to the financial statements important?

11.7 REVENUES

As discussed previously, revenues represent both the cash received to date and the unpaid obligations of payers for services provided during the period. For healthcare businesses, revenues result mostly from the provision of patient services, although some revenues result from nonoperating (financial) activities, such as interest earned on investments and contributions (for not-for-profit providers).

Revenues can be shown on the income statement in several different ways. In fact, there is more latitude in the construction of the income statement than there is in the balance sheet, so the income statements of different healthcare providers tend to vary somewhat in presentation. Park Ridge Homecare breaks its revenues into two sections: operating revenues and nonoperating revenues (nonoperating income). However, other formats can be used. (See Problems 11.2 and 11.3, as well Table 13.1, for examples of income statements of other types of providers.)

Park Ridge Homecare reported *net patient service revenue* of $4,042,000 for 2008. The key terms here are net and patient service. This line contains revenues that stem exclusively from the provision of patient services, as opposed to revenues from other sources such as cafeteria sales, charitable contributions, or interest earned on securities investments. The term "net" signifies that the amount shown is less than the clinic's gross charges for the services provided.

Net patient service revenue
The amount of revenue collected or expected to be collected as a direct result of providing patient services.

Chargemaster
A provider's official list of charges (prices) for goods and services rendered.

Park Ridge Homecare, like all healthcare providers, has a *chargemaster* that contains the charge code and gross price for each service that it provides. However, the chargemaster price rarely represents the amount the provider expects to be paid for a particular service.

For example, the chargemaster price for a routine home visit might be $80, but the contract with a particular payer might specify a reimbursement amount of only $50, which reflects a discount of $30. Discounts are accounted for before the revenue is recorded on the income statement, so the patient service revenue amounts shown on the income statement are net of discounts. For this home visit, the amount of net patient service revenue reported on Park Ridge's income statement would be $50, rather than the $80 chargemaster "price."

Charity (indigent) care
Care provided to patients who do not have the capacity to pay.

In addition to services provided to paying patients, some services have been provided as *charity care* to indigent patients who do not have the ability to pay for services provided. Park Ridge has no expectation of ever collecting for these services, so, like discounts, charges for charity care services are not reflected in the $4,042,000 net patient service revenue reported for 2008.

Bad debt losses
Revenue that is expected, but never collected, from patients (or third-party payers) who do have the capacity to pay.

Finally, some revenues that are expected to be collected and hence reported as net patient service revenue will never be realized and ultimately will become *bad debt losses*. To recognize that Park Ridge does not really expect to collect the entire $4,024,000 net patient service revenue reported, it lists $46,000 as a 2008 expense item (provision for bad debts). (This expense item is discussed in more detail in the next section.)

Note the distinction between charity care and bad debt losses. Charity care represents services that are provided to patients who do not have the capacity to pay. Bad debt losses result from the failure to collect for services provided to patients or third-party payers who do have the ability to pay.

A description of the policies regarding discounts and charity care will often appear in the footnotes to the financial statements. To illustrate, Park Ridge's financial statements include the following footnote information:

◆   *Net patient service revenue.* Net patient service revenue represents the estimated net realizable amounts from patients, third-party payers, and others for services rendered. Approximately 58 percent of net patient service revenue in 2008 and 37 percent in 2007 was derived from federal and state reimbursement programs.

◆   *Charity care.* Park Ridge Homecare has a policy of providing charity care to patients who are unable to pay. Such patients are identified on the basis of financial information obtained from the patient and subsequent analysis. Because Park Ridge Homecare does not expect payment from these patients, estimated charges for charity care are not included in revenue. Charity care represented approximately 6 percent of visits in 2008 and 5 percent of visits in 2007.

Even though Park Ridge ultimately expects to receive all of its reported net patient service revenue not yet collected (less realized bad debt losses), the clinic did not actually receive $4,042,000 in cash payments in 2008. Rather, some of the revenue for services provided toward the end of the year has not yet been collected. As discussed in Chapter 12, the yet-to-be-collected portion of the net patient service revenue appears on the balance sheet (Table 12.1) as net patient accounts receivable. In addition, some of the revenue reported for services provided toward the end of 2007 (hence reported for 2007) was not collected until 2008. The point here is that the actual cash revenues collected for 2008 will likely differ from the amount reported on the income statement.

In a fee-for-service environment, providers offer healthcare services that are paid for on the basis of utilization. Park Ridge operates primarily as a fee-for-service provider, so its patient service revenue is reported as shown in Table 11.1. Revenue associated with capitation contracts is often called *premium revenue* when reported on the income statement. If the provider has almost all capitated revenue, it may replace the patient service revenue entry, as reported by Park Ridge, with premium revenue.

Other providers, those with significant amounts of both fee-for-service and capitation revenue, may report both patient service revenue and premium revenue on the income statement. The key difference is that patient service revenue is reported when services are provided, but premium revenue is reported at the start of each contract payment period—typically, the beginning of each month. Thus, premium revenue implies an obligation on the part of the reporting organization to provide future services, while patient service revenue represents an obligation on the part of payers to pay the reporting organization for services already provided.

Most healthcare organizations have some revenue related to patient service operations that does not result directly from treating patients. This revenue, which stems from such activities as parking garages and cafeteria services, is reported in the revenue section as *other operating revenue*. In 2008, Park Ridge reported $27,000 of such revenue.

Park Ridge's total revenues, which in this format all stem from operations, is the sum of its net patient service revenue and other operating revenue. For 2008, this amount was $4,069,000.

Premium revenue
Revenue arising from capitated patients as opposed to fee-for-service patients.

Other operating revenue
Revenue that is related to patients but not directly tied to the provision of patient services. One common example for hospitals is cafeteria revenue.

HISTORICAL PERSPECTIVE: Gross Revenues Versus Net Revenues

Until 1996, in the revenue section of the income statement, healthcare providers reported both gross patient service revenue based on chargemaster prices and deductions from revenue for contractual discounts and charity care. This made the

(Continued)

HISTORICAL PERSPECTIVE: Gross Revenues Versus Net Revenues

revenue reporting for healthcare providers different from businesses in virtually every other industry.

For example, airlines have a set of full fares, such as $1,500 for a round-trip coach ticket from New York to Chicago. Most travelers in coach do not pay this fare, however. Rather, they pay restricted excursion fares that could be as low as $200. When an airline prepares its income statement, it does not list revenues at full fares and then subtract an allowance for discount fares. What it shows on the income statement are only those revenues that it actually expects to receive. For reporting consistency across industries, healthcare providers eventually were forced to report revenues the same way as everyone else—net of all discounts and charity care.

Under the old guidance, a healthcare provider's charity care was reported as a deduction to gross patient service revenue directly on the income statement. Thus, if $500 worth of charity services were provided to an indigent patient, the income statement would include this $500 in gross patient service revenue, but then deduct the $500 as charity care, resulting in $0 net patient service revenue for those services. This accounting treatment allowed providers, particularly those with not-for-profit status, to highlight the amount of charity care provided.

Today, a broad description of the organization's charity care policy, along with an estimate of the value of such care provided, is contained in the footnotes to the financial statements.

(?) SELF-TEST QUESTIONS

1. What categories of revenue are reported on the income statement?

2. Briefly, what is the difference between gross patient service revenue and net patient service revenue? Between patient service revenue and other operating revenue?

3. Describe how the following types of revenue are reported on the income statement: (a) discounts from charges, (b) charity care, and (c) bad debt losses.

11.8 EXPENSES

To produce revenues (and nonoperating income), businesses must incur expenses. As shown in Table 11.1, Park Ridge Homecare reports its expenses in categories such as salaries and benefits, supplies and drugs, and insurance.

The number and nature of expense items reported on the income statement, which depends on the nature and complexity of the organization, can vary widely. For example, some businesses (typically, small) may report only two categories of expenses: healthcare services and administration. Park Ridge takes a middle-of-the-road approach to the number of expense categories. Most readers of financial statements would prefer more rather than less because more insights can be gleaned if an organization reports revenues and expenses both by service breakdown (say, inpatient versus outpatient) and by type (say, salaries versus supplies).

Park Ridge is typical of most healthcare providers in that the dominant portion of its cost structure (almost 70 percent) is related to labor. It reported salaries and benefits of $2,714,000 for 2008. The detail of how these costs are broken down by department or contract, or the relationship of these expenses to volume, typically is not included in the financial statements. However, some organizations provide additional details on expenses in the footnotes to the financial statements.

The expense item titled supplies and drugs represents the cost of supplies (primarily medical) used in providing patient services. Park Ridge does not order and pay for supplies when a particular patient visit requires them. Rather, the business's managers estimate the usage of individual supply items, order them ahead of time, and then maintain a medical supplies inventory. (As discussed in Chapter 12, the amount of supplies on hand is reported on the balance sheet.)

The income statement expense listing for supplies and drugs represents the cost of the items actually consumed in providing patient services. Thus, the expense reported for supplies and drugs does not reflect the actual cash spent on inventory purchases. In theory, Park Ridge could have several years' worth of inventories at the beginning of 2008, could have used some of these items without replenishing the stocks, and hence might not have actually spent one dime of cash on supplies and drugs during that year.

Park Ridge uses commercial insurance to protect against many risks, including both property risks, such as fire and damaging weather, and liability risks, such as managerial malfeasance and professional (medical) liability. The cost of this protection is reported on the income statement as insurance expense.

The next expense category on Park Ridge's income statement is provision for bad debts. As discussed earlier, the clinic reports as revenue in each year the charges for services provided minus discounts and charity care. Thus, in theory, it either collected (or expects to collect) a total of $4,042,000 for patient services provided in 2008. However, past experience indicates that the business will not collect every dollar reported on the income statement, even though the payers are assumed to have the ability to pay.

Depreciation expense stems from the purchase of long-lived assets such as buildings and equipment. Because such assets create revenues over many years, it makes little sense to list their entire cost in the year of purchase as an expense. To more closely match the cost of a long-lived asset with the revenues that it is expected to produce, the cost is spread over the asset's expected useful life. For example, assume that an x-ray machine costs $100,000 in 2008 and is expected to have a five-year useful life and a salvage value of $25,000. For income statement purposes, the $100,000 cost, less the $25,000 salvage value estimate, would be spread over five years, so $75,000 / 5 = $15,000 would be expensed in each of the next five years (from 2009 through 2013). The $15,000 amortized (spread over many years) cost of the x-ray machine when expensed (listed) on the income statement is called depreciation expense.

Of the reported net patient service revenue, Park Ridge expects that $46,000 will never be collected. Thus, the clinic has already collected, or expects to collect, $4,042,000 − $46,000 = 3,996,000 for patient services provided in 2008. With bad debt losses running at about $46,000 / $4,024,000 = 0.011 = 1.1% of net patient service revenue, Park Ridge Homecare is not losing a high percentage to "deadbeat" payers. Still, margins are thin on healthcare services, so the business's collection procedures should be reviewed to ensure that they are effective. (As discussed in Chapter 7, one of the goals of receivables management is to reduce the amount of bad debt losses.)

The next expense category—depreciation—requires closer examination. Like virtually all businesses, Park Ridge requires long-lived assets such as buildings and equipment to provide goods and services. When these assets were initially purchased, Park Ridge did not report their purchase price as an expense on the income statement, but they were listed on the balance sheet as property and equipment owned by the business.

The logic of not reporting the cost of such assets when purchased is that it would be improper to allocate the acquisition costs of long-lived assets to a single accounting period because these assets are used to produce revenues for many years. A more pragmatic reason for not reporting long-lived asset costs when they occur is that such outlays would have a severe impact on reported profitability in years when large amounts are purchased. Furthermore, reported profitability would fluctuate widely from year to year on the basis of the amount of such assets acquired.

To match the cost of long-lived assets to the revenues produced by such assets, accountants use the concept of **depreciation expense,** which amortizes (spreads out) the cost of a long-lived asset over many years. Note that most people use the terms cost and expense interchangeably. To accountants, however, the terms can have different meanings. Depreciation expense is a good example. Here, the cost is the actual cash outlay for a long-lived asset, while the expense is the allocation of that cost over time.

The calculation of depreciation expense is somewhat arbitrary, so the amount of depreciation expense applied to a long-lived asset in any year generally is not closely related to the actual usage of the asset or its loss in market value.

To illustrate, Park Ridge owns a piece of diagnostic equipment that it uses infrequently. In 2007, the equipment was used 23 times, while in 2008 it was used only 9 times.

Still, the depreciation expense associated with this equipment was the same $1,725 in both years. Also, Park Ridge owns another piece of equipment that could be sold today for about the same price that the business paid for it four years ago, yet each year the clinic reports a depreciation expense for that equipment, which implies loss of value.

Depreciation expense, like all other financial statement entries, is calculated in accordance with GAAP. The calculation typically uses the *straight-line method*—that is, the depreciation expense is obtained by dividing the cost of the asset (less its estimated *salvage value*) by the number of years of its estimated useful life. The result is the asset's annual depreciation expense, which is the charge that is reflected in each year's income statement over the estimated life of the asset and, as discussed in Chapter 12, accumulated over time on the balance sheet.

The term straight-line stems from the fact that the depreciation expense is constant in each year, and hence the implied value of the asset declines evenly (like a straight line) over time. How is the useful life of a long-lived asset determined? Well, accountants use tables that list the useful lives of various classes of assets. For example, certain medical equipment has a five-year useful life, while office furniture has a 20-year life.

The final expense line on the income statement reports interest expense. Park Ridge had an obligation to pay its lenders $16,000 in interest expense for debt capital supplied during 2008. Not all of the interest expense reported was paid in 2008 because Park Ridge typically pays interest monthly or semiannually, and hence some portion of the interest owed on 2008 borrowings will not be paid until 2009.

The amount of interest expense reported by an organization is influenced primarily by its capital structure, which reflects the amount of debt that it uses. Also, interest expense is affected by the borrower's creditworthiness, its mix of long-term and short-term debt, and the impact of inflation expectations on the general level of interest rates. (These factors are covered in Chapter 8.)

In closing our discussion of expenses, note that many income statements contain a catchall expense category labeled other. Listed here are general and administrative expenses that are too small to list separately, including items such as marketing expenses and external auditor's fees. Although organizations cannot possibly report every expense item separately, it is frustrating for readers of financial statements to come across a large, unexplained expense item. Thus, income statements that include the "other" category often add a footnote that provides additional detail.

Straight-line method
A method for calculating the depreciation expense of a long-lived asset that assumes the loss of value is constant over time (follows a straight line).

Salvage value
The estimated value of a long-lived asset at the end of its useful life.

? SELF-TEST QUESTIONS

1. What is an expense?
2. Briefly, what are some of the commonly reported expense categories?
3. Explain the rationale behind the provision for bad debts?
4. What is the logic behind depreciation expense, and how is it calculated?

Operating income measures the profitability of a healthcare business's core activities—the provision of patient services and those activities that are directly related. It eliminates any income resulting from non-patient-service–related sources, such as contributions and securities investments. Many analysts consider operating income to be the most important income statement measure of a healthcare business's profitability. After all, if an organization cannot make a profit on its core business, its financial sustainability is in doubt.

11.9 OPERATING INCOME

Although the reporting of revenues and expenses is clearly important, the most important information on the income statement is profitability. As shown in Table 11.1, two different profit measures can be reported on the income statement. (Not all healthcare organizations report both measures; some report only the final measure—net income.)

The first profitability measure reported by Park Ridge Homecare is **operating income**, calculated in Table 11.1 as total revenues minus total expenses. The precise calculation is tied to the format of the income statement, but the general idea of operating income is to focus on revenues and expenses that are related to operations (the provision of patient services).

Because reported total revenues in Table 11.1 are all related to patient services, operating income measures the profitability of core operations (patient services and related endeavors). Many healthcare providers, especially large ones, have significant revenues that stem from non–patient-service-related activities, so it is useful to report the inherent profitability of the core business separately from the overall profitability of the enterprise.

Park Ridge reported $140,000 of operating income in 2008, which means that the provision of home health care services and directly related activities generated a profit of $140,000. Operating income is an important measure of a healthcare business's profitability because it focuses on the core activities of the business. Some healthcare businesses report a positive net income (net income is discussed in a later section) but a negative operating income (an operating loss). This situation is worrisome, because a business is on shaky financial ground if its core operations are losing money, especially if it does so year after year.

Note that the operating income reported on the income statement is defined by GAAP and represents an estimate of the long-run operating profitability of the business. It has some shortcomings—for one, it does not represent cash flow—that are similar to the shortcomings related to net income discussed in a later section. Still, measuring the profitability of a business is critical to understanding its financial status.

? SELF-TEST QUESTIONS

1. What is operating income?

2. Why is operating income such an important measure of profitability?

11.10 NONOPERATING INCOME

The next section of the income statement lists *nonoperating income*. As mentioned earlier, reporting the revenues of operating and nonoperating activities separately is useful. The revenues from operating activities were reported in the revenue section of Table 11.1. Now, Park Ridge Homecare's income statement reports the income (revenues) generated from activities unrelated to the provision of healthcare services.

The first category of nonoperating income listed for Park Ridge is contributions. Many not-for-profit organizations, especially those with large, well-endowed foundations, rely heavily on charitable contributions, as well as earnings on securities investments, as a revenue source. Those charitable contributions that can be used immediately (spent now) are reported as nonoperating income. However, contributions that create a permanent endowment fund, and hence are not available for immediate use, are not reported as nonoperating income.

The second category of nonoperating income is investment income, which stems from two primary sources:

1. Healthcare businesses usually have funds available that exceed the minimum necessary to meet current cash expenses. Because cash earns no interest, these "excess" funds usually are invested in short-term interest-earning securities, such as Treasury bills or money market mutual funds. Sometimes these invested funds can be quite large—say, when a business is building up cash to make a tax payment or to start a large construction project. Also, prudent businesses keep a reserve of funds on hand to meet unexpected emergencies. The interest earned on such funds is listed as investment income.

2. Not-for-profit businesses may have a large amount of endowment fund contributions. When these contributions are received, they are not reported as income because the funds are not available to be spent. However, the income from securities purchased with endowment funds is available to the healthcare organization, and hence this income is reported as nonoperating (investment) income.

In total, Park Ridge reported $23,000 of nonoperating income for 2008, consisting of $10,000 in spendable contributions and $13,000 earned on the investment of excess cash and endowments. Nonoperating income is not central to the core business, which is providing healthcare services. Over-reliance on nonoperating income could mask operational inefficiencies that, if not corrected, could lead to future financial problems. Note that the costs associated with creating nonoperating income are not separately reported. Thus, the expenses associated with soliciting contributions or investing excess cash and endowments are mixed in with the operating expenses listed in the expense section of the income statement.

Nonoperating income
The income of a healthcare provider that is not related to the provision of patient services. The two most obvious examples are income from securities investments and charitable contributions (for not-for-profit businesses).

Finally, note that the income statements of some providers do not contain a separate section titled nonoperating income. Rather, nonoperating income is included in the revenue section that heads the income statement. In this situation, total revenues include both operating and nonoperating revenues.

(?) SELF-TEST QUESTIONS

1. What is nonoperating income?

2. Why is nonoperating income reported separately from revenues? Is this always the case?

11.11 NET INCOME

The second profitability measure reported by Park Ridge Homecare is **net income**, which on Table 11.1 is equal to Operating income + Total nonoperating income. Park Ridge reported net income of $163,000 for 2008: $140,000 + $23,000 = $163,000. (Not-for-profit organizations use the term excess of revenues over expenses in place of net income, but we will call this measure net income.)

(!) CRITICAL CONCEPT
Net Income

Net income measures the total profitability of a business, including both operating and nonoperating income. Although operating income is an important profitability measure because it focuses on a healthcare business's core operations, the financial condition of the business ultimately depends on overall profitability, which is reported as net income. Healthcare providers can lose money on core operations, yet still be "above water" financially if operating losses are covered by nonoperating income. However, this is not a desirable situation in the long run.

Because of its location on the income statement and its importance, net income is referred to as the bottom line. In spite of the fact that Park Ridge is a not-for-profit organization, it still must make a profit. If the business is to offer new services in the future, it must earn a profit today to produce the funds needed for new assets. Furthermore, because of inflation, Park Ridge could not even replace its existing assets as they wear out or become obsolete without the funds generated by positive profitability. Thus, turning a profit is essential for all businesses, including not-for-profits.

What happens to a business's net income? For the most part, it is reinvested in the business. Not-for-profit corporations must reinvest all earnings in the business. An investor-owned corporation, on the other hand, may return a portion or all of its net income to owners in the form of dividend payments. The amount of profits reinvested in an investor-owned business, therefore, is net income minus the amount paid out as dividends. (Some for-profit businesses distribute profits to owners in the form of bonuses, which often occurs in medical practices. However, when this is done, the distribution becomes an expense item that reduces net income rather than a distribution of net income. The end result is the same—profits are distributed to owners—but the reporting mechanism is different.)

Note that both operating income and net income measure profitability as defined by GAAP. In establishing GAAP, accountants have created guidelines that attempt to measure the economic income of a business, which is a difficult task because economic gains and losses often are not tied to easily identifiable events.

Furthermore, some of the income statement items are estimates (e.g., provision for bad debt losses) and others (e.g., depreciation expense) do not represent actual cash revenues or costs. Because of accrual accounting and other factors, the fact that Park Ridge reported net income of $163,000 for 2008 does not mean that the business experienced a net cash inflow of that amount. This point is discussed in greater detail in the next section.

(?) SELF-TEST QUESTIONS

1. Why is net income called the bottom line?

2. What is the difference between net income and operating income?

(*) INDUSTRY PRACTICE Sources of Hospital Profitability

Ask the average healthcare manager this question: Do hospitals make money? Most would answer, "yes, but not very much." Follow up with this question: How do hospitals make money? The answers here might differ somewhat, but in general, most responses would be, "by providing patient services." Here are the results of a recent study on the components of hospital profitability.

Hospital revenues, and hence profits, come from many sources. But, in general, the revenue sources can be broken down into three major categories:

• *Patient service revenue.* The most obvious source of revenue stems from the provision of patient services. Hospitals generally provide both inpatient and outpatient services, including emergency, ancillary, and other patient services. The

(Continued)

monies received from patients and insurers for these services constitute the largest source of hospital revenue. About 94 percent of hospital total revenues are generated by patient services.

• *Other operating revenue.* The second source of revenue comes from activities that are related to hospital operations but do not stem directly from the provision of patient services. Examples here include cafeteria sales and parking garage revenues. Other operating revenue constitutes 1.5 percent of hospital total revenues.

• *Nonoperating revenue.* The third source of revenue stems from activities that are totally unrelated to operations. The primary sources in this category are earnings on financial investments and unrestricted contributions. Nonoperating revenue accounts for about 4.5 percent of total revenues.

What is the contribution of each revenue source to overall profitability? Patient service revenue contributes about 27 percent of the total before-tax profitability, or less than one-third. Other operating revenue contributes 33 percent, while nonoperating revenue contributes 40 percent. Thus, the largest contributor, on average, to a hospital's total profitability is nonoperating revenue, while other operating revenue contributes somewhat more to profitability than does patient service revenue. Combined, non–patient-service-related (nonoperating) revenue accounts for 73 percent of the total profitability of an average hospital.

The largest contributor, by far, to other operating revenue is cafeteria (non-inpatient food) services. Other significant sources are gift shop revenue and parking revenue. The largest source of nonoperating revenue is investment income, followed by revenue from physician office rentals and unrestricted contributions.

Although the specific contribution of patient service versus non–patient-service revenue varies by ownership, non–patient-service revenue clearly contributes substantially to hospital profitability. In fact, not-for-profit hospitals would be barely profitable without the contribution of non–patient-service revenue. Fur-

---

thermore, for-profit hospitals, when income taxes are considered, would have their total profits cut by slightly more than half were it not for the contribution of non–patient-service revenue.

These results confirm the conventional wisdom that holds that the profit earned on patient services is very thin or, for many hospitals, even negative. Thus, without non–patient-service revenue, most hospitals would be facing a difficult financial future.

Note: This industry practice is based on research conducted in 2008 by Niccie L. McKay and Louis C. Gapenski of the University of Florida. Publication forthcoming in *Health Care Management Review.*

11.12 NET INCOME VERSUS CASH FLOW

As stated previously, the income statement reports total profitability as net income, which is determined in accordance with GAAP. Although net income is an important measure of profitability, an organization's financial condition, at least in the short run, depends more on the actual cash that flows into and out of the business than it does on reported profitability. Thus, occasionally a business will go bankrupt even though its net income has historically been positive. More commonly, many businesses that have reported negative net incomes (net losses) for several years have survived with little or no financial damage.

How can these things happen? The problem is that the income statement is like a mixture of apples and oranges. Consider Table 11.1. Park Ridge Homecare reported total revenues of $4,069,000 for 2008. Yet, even if we assume no bad debt losses, this is not the amount of cash that was actually collected during the year, because some of these revenues will not be collected until 2009. Furthermore, some revenues reported for 2007 were actually collected in 2008, but these do not appear at all on the 2008 income statement. Thus, because of accrual accounting, reported revenue is not the same as cash revenue.

The same logic applies to expenses; few of the values reported as expenses on the income statement are the same as the actual cash outflows. To make matters even worse, not one cent of depreciation expense was paid out as cash. Depreciation expense is an accounting reflection of the cost of long-lived assets, but Park Ridge did not actually pay out $21,000 in cash to someone called the "collector of depreciation." The actual cash outlays

Noncash expenses
Expenses that are listed on the income statement that do not represent cash outlays. The most prominent noncash expense is depreciation.

associated with reported depreciation expense occurred in past years when the long-lived assets were purchased.

Can net income be converted to net cash flow—the actual amount of cash generated during the year? As a rough estimate, net cash flow can be thought of as net income plus *noncash expenses*. Thus, the net cash flow generated by Park Ridge in 2008 is not merely the $163,000 reported net income, but this amount plus the $21,000 shown for depreciation, for a total of $184,000. Depreciation expense must be added back to net income to estimate net cash flow because initially it was subtracted from revenues to obtain net income even though there was no associated cash outlay.

Here is another way of looking at cash flow versus accounting income: If Park Ridge showed zero net income for 2008, it would still be generating cash of $21,000 because that amount was listed as an expense but not actually paid out in cash. The idea behind the income statement treatment of depreciation is that Park Ridge would be able to set aside the depreciation amount, which is above and beyond its actual operating expenses, this year and in future years.

Eventually, the accumulated total of depreciation cash flow would be used by Park Ridge to replace its existing assets as they wear out or become obsolete. Thus, the incorporation of depreciation expense into the cost, and ultimately the price structure, of services provided is designed to ensure the ability of a business to replace its buildings and equipment as needed, assuming that they could be purchased at their historical cost. To be more realistic, businesses must plan to generate net income, in addition to the accumulated depreciation funds, sufficient to replace existing assets in the future at inflated costs or to expand (grow) the business.

Understand that because of accrual accounting, the $184,000 net cash flow calculated here is only an estimate of actual cash flow for 2008, because almost every item of revenues and expenses listed on the income statement does not equal its cash flow counterpart. The greater the difference between the reported values and cash values, the less reliable is the net cash flow estimate. The value of knowing the precise amount of cash generated or lost has not gone unnoticed by accountants. In Chapter 12, you will learn about the statement of cash flows, which can be thought of as an income statement that is recast to focus on cash flow.

? SELF-TEST QUESTIONS

1. Why is there a difference between net income and cash flow?

2. How can income statement data be used to estimate cash flow?

3. Why do not-for-profit businesses need to make a profit?

11.13 INCOME STATEMENTS OF INVESTOR-OWNED FIRMS

What do the income statements of investor-owned firms look like? The financial statements of investor-owned firms and not-for-profit businesses are generally similar, except for those transactions, such as tax payments, that are applicable only to one form of ownership. Because the transactions of all healthcare organizations in the same core business are similar, ownership plays only a minor role in the presentation of financial statement data. For the most part, the differences involve labeling (i.e., net income versus excess of revenues over expenses). In reality, more differences exist in financial statements because of lines of business (e.g., hospitals versus nursing homes versus managed care plans) than because of ownership.

? SELF-TEST QUESTION

1. Are there appreciable differences in the income statements of not-for-profit and investor-owned businesses?

11.14 A LOOK AHEAD: FINANCIAL CONDITION ANALYSIS

Chapter 13 details the techniques used to analyze financial statements to gain insights into a business's financial condition. At this point, however, it is worthwhile to introduce *ratio analysis*, one method used in financial condition analysis. In ratio analysis, values found on the financial statements are combined to form ratios that have economic meaning and hence help managers and investors interpret the numbers.

To illustrate, *total profit margin*, usually just called *total margin*, is defined as net income divided by total (all) revenues. For Park Ridge Homecare, net income for 2008 was $163,000, while total (all) revenues were $4,069,000 + $23,000 = $4,092,000, so the total margin was $163,000 / $4,092,000 = 0.040 = 4.0%. Thus, each dollar of total revenues produced 4.0 cents of total profit (net income). By implication, the production of each dollar of revenues required 96.0 cents of expenses.

The total margin is a measure of expense control; for a given amount of revenues, the higher the net income, and hence total margin, the lower the expenses. If the total margin for other home health businesses were known, judgments about how well Park Ridge is doing in the area of expense control, relative to its peers, could be made.

Note that the *operating margin* for 2008 was Operating income / Operating revenues = $140,000 / $4,069,000 = 0.034 = 3.4%. (On Park Ridge's income statement, operating revenues are labeled as total revenues.) Thus, in 2008, 85 percent (3.4% / 4.0%) of the overall profitability of the business was generated by the provision of healthcare services (operations), while 15 percent stemmed from nonoperating sources (contributions and investment income).

Ratio analysis
The process of creating and analyzing ratios from the data contained in a business's financial statements and elsewhere to help assess financial condition.

Total (profit) margin
Net income divided by all (both operating and nonoperating) revenues. It measures the amount of total profit per dollar of revenues.

Operating margin
Operating income divided by operating revenues. It measures the amount of profit per dollar of operating revenues and hence focuses on the core activities of a business.

Park Ridge's total margin for 2007 was $99,000 / $2,747,000 = 0.036 = 3.6%, so the total margin increased from 2007 to 2008. In effect, Park Ridge's revenues increased faster than its expenses, which resulted in increasing profitability as measured by total margin. Managers should identify the conditions that contributed to the increase in profitability and attempt to continue this positive trend into 2009.

A complete discussion of ratio analysis can be found in Chapter 13. The discussion here, along with a brief visit in Chapter 12, is intended to give you a preview of how financial statement data can be used to make judgments about a business's financial condition.

(?) SELF-TEST QUESTIONS

1. Explain how ratio analysis can be used to help interpret income statement data.

2. What is the total margin, and what does it measure?

3. How does the total margin differ from the operating margin?

THEME WRAP-UP   CONSTRUCTING AN INCOME STATEMENT

As Lori considers opening another home health care business, she wonders if the financial resources of her existing facility, Park Ridge Homecare, can be used as a "springboard" to support the second location. After reviewing two years worth of Park Ridge's income statements, Lori (and you) has learned a fair amount about the revenues, expenses, and profitability of the business.

The business significantly increased its revenues from 2007 to 2008, but, at the same time, its cost of providing services (expenses) also increased. The net result was an almost doubling of operating income from $71,000 in 2007 to $140,000 in 2008. The largest revenue source was patient services, while the largest expense was for salaries and benefits.

Because Park Ridge also had nonoperating income in 2007 and 2008, its net income (excess of revenues over expenses) was greater than its operating income. In total, the business generated $163,000 + $99,000 = $262,000 in net income over the two-year period. The business's estimated cash flow was even greater, because a noncash charge (depreciation) was subtracted as an expense even though no cash transaction occurred. Thus, operating and nonoperating revenues provided the business with income that it can use in the future to improve and/or expand its services.

Although Lori now has a clearer picture of Park Ridge's profit status, she still does not have sufficient information to make a sound judgment about its ability to financially support a second location. For example, how much cash does Park Ridge Homecare have on hand? Does the business have any savings available to help finance a new location? Where is the business's cash coming from, and what is it used for?

To learn the answers to these questions, Lori needs to examine Park Ridge's two other financial statements: the balance sheet and statement of cash flows. These statements are the focus of Chapter 12.

Key Concepts

This chapter lays out the basics of financial reporting and the income statement. Here are the key concepts:

➤ The field of *financial accounting* involves identifying, measuring, recording, and communicating the economic events and status of an organization.

➤ The financial status of an organization is reported by a set of financial statements. The three most important statements are the *income statement*, the *balance sheet*, and the *statement of cash flows*.

➤ The predominant users of financial statement information are the business's *stakeholders*—parties (primarily managers and investors) who have a direct financial interest in the business.

➤ *Generally accepted accounting principles* (*GAAP*) establish the standards for financial measurement and reporting. Although these principles are sanctioned by the *Securities and Exchange Commission* (*SEC*), they are developed by other organizations.

➤ Under *cash accounting*, economic events are recognized when the financial (cash) transaction occurs. Under *accrual accounting*, economic events are recognized when the obligation to make payment occurs. GAAP require that businesses use accrual accounting because it provides a better picture of a business's true financial status.

➤ The *income statement* reports on an organization's operations over a period of time. Its basic structure consists of *revenues*, *expenses*, and *profitability*.

➤ *Revenues* are monies collected or expected to be collected by the business. Revenues are broken down into categories—often, *net patient service revenue* and *other operating revenue*.

➤ *Expenses* are the economic costs associated with generating revenues.

➤ *Operating income* is the dollar amount of profit earned from patient services and other sources directly related to patient services.

➤ *Nonoperating income* represents income (revenue) from sources unrelated to patient services, such as contributions and earnings on securities investments.

➤ *Net income*, or *excess of revenues over expenses* for not-for-profits, is the dollar amount of total profit earned from both patient service operations and nonoperating sources.

➤ Because the income statement is constructed using accrual accounting, net income does not represent the actual amount of cash that has been earned or lost during the reporting period. To estimate *cash flow*, noncash expenses (primarily depreciation) must be added back to net income.

➤ The income statements of investor-owned and not-for-profit businesses tend to look alike. However, the income statements of healthcare organizations in different lines of business can vary in format. The good news is that all income statements have essentially the same economic content.

➤ *Ratio analysis,* which combines values that are found in the financial statements, helps managers and investors interpret the data with the goal of making judgments about the financial condition of the business.

In Chapter 12, our discussion continues with the remaining two statements: the balance sheet and statement of cash flows.

END-OF-CHAPTER QUESTIONS

11.1 a. What is a stakeholder?

b. What stakeholders are most interested in the financial condition of a healthcare business?

11.2 a. What are generally accepted accounting principles (GAAP)?

b. What is the purpose of GAAP?

c. What organizations are involved in establishing GAAP?

11.3 Explain the difference between cash accounting and accrual accounting.

11.4 Briefly describe the format of the income statement.

11.5 a. What is the difference between gross revenues and net revenues? (Hint: Think about discounts and charity care.)

b. What is the difference between patient service revenue and other operating revenue?

c. What is the difference between charity care and bad debt losses? How is each handled on the income statement?

11.6 a. What is meant by the term expense?

b. What is depreciation expense, and what is its purpose?

c. What are some other categories of expenses?

11.7 a. What is operating income?

b. What is net income, and how does it differ from operating income?

c. Why is net income called the bottom line?

d. What is the difference between net income and cash flow?

e. Is financial condition more closely related to net income or to cash flow?

END-OF-CHAPTER PROBLEMS

11.1 Entries for the Warren Clinic 2008 income statement are listed below in alphabetical order. Reorder the data in the proper format.

Bad debt expense	$ 40,000
Depreciation expense	90,000
General/administrative expenses	70,000
Interest expense	20,000
Interest income	40,000
Net income	30,000
Other revenue	10,000
Patient service revenue	440,000
Purchased clinic services	90,000
Salaries and benefits	150,000
Total revenues	490,000
Total expenses	460,000

11.2 Consider the following income statement:

BestCare HMO

Statement of Operations

Year Ended June 30, 2008

(in thousands)

Revenue:	
Premiums earned	$26,682
Coinsurance	1,689
Interest and other income	242
Total revenues	$28,613
Expenses:	
Salaries and benefits	$ 15,154
Medical supplies and drugs	7,507
Insurance	3,963
Provision for bad debts	19
Depreciation	367
Interest	385
Total expenses	$27,395
Net income	$ 1,218

a. How does this income statement differ from the one presented in Table 11.1?

b. Did BestCare spend $367,000 on new fixed assets during fiscal year 2008? If not, what is the economic rationale behind its reported depreciation expense?

c. Explain the provision for bad debts entry.

d. What is BestCare's total margin? How can it be interpreted?

11.3 Consider this income statement:

Green Valley Nursing Home, Inc.
Statement of Income
Year Ended December 31, 2008

Revenue:	
Resident services revenue	$3,163,258
Other revenue	106,146
Total revenues	$3,269,404
Expenses:	
Salaries and benefits	$1,515,438
Medical supplies and drugs	966,781
Insurance and other	296,357
Provision for bad debts	110,000
Depreciation	85,000
Interest	206,780
Total expenses	$3,180,356
Operating income	$ 89,048
Provision for income taxes	31,167
Net income	$ 57,881

a. How does this income statement differ from the ones presented in Table 11.1 and Problem 11.2?

b. Why does Green Valley show a provision for income taxes while the other two income statements did not?

c. What is Green Valley's total (profit) margin? How does this value compare with the values for Park Ridge Homecare Clinic and BestCare?

d. The before-tax profit margin for Green Valley is operating income divided by total revenues. Calculate Green Valley's before-tax profit margin. Why may this be a better measure of expense control when comparing an investor-owned business with a not-for-profit business?

11.4 Great Forks Hospital reported net income for 2008 of $2.4 million on total revenues of $30 million. Depreciation expense totaled $1 million.

a. What were total expenses for 2008?

b. What were total cash expenses for 2008? (Hint: Assume that all expenses, except depreciation, were cash expenses.)

c. What was the hospital's 2008 cash flow?

11.5 Brandywine Clinic, a not-for-profit business, had revenues of $12 million in 2008. Expenses other than depreciation totaled 75 percent of revenues, and depreciation expense was $1.5 million. All revenues were collected in cash during the year and all expenses other than depreciation were paid in cash.

a. Construct Brandywine's 2008 income statement.

b. What were Brandywine's net income, total profit margin, and cash flow?

c. Now, suppose the company changed its depreciation calculation procedures (still within GAAP) such that its depreciation expense doubled. How would this change affect Brandywine's net income, total profit margin, and cash flow?

d. Suppose the change had halved, rather than doubled, the firm's depreciation expense. Now, what would be the impact on net income, total profit margin, and cash flow?

11.6 Assume that Mainline Healthcare, a for-profit corporation, had exactly the same situation as reported in Problem 11.5. However, Mainline must pay taxes at a rate of 40 percent of pretax income. Assuming that the same revenues and expenses reported for financial accounting purposes would be reported for tax purposes, redo Problem 11.5 for Mainline.

CHAPTER 12

REPORTING ASSETS, FINANCING, AND CASH FLOWS

UNDERSTANDING THE BALANCE SHEET AND THE STATEMENT OF CASH FLOWS

Lori Gibbs, founder of Park Ridge Homecare, is considering opening a second location of her home health care business. Rather than start from scratch, she wants to use the resources of the existing organization as a financial springboard. Her task at hand is to assess the financial condition of the current business to determine whether or not it can support the opening of a new enterprise.

So far, Lori knows this: Over the past two years, Park Ridge generated $262,000 in net income (earnings). Its estimated cash flow was even greater, because a noncash charge (depreciation) was subtracted as an expense on the income statement even though no cash transaction occurred. However, she does not know if these earnings have already been spent or are still available to help fund the new business. To find out more about these earnings, plus other information relevant to Park Ridge's financial condition, Lori set out to study two other financial statements: the balance sheet and statement of cash flows.

By the end of the chapter, you will see how a business reports assets, financing, and cash flows.

LEARNING OBJECTIVES

After studying this chapter, you will be able to

➤ Explain the purpose of the balance sheet.

➤ Describe the organization and contents of the balance sheet, including the basic accounting equation.

➤ State the purpose of the statement of cash flows.

➤ Detail the contents of the statement of cash flows and the way it differs from the income statement.

➤ Discuss the interrelationships among the income statement, balance sheet, and statement of cash flows.

12.1 INTRODUCTION

As discussed in Chapter 11, the income statement contains information about an organization's revenues, expenses, and profitability. But it does not provide data related to what assets a business owns or how those assets are financed. Those specifics are contained in the balance sheet, another kind of financial statement.

Furthermore, investors and managers recognize that financial condition, especially in the short run, is more related to the actual flow of cash into and out of a business than to economic income as reported on the income statement. The statement of cash flows focuses on this important determinant of financial condition.

Understanding the composition of each of the three financial statements (income statement, balance sheet, and statement of cash flows) is essential, but it is similarly critical to be aware of how these statements fit together. Thus, throughout this chapter, we emphasize the interrelationships among the statements.

12.2 BALANCE SHEET BASICS

Whereas the income statement reports the results of operations over a period of time, the **balance sheet** presents a snapshot of a business's assets and financing at a given point in time. The balance sheet changes every day as a business increases or decreases its assets, or changes the composition of its financing. Note that the balance sheet, unlike the income statement, reflects a business's financial position as of a given date, so the data typically become invalid one day later, even when both dates are in the same accounting period.

CRITICAL CONCEPT
Balance Sheet

The balance sheet is one of the three primary financial statements. Unlike the income statement, which reports the results of operations over some period of time (often a year), the balance sheet reports the financial position of a business at a single point in time. Specifically, the balance sheet lists the assets (resources) of a business and the claims against those assets (obligations), or how the assets are financed. The balance sheet has three basic sections: total assets, total liabilities, and equity. Perhaps the most important feature of this financial statement is that it must balance. Specifically, Total assets = Total liabilities + Equity.

Healthcare providers with seasonal demand, such as a walk-in clinic in Fort Lauderdale, Florida, have especially large changes in their balance sheets during the year. For such businesses, a balance sheet constructed in February can look quite different from one prepared in August. Also, businesses that are growing rapidly will have significant changes in their balance sheets over relatively short periods of time.

The balance sheet lists, as of the end of the reporting period, the resources of an organization and the claims against those resources. In other words, the balance sheet reports the assets of an organization and how those assets are financed. The balance sheet has the following basic structure:

Assets
Current (short-term) assets
Long-term assets

Total assets

Liabilities and Equity
Current (short-term) liabilities
Long-term liabilities
Equity

Total liabilities and equity

The upper section (assets) lists all the resources (in dollar terms) owned by the organization. In general, assets are broken down into categories that distinguish short-lived assets from long-lived assets. The lower section (liabilities and equity) lists the claims (again in dollar terms) against these resources. By claims, we mean that if the business closes and the assets are sold, the funds obtained would have to be distributed to the claimants listed in the lower section.

In essence, the lower section reports the sources of financing (capital) used to acquire the assets listed in the upper section. The sources of capital are divided into two broad categories: liabilities (which are financial obligations fixed by contract) and equity (which is a residual claim that depends on asset values and the amount of liabilities). As with assets, liabilities are listed by maturity (short term versus long term).

Perhaps the most important characteristic of the balance sheet is that it must balance—that is, the total of the upper section must equal the total of the bottom section. This relationship, called the *basic accounting equation*, can be expressed in equation form:

Basic accounting equation
The relationship between balance sheet accounts that requires the balance sheet to balance. That is, total assets must equal total liabilities plus equity.

$$\text{Total assets} = \text{Total liabilities} + \text{Equity}.$$

Because liability claims are paid before equity claims if a healthcare organization is liquidated, liabilities are shown before equity, both on the balance sheet and in the basic accounting equation.

Note that the basic accounting equation can be rearranged:

$$\text{Equity} = \text{Total assets} - \text{Total liabilities}.$$

This format reinforces the concept that equity represents an ownership (residual) claim against the total assets of the business and also the fact that equity can be negative.

To illustrate, suppose a for-profit business has $100,000 in total assets financed by $50,000 in debt financing (total liabilities) and $50,000 in ownership (equity) financing. If a business writes down (decreases) the value of some of its assets because they become obsolete, its liabilities are unaffected because these amounts are still owed to creditors and others. If total assets are written down so much that their value drops below that of total liabilities, then the equity reported on the balance sheet becomes a negative amount.

In our example, if total assets are now considered to be worth only $40,000 but the business still owes its lenders $50,000, the only way for the basic accounting equation to hold is to have a negative equity value; in this situation, -$10,000. Negative equity, which can also result from a long period of losses (negative net income), is relatively rare and reflects an ominous financial situation.

Table 12.1 contains Park Ridge Homecare's balance sheet, which follows the basic structure discussed above. The title of the balance sheet reinforces the fact that the data are presented for the entire business. The balance sheet is not going to provide much information, if any, about the subparts of an organization, such as departments or service lines. Rather, the balance sheet will provide an overview of the economic position of the organization as a whole.

The timing of the balance sheet is apparent in the title. The data are reported for 2008 and 2007 as of December 31. Whereas Park Ridge's income statement indicates the data were for the years ended on December 31, the balance sheet merely indicates a closing date. This minor difference in terminology reinforces the fact that the income statement reports operational results over a period of time, while the balance sheet reports financial position at a single point in time. Finally, the amounts reported on Park Ridge's balance sheet, just as on its income statement, are expressed in thousands of dollars.

The format of the balance sheet emphasizes the basic accounting equation. For example, as of December 31, 2008, Park Ridge Homecare had a total of $1,181,000 in assets that were financed by a total of $1,181,000 of liabilities and equity. Besides this obvious confirmation that the balance sheet balances, this statement indicates that the total assets of Park Ridge were valued, according to GAAP (generally accepted accounting principles), at $1,181,000.

The lower section of the balance sheet reflects the manner in which Park Ridge raised the capital needed to acquire its $1,181,000 in assets. Liabilities and equity represent claims against the assets of the business by various classes of creditors, other claimants with fixed claims, and owners. Creditors and other claimants have first priority in claims for $703,000, while the owners (which in the case of not-for-profit Park Ridge means the community at large) follow with a residual claim of $478,000.

If, for some reason, Park Ridge went out of business on December 31, 2008, and if its assets were sold for exactly $1,181,000, liability holders would receive $703,000 of

	2008	2007
ASSETS		
Current Assets:		
Cash and cash equivalents	$ 74	$ 41
Short-term investments	147	137
Accounts receivable, net	727	476
Inventories	27	22
Total current assets	$ 975	$ 676
Investments	$ 125	$ 100
Property and Equipment:		
Medical and office equipment	$ 56	$ 54
Vehicles	70	47
Total	$ 126	$ 101
Less: Accumulated depreciation	(45)	(24)
Net property and equipment	$ 81	$ 77
Total assets	$1,181	$ 853
LIABILITIES AND EQUITY		
Current Liabilities:		
Notes payable	$ 13	$ 13
Accounts payable	40	21
Accrued expenses	496	337
Total current liabilities	$ 549	$ 371
Long-term debt	154	167
Total liabilities	$ 703	$ 538
Equity (net assets)	$ 478	$ 315
Total liabilities and equity	$1,181	$ 853

the proceeds, and the remaining $478,000 would go back to the community. (As a not-for-profit organization, any proceeds from the sale or liquidation of the business must be used for charitable purposes.)

If the assets were worth less than $1,181,000 (but more than $703,000), the liability holders would still get their $703,000, but the amount remaining to be returned to the community would be reduced. Conversely, sale of the assets for more than $1,181,000 would create a greater amount for the community.

? SELF-TEST QUESTIONS

1. What is the purpose of the balance sheet?

2. What are the three major sections of the balance sheet?

3. What is the basic accounting equation, and what information does it provide?

Current assets
Cash and assets that are expected to be converted into cash within one accounting period (often a year). Examples of noncash current assets include short-term investments, receivables, and inventories.

12.3 ASSETS

Assets either possess or create economic benefit for the organization. Table 12.1 contains three major categories of assets: current assets, investments, and property and equipment. The following sections describe each asset category in detail.

CURRENT ASSETS

Current assets include cash and other assets that are expected to be converted into cash within one accounting period, which in this example is one year. For Park Ridge Homecare, current assets totaled $975,000 at the end of 2008.

Suppose that the short-term investments were converted into cash as they matured; the receivables were collected; and the inventories were used, billed to patients, and collected—all at the values stated on the balance sheet. With all else the same, Park Ridge would have $975,000 in cash at the end of 2009. Of course, all else will not be the same, so Park Ridge's 2009 reported cash balance will undoubtedly be different from that amount. Still, this little exercise reinforces

! CRITICAL CONCEPT
Assets

The assets of a business represent items of value owned by the business. Some items are tangible (can be touched and felt), such as buildings, equipment, cash, and supplies inventories. Also included in tangible assets are those that are financial in nature, such as securities investments and monies owed to the business for services rendered (accounts receivable). Intangible assets include such items as the value of a trademark (think Coca-Cola) or the value created by research and development efforts. Assets are listed on the balance sheet in order of liquidity, or the speed at which they are converted to cash. Thus, cash itself is listed first, and long-lived physical assets (property and equipment) are listed last.

the concept behind the current asset category: the assumption that these assets will be converted into cash during the next accounting period.

The conversion of current assets into cash is expected to provide some or all of the funds needed to pay off the $549,000 in current liabilities outstanding at the end of 2008 as they become due in 2009. At the end of 2008, Park Ridge had $975,000 − $549,000 = $426,000 more in current assets than in current liabilities. In general, the greater this difference, the better, because more funds are expected to be converted into cash during the next year than will be required to "pay the bills" that are expected to become due.

Within Park Ridge's current assets, there is $74,000 in **cash and cash equivalents,** an account that represents actual cash in hand plus money held in commercial checking accounts plus securities investments with a maturity of three months or less (such as money market mutual funds). There is also $147,000 of *short-term investments* (sometimes called *marketable securities*), which represent investments in highly liquid, low-risk securities such as U.S. Treasury bills that have maturities greater than three months but less than one year. Note that cash equivalents and short-term investments are similar in nature; they differ only slightly in maturity.

Organizations hold cash equivalents and short-term investments because cash and funds held in commercial checking accounts earn no interest. Thus, businesses should hold only enough cash and checking account balances to pay their recurring operating expenses; any funds on hand in excess of immediate needs should be invested in safe, short-term, easily sellable, interest-bearing securities.

> **⊘ CRITICAL CONCEPT**
> Cash and Cash Equivalents
>
> Cash and cash equivalents make up the first current asset account listed on a business's balance sheet. Cash is actual (petty) cash plus the amount of money held in commercial checking accounts, so cash is immediately (more or less) available for disbursement. Cash equivalents are those securities investments that have a maturity of 90 days or less, such as money market funds and short-term Treasury securities. Such funds can be quickly converted into cash at known prices. The cash and cash equivalents account is the most liquid of a business's balance sheet accounts; that is, it consists of either cash or securities that can be turned quickly into cash at a known price.

In addition to holding excess cash, short-term investments are built up periodically to meet projected nonoperating cash outlays, such as tax payments, investments in property and equipment, and legal judgments. Even though short-term investments pay relatively low interest, any return is better than none, so such investments are preferable to cash and checking account holdings.

Accounts receivable represents money owed to Park Ridge for services that have already been provided. As discussed in Chapters 3 and 7, third-party payers make most payments for healthcare services, and these payments often take weeks or months to be billed, processed, and ultimately paid. The accounts receivable balance of $727,000 represents monies owed to the business for services rendered in 2008 that have not yet been received. Note that the $727,000 amount is net of allowances for discounts, charity care, and bad debt losses. In other words, the amount listed represents the actual amount expected to be collected. Thus, the presentation on the balance sheet is consistent with the Chapter 11 discussion concerning net patient service revenue.

The $727,000 net receivable amount listed on the balance sheet stems from the income statement's 2008 net patient service revenue of $4,024,000 (see Table 11.1 in Chapter 11). Here's the logic: A total of $4,024,000 was billed to patients and payers during 2008. Of this amount, $46,000 is shown as a provision for bad debts on the income statement. This bad debt expense represents Park Ridge's best estimate, based on past experience, of the total dollar amount of net patient service revenue that will never be collected. Thus, Park Ridge actually expected to receive $4,024,000 – $46,000 = $3,978,000 in revenues (reimbursement) for services provided during 2008.

The fact that $727,000 of the net patient service revenue remains to be collected suggests that the difference between $3,978,000 and $727,000, which totals $3,251,000, was collected during 2008. Where is this collected cash? It could be anywhere. Most of it went right out the door to pay operating expenses, primarily for salaries and benefits. Some of the collected cash may have been spent on new equipment or on inventories that have not yet been used, and hence may be sitting in one of the asset accounts on the balance sheet.

If the business were to close its doors on the last day of 2008, its accounts receivable balance of $727,000 would fall to zero when the entire amount was eventually collected (except for any errors in the bad debt forecast). However, if Park Ridge continues as an ongoing enterprise, the receivables balance really never falls to zero because while Park Ridge's collections are lowering it, new services are constantly being provided that create new billings, and hence new receivables, that are added to this balance.

The final current asset on Table 12.1, inventories, primarily reflects Park Ridge's investment in medical supplies, including drugs. The value of supplies on hand at the end of 2008 was $27,000. As with the cash account, it is not in a business's best interest to hold excessive inventories. A certain level of supplies is necessary to meet immediate expected needs and to maintain a safety stock to guard against unexpected surges in usage. Any inventories held that are above this level create unnecessary costs. Thus, many healthcare organizations limit their investment in inventories through aggressive inventory management techniques, as discussed in Chapter 7.

It should be obvious that the primary purpose of the current asset accounts is to support the operations of the organization. However, current assets do not generate high returns. For example, cash earns no return, and short-term investments generally earn relatively low returns. The receivables account does not earn interest income nor does it generate new patient service revenue, and inventories represent dollar amounts invested in items sitting on shelves, which earn no return until patients are billed for their use. Because of the low (or zero) return earned on current assets, businesses try to minimize the amounts in these accounts but ensure that the levels on hand are sufficient to keep operations running smoothly.

The importance of converting inventories, accounts receivable, and cash into securities investments as quickly as possible, and hence turning zero-return assets into some-return assets, cannot be overemphasized. Under most reimbursement methods, providers must first build the current assets necessary to provide the services; then actually do the work; and some time later (often 50 days or more), get paid.

INVESTMENTS (LONG TERM)

Financial asset
A security (piece of paper) such as a stock or bond that gives the holder a claim against the issuing business's cash flows.

The second major asset category is investments. Because these investments are not listed under current assets, they represent the money Park Ridge has invested in various forms of long-term (maturities that exceed one year) securities. Note that this account represents investments in long-term *financial assets*, as opposed to investments in *real assets*, which are listed next on the balance sheet as property and equipment. The $125,000 reported at the end of 2008 represents the amount that the business has invested in stocks, bonds, and other securities that have a longer maturity than its short-term investments (less than one year) and that it is hoped will provide a higher return.

Real asset
Property and equipment, such as land, buildings, and machines, used to create a business's cash flows.

The income earned on near cash, short-term, and long-term investments is reported on Park Ridge's income statement as investment income. As discussed in Chapter 11, Park Ridge reported investment income of $13,000 for 2008. A footnote often will reveal the details of the types of security investments held by the organization. For example, Park Ridge reported the following information in the footnotes: "Investments consist of U.S. Treasury obligations that are reported at fair (market) value on the balance sheet. Investment income is reported on the income statement unless restricted by donor."

Not-for-profit organizations often carry large amounts of long-term securities investments. Eventually, the funds that Park Ridge invested in long-term securities investments will be used to purchase buildings and equipment and other real assets that provide new or improved services to its patients.

In contrast, investor-owned businesses usually do not build up such reserves. Any cash flow above the amount needed for near-term reinvestment in the business would likely be returned to owners, primarily as dividends. When additional capital is needed for property and equipment purchases, an investor-owned business simply accesses the capital (debt and equity) markets for additional financing.

PROPERTY AND EQUIPMENT (FIXED ASSETS)

The third asset category is **property and equipment**, often called **fixed assets**. Fixed assets, as compared to current assets, and even compared to long-term securities investments, are highly illiquid (cannot easily be bought and sold) and are used over relatively long periods of time. Whereas the levels of current assets rise and fall spontaneously with the organization's level of operations, fixed assets (land, buildings, and equipment) are normally maintained at a level sufficient to handle peak patient demand.

Fixed assets are listed at historical cost (the purchase price) minus accumulated depreciation as of the date of the balance sheet. *Accumulated depreciation* represents the total dollars of depreciation that have been expensed on the income statement against the historical cost of the organization's fixed assets. (Depreciation expense, which is an income statement item, was discussed in Chapter 11.)

Numerically, the amounts of depreciation expense reported on the income statement each year are accumulated over time to create the accumulated depreciation account on the balance sheet. Then, the accumulated depreciation amount is subtracted from the historical cost to obtain net fixed assets (net property and equipment), which is the balance sheet value of a business's property and equipment.

Park Ridge lists two categories of property and equipment: medical and office equipment (with a cost of $56,000) and vehicles (with a cost of $70,000), for a total acquisition cost of $126,000. But the accumulated depreciation amount on these assets was $45,000, so the net property and equipment balance was $126,000 – $45,000 = $81,000 at the end of 2008. (The accumulated depreciation amount is shown as a negative number because it is subtracted on the balance sheet.)

Note that the historical cost of these assets (gross property and equipment) was $126,000. Some of the fixed assets were purchased in 2008 and some earlier, but the total acquisition cost of all the fixed assets used by Park Ridge on December 31, 2008, was $126,000. The accumulated depreciation on these assets through December 31, 2008 was $45,000, which accounts for that portion of the value of the assets that was "spent" in producing income.

The difference, or net, of $81,000, reflects the remaining **book value** of the business's fixed assets. Often, a more detailed explanation of the fixed asset accounts is found in the footnotes.

As mentioned earlier, the connection of the balance sheet net property and equipment account to the income statement is through depreciation expense. The accumulated depreciation of $45,000 reported at the end of 2008 is $21,000 greater than the 2007 amount of $24,000. This increase in accumulated depreciation on the balance sheet reflects

---

> ⓘ **CRITICAL CONCEPT**
> Property and Equipment (Fixed Assets)
>
> The property and equipment account on the balance sheet lists a business's land; buildings; and equipment, including vehicles, office furniture, and computers. Such physical assets have lives greater than one year and are fundamentally different from short-term assets, which are converted into cash in a relatively short time. The categories of assets that are listed as property and equipment often are called fixed assets because they are "left in place" to produce income as opposed to, say, inventories, which are consumed to produce income. Fixed assets are listed on the balance sheet at historical cost minus the cumulative amount of depreciation taken on the listed assets. The result—net property and equipment—is the book value of a business's fixed assets.

Accumulated depreciation
The total amount of depreciation expensed over time against the fixed assets listed on the balance sheet.

Gross fixed assets
The historical cost of a business's fixed assets (property and equipment), as opposed to net fixed assets, which is the historical cost minus accumulated depreciation.

> ⓘ **CRITICAL CONCEPT**
> Book Value
>
> This is the value of a business's assets as reported on the balance sheet. Note that an asset's book value might be quite different from its current, or market, value. For example, an inventory item might be obsolete and might be worthless, but until disposed of it typically would be carried on the balance sheet at cost. Or, because of inflation, a business's property and equipment may be worth far more than the depreciated (net) value reported on the balance sheet.

the $21,000 in depreciation expense reported on the 2008 income statement.

Depreciation, even though it rarely reflects the true change in value of a fixed asset over time, at least ensures an orderly recognition of value loss. Occasionally, assets experience a sudden, unexpected loss of value. One example is when changing technology instantly makes a piece of diagnostic equipment obsolete and hence worthless. When this occurs, the asset that has experienced the decline in value is written off, which means that its value on the balance sheet is reduced (perhaps to zero) and the amount of the reduction is taken as an expense on the income statement.

> ⓘ **SELF-TEST QUESTIONS**
>
> 1. What are the three major categories of asset accounts?
>
> 2. What is the primary difference between current assets and the remainder of the assets listed on the balance sheet?
>
> 3. What is accumulated depreciation, and how does it tie in to the income statement?

Capital
The funds used to finance a business.

12.4 LIABILITIES

As shown in Table 12.1, liabilities and equity make up the lower section of the balance sheet. Together, they represent the *capital* that a business has raised to acquire the assets shown in the upper section of the balance sheet. Again, by definition, total liabilities and equity must equal total assets. Another way of looking at this is that every dollar of assets listed in the upper section of the balance sheet must be matched by a dollar of capital from the lower section.

Liabilities represent financing, provided by individuals and businesses that have claims against the organization, that is fixed by contract. For example, employees may have unpaid wages and salaries, tax authorities may have unpaid taxes, and vendors may have unpaid bills for supplies or equipment sold to the business. (Even not-for-profit organizations, which do not pay income taxes, typically have unpaid payroll and withholding taxes on their employees.)

However, the largest liability claims typically are by creditors (lenders) who supplied debt capital to the business, often in the form of bank loans or bonds (for large businesses). Most creditors' claims are against the total assets of the organization (unsecured), rather than tied to specific assets that were used as collateral for the loan (secured).

In the event of default (nonpayment of interest or principal) by the borrower, creditors have the right to force the business into bankruptcy, with liquidation as a possible consequence. If liquidation occurs, the law requires that any proceeds be used first to satisfy liability claims before any funds can be paid to owners or, in the case of not-for-profits, used for charitable purposes. Furthermore, the dollar value of each liability claim is fixed by the amount shown on the balance sheet, while the owners, including the community at large for not-for-profit organizations, have a claim to the residual proceeds of the liquidation rather than to a fixed amount.

CRITICAL CONCEPT
Liabilities

Liabilities represent the payment obligations of a business. Thus, liabilities stem from many sources. Perhaps the most obvious liability is money owed to lenders for furnishing debt capital. Typically, borrowers must pay lenders interest and must, at some point, repay the principal amount. These debt obligations are listed as liabilities on the balance sheet. Other liabilities include monies owed to suppliers, employees, and tax authorities. The difference between liabilities and equity is that liabilities are contractual obligations that must be paid, or severe consequences can result, including the hospital being forced into bankruptcy. Businesses, even for-profit ones, have no contractual obligations to make payments to their suppliers of equity capital.

Like assets, the balance sheet presentation of liabilities follows a logical format. Current liabilities, which are those liabilities that fall due (must be paid) within one accounting period (one year in this example), are listed first. Long-term debt, distinguished from short-term debt by having maturities greater than one accounting period, is listed second.

As shown in Table 12.1, Park Ridge Homecare had total liabilities at the end of 2008 of $703,000, which consisted of two parts: total current liabilities of $549,000 and total long-term debt of $154,000. The following sections describe each liability account in detail.

Current liability
A payment obligation (liability) of a business that is due in the next accounting period, often one year.

Notes payable
The balance sheet name typically used for a business's short-term debt.

CURRENT LIABILITIES

Current liabilities are liabilities that must be paid within one accounting period (one year, in this example). Many healthcare businesses use both short-term and long-term debt financing. Short-term debt, with a maturity of less than one year, usually takes the form of a bank loan and generally is used to finance temporary (seasonal) asset needs. When listed on the balance sheet, short-term debt typically is called *notes payable*. We see that Park Ridge Homecare had $13,000 of short-term debt outstanding at the end of 2008.

Accounts payable represent payment obligations to vendors (suppliers) that have been incurred as of the balance sheet date but that have not yet been paid. Often, suppliers

Accounts payable
Monies owed to vendors for purchased supplies. Payables arise when vendors offer credit terms that allow the buyer to pay some time (say, 30 days) after the supplies have been purchased.

offer their customers credit terms, which allow payment sometime after the purchase is made—say, 30 days. By allowing Park Ridge to pay 30 days after the supplies have been received, the supplier is acting as a creditor. The balance sheet tells us that suppliers, at the end of 2008, had extended Park Ridge $40,000 worth of such credit.

Wages and benefits due to employees, interest due on debt financing, accrued utilities expenses, and similar items are included on the balance sheet as *accrued expenses (accruals)*. Let's use Park Ridge's employees to illustrate the logic behind accruals.

The staff earns wages and benefits on a daily basis as the work is performed. However, the business pays its workers every two weeks. Therefore, other than on paydays (assuming no lag), it owes its staff some amount of salaries for work performed. Whenever the obligation to pay wages extends into the next accounting period, an accrual is created on the balance sheet. This obligation, as well as taxes due to government authorities and interest due to lenders, appears on Park Ridge's balance sheet as an accrual. At the end of 2008, the business owed $496,000 to its employees, creditors, and tax authorities (withholding and payroll taxes).

At the end of 2008, current liability accounts provided a total of $549,000 in financing for Park Ridge. In effect, these funds represent "loans" provided to the business by lenders, suppliers, employees, and taxing authorities that must be paid in 2009. In fact, most of these obligations must be paid in a much shorter time than one year; many are due just a few days or weeks into the year.

LONG-TERM DEBT

The *long-term debt* section of Table 12.1 represents debt financing to the organization with maturities of more than one year. The long-term debt section lists any debt owed to banks and other creditors, such as bondholders, as well as obligations under certain types of lease arrangements. Usually, detailed information relative to the specific characteristics of the long-term debt is disclosed in the footnotes to the financial statements. For example, the footnotes to Park Ridge's financial statements indicate that the business's long-term debt consists of a bank loan with a 10 percent interest rate that matures in 2018.

At the end of 2008, Park Ridge had total liabilities—combined current liabilities and long-term debt—of $703,000. As discussed in the next section, Park Ridge reported $478,000 in equity, for total financing (which must equal total assets) of $1,181,000. Thus, based on the values recorded on the balance sheet (book values), Park Ridge uses more debt financing than equity financing.

The choice between debt and equity financing is discussed in Chapter 8. Also, Chapter 13 covers alternative ways to measure the amount of debt financing that an organization uses and its effect on the business's financial condition.

Accrued expenses (accruals)

Monies owed to various parties, such as to employees for services rendered. Also includes interest owed to lenders and tax obligations.

Long-term debt

Debt financing that has a maturity greater than one accounting period.

? SELF-TEST QUESTIONS

1. What are liabilities?

2. What are some of the accounts that would be classified as current liabilities?

3. Use an example to explain the logic behind accruals.

4. What is the difference between notes payable and long-term debt?

12.5 EQUITY (NET ASSETS)

On the balance sheet, the equity (ownership) claim on an organization's assets is called *net assets* when the organization has not-for-profit status. As the term "net" implies, net assets represent the dollar value of assets remaining when a business's liabilities are stripped out.

However, as detailed in Chapter 2, the healthcare industry has a wide variety of ownership types, which results in different terminology being used for the equity section of the balance sheet. To keep things manageable, we will use the term **equity** to specify nonliability (ownership) capital.

To determine what belongs to the owners, whether explicitly recognized in for-profit businesses or implied in not-for-profit organizations, fixed claims (liabilities) are subtracted from the value of the business's assets. The remainder, the equity, represents the residual value of the assets of the organization.

Park Ridge Homecare's equity increased by $163,000 from 2007 to 2008, which is the same amount that it reported as net income (excess of revenues over expenses) for 2008. This connection between the bottom line of the income statement and the equity section of the balance sheet is a mathematical necessity. In the case of not-for-profit businesses, there is simply nowhere else for those earnings to go. This highlights a second connection between the balance sheet and the income statement; the first was depreciation.

Park Ridge's balance sheet balances because the increase in equity of $163,000 was matched by

> **Net assets**
> The label used to designate the equity on a not-for-profit organization's balance sheet.

! CRITICAL CONCEPT
Equity

Equity represents the value of a business that remains when the value of its liabilities is subtracted from asset value. Perhaps the best way to look at this is in terms of home ownership. Suppose you own a home that is worth $200,000 today. But you have a mortgage on the home with a $150,000 balance. In this situation, the balance sheet for the home would look like this:

Assets	
Home	$200,000
Total assets	$200,000

Liabilities and Equity	
Mortgage	$150,000
Equity	50,000
Total liabilities	
and equity	$200,000

(Continued)

The $50,000 represents the value of the home to the owner. If you sold the home today for $200,000 and paid off the mortgage balance of $150,000, you could pocket $50,000. Of course, you would have no place to sleep!

A business's equity is similar. If a business sold off its assets and realized the exact amounts listed on the balance sheet and then used the proceeds to pay off its liabilities, the amount in the equity section would be left. If the business were for-profit, this amount would be distributed to the owners. If the business were not-for-profit, the amount would belong to the community at large and would have to be used for some charitable purpose.

Note that this balance sheet was created using market values. That is, the $200,000 value of the home is an estimate of its price if sold today, as opposed to book values, which are created following accounting rules (GAAP).

Also, note what would happen if the value of your home dropped to $150,000. Your equity value would drop to $0; you would be wiped out. Even worse, what would happen if the value dropped to $125,000? To make the balance sheet balance, your equity balance would have to be −$25,000. Now you owe more on the home than it is worth, which is called being "under water."

a like increase in assets, along with asset increases that resulted from other financing. The asset increases might be in cash, receivables, fixed assets (property and equipment), or some other account.

The key point is that the equity account is not a store of cash. As Park Ridge earns profits that increase the equity account, these funds are invested in supplies, property and equipment, and other assets to provide future services that would likely generate even larger profits in the future. Park Ridge's total assets grew by $1,181,000 − $853,000 = $328,000 in 2008, which was supported by an increase in total liabilities of $703,000 − $538,000 = $165,000 and an increase in equity (net assets) of $163,000. Thus, the increase in the lower section of the balance sheet, $165,000 + $163,000 = $328,000, was the same as the increase in the upper section. After all, the balance sheet must balance!

Thus far, the discussion of the balance sheet has focused on Park Ridge Homecare, a not-for-profit corporation. In general, the asset and liability sections of the balance sheet are much the same, regardless of ownership status. The equity section tends to differ in presentation for different types of ownership because the forms of equity differ. That is the bad news. The good news is that the economic substance of the equity section remains the same.

? **SELF-TEST QUESTIONS**

1. What is equity (net assets)?

2. What is the relationship between the equity account on the balance sheet and earnings (net income) reported on the income statement?

✳ INDUSTRY PRACTICE The Average Home Health Care Business

When financial statements are created for entire industries, as opposed to individual businesses, it is most useful to express the balance sheet accounts and income statement items in percentages rather than in dollars. That way, easy comparison can be made between a specific business (e.g., Park Ridge Homecare) and "the industry." (Financial statements that are expressed in percentages rather than dollars are called common size statements.)

The average home health care business has a common size income statement that looks like this:

Total revenues	100.0%
Operating expenses	90.3
Operating profit	9.7%
All other expenses	2.9
Profit before taxes	6.8%

Notice that this format does not match the format of Park Ridge Homecare's income statement given in Table 11.1. Unfortunately, industry-wide data, which come from many sources, typically are summarized using a more generic format than specified by GAAP. That's just a fact of life.

The bottom line for the industry is that the average home health care business makes 6.8 percent (6.8 cents) before taxes on every dollar of revenue. But let's not get too far ahead of ourselves; we will analyze Park Ridge's financial condition in detail in Chapter 13. However, remember from Chapter 11 that Park Ridge had a total margin—defined as total profits divided by total revenues—of 4.0 percent. Furthermore, the average 6.8 percent profit before taxes for the industry is equivalent to total margin for a not-for-profit business. Thus, as measured by total margin, Park Ridge is not as profitable as the average home health care business.

(Continued)

✱ INDUSTRY PRACTICE The Average Home Health Care Business

Here is what the average home health care business balance sheet looks like:

ASSETS

Current Assets:

Cash and cash equivalents	12.4%
Receivables	45.1
Inventories	1.8
Other current assets	3.3
Total current assets	62.6%

Fixed assets	21.9%
Other long-term assets	15.5
Total long-term assets	37.4%

Total assets	100.0%

LIABILITIES AND EQUITY

Current Liabilities:

Short-term debt	9.2%
Accounts payable	11.3
Other short-term expenses	19.1
Total current liabilities	39.6%

Long-term debt	33.8
Total liabilities	73.4%

Equity	26.6%

Total liabilities and equity	100.0%

Note that Park Ridge had a debt ratio—defined as total debt (total liabilities) divided by total assets—of 59.5 percent in 2008. The average home health care

12.6 FUND ACCOUNTING

One unique feature of many not-for-profit balance sheets is that they classify certain asset and equity accounts as being *restricted accounts*. When a not-for-profit organization receives contributions that donors have indicated must be used for a specific purpose, the organization must create multiple funds to account for its assets and equity. Each fund typically has assets, liabilities, and an equity balance.

Because the balance sheet of an organization that receives restricted contributions is separated into restricted and unrestricted funds, this form of accounting is called **fund accounting.** Only contributions to not-for-profit organizations are tax deductible to the donor, and hence few contributions are made to investor-owned healthcare businesses. Thus, fund accounting is only applicable to not-for-profit organizations.

Restricted contributions and gifts impose legal and fiduciary responsibilities on healthcare organizations to carry out the written wishes of donors. Thus, numerous rules are associated with fund accounting, but they will not be discussed here as they go well beyond the scope of this book.

The good news is that GAAP encourage organizations that use fund accounting to present balance sheets to outside parties that have roughly

Restricted account
An account whose funds are restricted to specific uses by donors or by management designation.

CRITICAL CONCEPT
Fund Accounting

Fund accounting involves the separation of balance sheet accounts into separate "funds" by designated purpose. Thus, an investment account shown on the balance sheet might be labeled as restricted, meaning that the dollar amount of that account must be used for a specific purpose, which often is designated by donors. Another investment account might be labeled as unrestricted, meaning it is available for any use deemed appropriate by management. Fund accounting typically is used by not-for-profits and charities, although such businesses are encouraged to also create a set of "regular" financial statements for public distribution.

the same look as shown in Table 12.1. Thus, with the exception of further breakdown into unrestricted and restricted accounts, such balance sheets have the same economic content as those prepared by businesses that do not use fund accounting.

Although Park Ridge Homecare's balance sheet does not designate any accounts as restricted, the notes to the financial statements indicate that $90,000 of the $478,000 reported net assets are restricted to specific activities. There is no indication in the footnotes of what assets were supported by this $90,000, but these funds likely have been invested in securities for some specific (designated) use.

? SELF-TEST QUESTIONS

1. What is fund accounting?

2. What type of a healthcare organization is most likely to use fund accounting?

3. Is there a significant difference in the economic content of balance sheets created by investor-owned and not-for-profit healthcare organizations?

12.7 THE STATEMENT OF CASH FLOWS

The balance sheet and income statement are traditional financial statements that have been required by GAAP for many years. In contrast, the **statement of cash flows** has only been required for for-profit businesses since 1989 and for not-for-profit businesses since 1995.

The statement of cash flows was created in response to demands by users for better information about a firm's cash inflows and outflows.

While the balance sheet reports the cash balance on hand at the end of the period, it does not provide details on why the cash account is greater or smaller than the previous year's value, nor does the income statement give detailed information on cash flows.

In addition to the problems of accrual accounting and noncash expenses discussed in Chapter 11, some cash raised by a business may not even appear on the income statement. For example, Park Ridge Homecare may have raised cash during 2008 by taking on more debt or by selling some equipment. Such flows, which are not shown on the income statement, affect a firm's cash balance.

! CRITICAL CONCEPT
Statement of Cash Flows

The statement of cash flows can be thought of as an income statement that has been converted from accrual accounting to cash accounting. In essence, the statement of cash flows reports where a business gets its cash and what it does with that cash. The statement is organized into three major sections: The first section focuses on operating flows, the second on capital investment flows, and the third on financing flows. In addition, there is a short section that reconciles the net cash flow reported on the statement to the change in the cash reported on the balance sheet.

Finally, the cash coming into a business does not just sit in the cash account. Most of it goes to pay operating expenses or to purchase other assets, or for investor-owned firms, some may be paid out as dividends. Thus, the cash account does not increase by the full amount of cash generated, and it would be useful to know how the difference was spent. The statement of cash flows details where cash resources came from and how they were used.

Park Ridge's 2008 and 2007 statements are presented in Table 12.2. To simplify the discussion, the data in the statement have been reduced; they are somewhat shorter and easier to comprehend than most real-world statements. Nevertheless, an understanding of the composition and presentation of Table 12.2 will give you an excellent appreciation for the value of the statement of cash flows. Also, note that an alternative format of this statement differs in how the operational cash flows are reported but not in overall structure.

	2008	2007
Cash Flows from Operating Activities:		
Cash received from patient services	$3,783	$2,590
Cash paid to employees and suppliers	(3,684)	(2,541)
Interest paid	(16)	(14)
Interest earned	13	6
Net cash from operations	$ 96	$ 41
Cash Flows from Investing Activities:		
Purchase of property and equipment	($ 25)	($ 19)
Net cash from investing activities	($ 25)	($ 19)
Cash Flows from Financing Activities:		
Securities purchases	($ 35)	($ 15)
Contributions	10	6
Repayment of long-term debt	(13)	0
Net cash from financing activities	($ 38)	($ 9)
Net increase (decrease) in cash and equivalents	$ 33	$ 13
Cash and equivalents, beginning of year	$ 41	$ 28
Cash and equivalents, end of year	$ 74	$ 41

TABLE 12.2
Park Ridge Home-care: Statements of Cash Flows Years Ended December 31, 2008 and 2007 (in thousands)

The format of the statement of cash flows makes it easy to understand why Park Ridge's cash position increased by $33,000 during 2008. In other words, the statement tells us Park Ridge's sources of cash and how this cash was used.

The statement is divided into three major sections: cash flows from operating activities, cash flows from investing activities, and cash flows from financing activities.

Cash Flows from Operating Activities

The first section focuses on the sources and uses of cash tied to operations. Of course, the most important source is cash received from the provision of patient services, so its value for 2008 ($3,783,000) is listed first.

Note that this is not the same amount as that listed for net patient service and other operating revenue on the income statement. As you know, income statement revenues follow accrual accounting guidelines, but the statement of cash flows follows cash accounting guidelines. Thus, Park Ridge "booked" $4,069,000 in operating revenues in 2008, but the cash collected in that year was only $3,783,000.

The next item in the section is cash paid to employees and suppliers. As we just discussed, because of accrual accounting, the total cash outlay in 2008 ($3,684,000) does not exactly match the total matching expenses listed on the income statement. The statement of cash flows focuses on the actual movement of cash into and out of a business, while the income statement centers on the obligations that create the cash flows. Note that the cash paid to employees and suppliers is enclosed in parentheses in Table 12.2. On the statement of cash flows, all outflows are shown in parentheses to differentiate them from inflows.

The items interest paid and interest earned are listed here as operating activities, which shows some leeway in formatting. These flows could also be listed in the financing activities section rather than the operating activities section.

When all the operating activities entries are totaled, Park Ridge reported $96,000 in net cash from operations for 2008. For a business, whether investor-owned or not-for-profit, to be financially sustainable, it must generate a positive cash flow from operations. Thus, at least for 2008 and 2007, Park Ridge's operations are doing financially what they should be doing—generating cash.

Furthermore, the business's cash flow from operations more than doubled from 2007 to 2008. Much of this was the result of an increase in volume, but other factors also played a role. Lori Gibbs, the founder of Park Ridge Homecare, should identify those factors that contributed to the increase and take appropriate action to ensure another increase in 2009. Unlike the situation reported by Park Ridge, a consistent negative net cash flow from operations sends a warning to managers and other stakeholders that the business may not be economically sustainable.

CASH FLOWS FROM INVESTING ACTIVITIES

The title of this section can be misleading because the emphasis here is on capital investing (property and equipment), not financial investing (securities).

As evidenced by the 2007 to 2008 change in total (gross) property and equipment derived from the balance sheets, Park Ridge spent $126,000 – $101,000 = $25,000 to acquire additional fixed assets. Thus, roughly one-quarter of the business's operating cash flow was spent on new property and equipment. This fact should not be alarming, especially for a not-for-profit business, as long as the investments are prudent. (Chapters 9 and 10 contain a great deal of insights into what makes a prudent capital investment, at least from a financial perspective.) Because there is only one line in this section, the total net cash from investing activities was also -$25,000 for 2008.

CASH FLOWS FROM FINANCING ACTIVITIES

This third section focuses on securities investments and financing flows. The changes in balance sheet accounts from 2007 to 2008 indicate that the business invested $10,000 in short-term investments and $25,000 in long-term investments (which require a use of cash). Thus, the first item in this section for 2008 is $35,000 in securities purchases (an outflow).

Also, the business received $10,000 in contributions in 2008 (an inflow) and spent $13,000 to repay long-term debt. On net, Park Ridge had a net cash outflow from financing activities of $38,000 in 2008. Thus, roughly one-third of the net cash flow from operations was used for financial activities.

NET INCREASE (DECREASE) IN CASH AND RECONCILIATION

After the three major sections, the next line in the statement of cash flows is the net increase (decrease) in cash and equivalents. This number is the sum of the totals from the three major sections. For Park Ridge in 2008, the net increase in cash and equivalents is $96,000 – $25,000 – $38,000 = $33,000.

Unlike the "bottom line" of the income statement, the change in cash line has limited value in assessing an organization's financial condition because it can be manipulated by financing activities. If an organization is losing cash on operations, but its managers want to report an increase in the cash account, in most cases they simply can borrow the funds necessary to show a net cash increase on the statement of cash flows. Thus, the net cash from operations line is a more important indicator of financial well-being than is the net increase (decrease) in cash line.

The net increase (decrease) in cash line is used to verify the correctness of the entries on the statement of cash flows. As shown in Table 12.2, the $33,000 increase in cash reported by Park Ridge for 2008 added to the $41,000 beginning-of-year cash balance totals $74,000. A check of the end-of-2008 cash balance shown in Table 12.1 confirms the amount calculated on the statement of cash flows.

In summary, the income statement focuses on accounting profitability, while the statement of cash flows follows the movement of cash—that is, where did the money come from, and how did the organization use it? The major concern for the income statement is economic profitability as defined by GAAP, while for the statement of cash flows, it is cash viability. Is the organization generating, and will it continue to generate, sufficient cash to meet both short-term and long-term needs?

(?) SELF-TEST QUESTIONS

1. How does the statement of cash flows differ from the income statement?

2. Briefly explain the three major sections on the statement of cash flows.

3. In your view, what is the most important piece of information reported on the statement of cash flows?

12.8 A LOOK AHEAD: FINANCIAL STATEMENT ANALYSIS

Debt ratio (or debt-to-assets ratio)
A ratio that measures the proportion of debt (versus equity) financing. Typically defined as total debt (liabilities) divided by total assets.

Here, we continue our discussion of ratio analysis (started in Chapter 11) using balance sheet data.

The *debt ratio* (or *debt-to-assets ratio*) is defined as total debt divided by total assets. Total debt can be defined several ways, depending on the use of the ratio, but for purposes here, assume that total debt includes all liabilities—that is, all non-equity capital. (An alternative would be to include only interest-bearing debt in our definition.) Using Table 12.1 data, Park Ridge Homecare's debt ratio at the end of 2008 was total debt (total liabilities) divided by total assets = $703,000 / $1,181,000 = 0.595 = 59.5%. This ratio reveals that each dollar of assets was financed by about 60 cents of debt and, by inference, about 40 cents of equity.

Park Ridge's debt ratio at the end of 2007 was $538,000 / $853,000 = 0.631 = 63.1%. Thus, the business decreased its proportional use of debt financing by roughly 3 percentage points in one year. That information is important to Park Ridge's managers and creditors. Also, note that judgments about Park Ridge's capital structure could not be made easily without constructing the debt ratio and other ratios; interpreting the dollar values directly is just too difficult.

? SELF-TEST QUESTIONS

1. Explain how ratio analysis can be used to help interpret balance sheet data.

2. What is the debt ratio, and what does it measure?

THEME WRAP-UP   UNDERSTANDING THE BALANCE SHEET AND THE STATEMENT OF CASH FLOWS

After reviewing Park Ridge Homecare's balance sheet and statement of cash flows, what have you (and Lori) learned about Park Ridge's financial ability to start a second location?

The business has nearly $350,000 in cash and securities investments. Of course, some cash must be held to meet day-to-day operating expenses and some of the securities investments are restricted, and hence could not be used to fund a new location. Still, some portion of the $350,000 could likely be used to help open a second facility.

According to the balance sheet, Park Ridge currently has $27,000 in inventories and $126,000 in gross fixed assets (vehicles and equipment), for a total gross investment of $153,000. Assuming that a start-up location would require about the same amount (or perhaps less initially) of these assets, it appears that the proposed business could be partially or wholly funded from Park Ridge's current securities investments.

Finally, the statement of cash flows indicates that Park Ridge has generated $137,000 of operating cash flow over the last two years of operations. This means that a new location, if it achieves the same potential as the existing business, would quickly generate a positive operating cash flow and hence would be more or less self-sustaining in a short time.

All-in-all, Lori's plan to use Park Ridge's resources to fund another location seems feasible. However, a complete financial statement analysis will yield the best possible picture of Park Ridge's financial condition, and hence its ability to support the opening of a new business. We will perform that analysis in Chapter 13.

KEY CONCEPTS

This chapter extends the discussion of financial statements to the balance sheet and the statement of cash flows. Here are the key concepts:

➤ The *balance sheet* provides a snapshot of the financial position of a business at a given point in time.

➤ The *basic accounting equation* specifies that assets must equal liabilities plus equity (total assets must equal total financing). When rearranged, the accounting identity reminds us that a business's equity is really a residual amount that represents the difference between assets and liabilities.

➤ *Assets* identify the resources (in dollar terms) owned by the organization. Assets are listed by *maturity* (order of when the assets are expected to be converted into cash). Current assets are expected to be converted into cash during the next accounting period—often, one year.

➤ *Liabilities* represent a business's payment obligations to employees, suppliers, tax authorities, and lenders. *Current liabilities*—those obligations that fall due within one accounting period—are listed first. *Long-term liabilities* (typically, debt with maturities greater than one accounting period) are listed second.

➤ *Equity* represents the residual (ownership) claim against a business's assets. Depending on the form of organization and ownership, this claim may be called *net assets* or something else.

➤ There are two *primary interrelationships* between the balance sheet and the income statement. First, the annual depreciation expense shown on the income statement accumulates on the balance sheet in the accumulated depreciation account. Second, all earnings from the income statement that are reinvested in the business accumulate on the balance sheet in the equity account.

➤ *Fund accounting* is used by organizations that have restricted contributions. This complicates internal accounting procedures and adds additional detail to the balance sheet. However, fund accounting does not alter the basic format of the balance sheet nor its economic interpretation.

➤ The *statement of cash flows* shows where an organization gets its cash from and how the cash is used. It combines information found on both the income statement and the balance sheet.

➤ The statement of cash flows has three major sections: *cash flows from operating activities*, *cash flows from investing activities*, and *cash flows from financing activities*.

➤ The "bottom line" of the statement of cash flows is the *net increase (decrease) in cash*. Although this amount is useful in verifying the accuracy of the statement, its economic content is not as meaningful as the statement's component amounts, particularly *net cash from operations*.

In Chapter 13, we focus on using the information in all three financial statements to assess a business's financial condition.

END-OF-CHAPTER QUESTIONS

12.1 a. What is the difference in timing between the income statement and the balance sheet?
  b. What is wrong with this statement: "The clinic's cash balance for 2008 was $150,000, while its net income on December 31, 2008, was $50,000."

12.2 a. What is the basic accounting equation?
  b. What is its implication for the numbers on a balance sheet?
  c. What does the basic accounting equation tell us about a business's equity?

12.3 a. What are assets?
  b. What are the three major categories of assets?

12.4 a. What makes an asset a current asset?
  b. Provide some examples of current assets.

12.5 a. On the balance sheet, what is the difference between long-term investments and property and equipment?
  b. What is the difference between gross fixed assets (gross plant and equipment) and net fixed assets?

c. How does depreciation expense on the income statement relate to accumulated depreciation on the balance sheet?

12.6 a. What is the difference between liabilities and equity?
      b. What makes a liability a current liability?
      c. Give some examples of current liabilities.
      d. What is the difference between notes payable and long-term debt?

12.7 What is the relationship between net income on the income statement and the equity section on a balance sheet?

12.8 What is fund accounting, and why is it important to some healthcare providers?

12.9 a. What is the statement of cash flows, and how does it differ from the income statement?
      b. What are the three major sections of the statement of cash flows?
      c. What is the most important line on the statement of cash flows?

END-OF-CHAPTER PROBLEMS

12.1 Middleton Clinic had total assets of $500,000 and an equity balance of $350,000 at the end of 2007. One year later, at the end of 2008, the clinic had $575,000 in assets and $380,000 in equity. What was the clinic's dollar growth in assets during 2008, and how was this growth financed?

12.2 San Mateo Healthcare had an equity balance of $1.38 million at the beginning of the year. At the end of the year, its equity balance was $1.98 million. Assume that San Mateo is a not-for-profit organization. What was its net income for the period?

12.3 Here is financial statement information on four not-for-profit clinics:

	Pittman	Rose	Beckman	Jaffe
December 31, 2007:				
Assets	$ 80,000	$ 100,000	g	$ 150,000
Liabilities	50,000	d	$ 75,000	j
Equity	a	60,000	45,000	90,000

December 31, 2008:

Assets	b	130,000	180,000	k
Liabilities	55,000	62,000	h	80,000
Equity	45,000	e	110,000	145,000

During 2008:

Total revenues	c	400,000	i	500,000
Total expenses	330,000	f	360,000	l

Fill in the missing values labeled a through l.

12.4 The following are selected entries for Warren Clinic for December 31, 2008, in alphabetical order. Create Warren Clinic's balance sheet.

Accounts payable	$ 20,000
Accounts receivable, net	60,000
Cash	30,000
Equity	230,000
Long-term debt	120,000
Long-term investments	100,000
Net property and equipment	150,000
Other assets	40,000
Other long-term liabilities	10,000

12.5 Consider the following balance sheet:

BestCare HMO

Balance Sheet

June 30, 2008

(in thousands)

Assets

Current Assets:

Cash and cash equivalents $ 2,737

Net premiums receivable	821
Supplies	387
Total current assets	$3,945
Net property and equipment	$5,924
Total assets	$9,869
Liabilities and Net Assets	
Accounts payable—medical services	$ 2,145
Accrued expenses	929
Notes payable	382
Total current liabilities	$3,456
Long-term debt	$4,295
Total liabilities	$ 7,751
Net assets—unrestricted (equity)	$ 2,118
Total liabilities and net assets	$9,869

a. How does this balance sheet differ from the one presented in Table 12.1 for Park Ridge Homecare?

b. What is BestCare's debt ratio? How does it compare with Park Ridge Homecare's debt ratio?

12.6 Consider this balance sheet:

Green Valley Nursing Home, Inc.

Balance Sheet

December 31, 2008

Assets

Current Assets:

Cash and cash equivalents	$ 105,737
Investments	200,000
Net patient accounts receivable	215,600
Supplies	87,655

Total current assets	$ 608,992
Property and equipment	$2,250,000
Less accumulated depreciation	356,000
Net property and equipment	$1,894,000
Total assets	$2,502,992

Liabilities and Shareholders' Equity

Current Liabilities:

Accounts payable	$ 72,250
Accrued expenses	192,900
Notes payable	180,000
Total current liabilities	$ 445,150
Long-term debt	$1,700,000

Shareholders' Equity:

Common stock, $10 par value	$ 100,000
Retained earnings	257,842
Total shareholders' equity	$ 357,842
Total liabilities and shareholders' equity	$2,502,992

a. How does this balance sheet differ from the ones presented in Table 12.1 and Problem 12.5?

b. What is Green Valley's debt ratio? How does it compare with the debt ratios for Park Ridge Homecare and BestCare?

CHAPTER 13

ANALYZING FINANCIAL CONDITION

TECHNIQUES FOR EVALUATING FINANCIAL STATEMENTS

Following Lori Gibbs's story, we have learned that over the past two years, Park Ridge Home-care generated $262,000 in net income (earnings) and currently has nearly $350,000 in cash and securities investments. In addition, the balance sheet indicates that the business has a total gross (pre-depreciation) investment in property, equipment, and inventories of $153,000.

If the second location would require about the same amount of start-up resources as is needed by Park Ridge today, then it appears that the organization's current securities investments could fund the new enterprise.

Also, by examining the statement of cash flows, Lori found out that, over the last two years of operations, Park Ridge has generated $137,000 of operating cash flow. This is good news. It shows that if the new location achieves the same potential as Park Ridge, it would quickly generate a positive operating cash flow and hence could sustain itself.

Lori's intention to use Park Ridge's success as a financial springboard for the new location appears feasible. At this point, a complete financial statement analysis should be performed. Doing so would generate the clearest picture of Park Ridge's current financial condition.

That is our task in this chapter.

LEARNING OBJECTIVES

After studying this chapter, you will be able to

➤ Explain the purpose of financial statement analysis.

➤ Describe the primary techniques used in financial statement analysis.

➤ Conduct basic financial statement analyses to assess the financial condition of a business.

➤ Discuss the problems associated with financial statement analysis.

13.1 INTRODUCTION

In the last two chapters, we presented an overview of a business's financial statements. The purpose of these statements is to provide relevant information about the operations and financial status of an organization. Now, we turn our attention to assessing financial condition: Does the organization have the financial capacity to perform its mission?

Although the information contained in the financial statements is logically organized and presented, to gain a better understanding of a business's financial condition it is necessary to "massage," or reformat, the financial statement data. Furthermore, data found outside of the financial statements can be used to provide additional insights. By using various techniques applied to a variety of data, analysts can make the best possible judgments about a business's financial capabilities.

In this chapter, we explore several analytical techniques used in financial condition analysis and the problems inherent in such analyses. Along the way, you will discover that such analyses generate a great deal of data. A significant problem in assessing financial condition is separating the important from the unimportant and presenting the results in a simple format that is easy to understand and monitor.

13.2 FINANCIAL STATEMENT ANALYSIS

Often, initial judgments about financial condition are made on the basis of **financial statement analysis,** which focuses on the data contained in a business's financial statements.

Financial statement analysis is applied both to historical data, which reflect the results of past managerial decisions, and to forecasted data, which provide the road map for the business's future. Therefore, managers use financial statement analysis not only to assess current condition but also to plan for the future.

Although financial statement analysis provides a wealth of information regarding financial condition, it often fails to provide insight into the operational causes of that condition. Thus, financial statement analysis typically is supplemented by an analysis of the business's operating data, such as occupancy rate, patient mix, length of stay, and productivity measures. (Some of these operational measures are discussed in Chapter 7.)

By examining operational data in conjunction with financial data, managers can easily identify factors that contributed to the assessed financial condition. Through such combined analyses, managers are better able to develop and implement strategies that ensure a sound financial condition in the future.

> ⊘ **CRITICAL CONCEPT**
> Financial Statement Analysis
>
> Financial statement analysis involves using financial statement data to make judgments about a business's financial condition. Several techniques can be used in financial statement analysis, and the most important is ratio analysis. Because financial statement analysis does not provide much information about the underlying operational factors that contribute to financial condition, often it is supplemented by an analysis of operating data. The results of a financial statement analysis usually are presented as a list of financial (and operational) strengths and weaknesses.

In this chapter, we continue to use Park Ridge Homecare, a not-for-profit home health care business, to illustrate financial statement analysis. However, all the techniques we present here can be applied to any healthcare organization, regardless of setting.

(?) SELF-TEST QUESTIONS

1. What is financial statement analysis, and what is its purpose?

2. Why is financial statement analysis typically accompanied by an operational analysis?

13.3 INTERPRETING THE STATEMENT OF CASH FLOWS

We begin our financial statement analysis of Park Ridge Homecare by examining the statement of cash flows, presented here in Table 13.1. We look at this statement first because it is constructed in a way that allows us to make judgments without having to reformat the data. (Consider this discussion to be a review of Chapter 12 material—it never hurts to cover basic concepts a second time.)

The statement of cash flows answers the following questions:

◆ Are the firm's core operations profitable?

◆ How much capital did the firm raise? How was this capital used?

◆ What impact did operating and financing decisions have on the business's cash position?

The top section of the statement shows cash generated by and used in operations. For Park Ridge, operations in 2008 provided $96,000 in net cash flow. The next section focuses on investments in fixed assets. Park Ridge spent $25,000 on capital expenditures in 2008. Is that a large or small amount?

The income statement (Table 11.1) reports a depreciation expense of $21,000, so the business spent only slightly more on fixed assets in 2008 than the amount expensed for wear and tear. Furthermore, according to the balance sheet (Table 12.1), the bulk of the fixed-assets addition was a $23,000 increase in vehicles. Thus, Park Ridge likely added a vehicle to its fixed-assets base, which appears to be a sound capital investment for a growing home care business.

The third section highlights the fact that Park Ridge received $10,000 in contributions in 2008 and used cash to pay off previously incurred debt and to invest in securities. As indicated by account changes on the balance sheet, the $35,000 investment in securities consisted of $10,000 in short-term investments and $25,000 in long-term investments. The net result of the business's financing activities was a net cash outflow from financing of $38,000.

TABLE 13.1
Park Ridge Home-
care: Statements of
Cash Flows
Years Ended
December 31,
2008 and 2007 (in
thousands)

	2008	2007
Cash Flows from Operating Activities:		
Cash received from patient services	$3,783	$2,590
Cash paid to employees and suppliers	(3,684)	(2,541)
Interest paid	(16)	(14)
Interest earned	13	6
Net cash from operations	$ 96	$ 41
Cash Flows from Investing Activities:		
Purchase of property and equipment	($ 25)	($ 19)
Net cash from investing activities	($ 25)	($ 19)
Cash Flows from Financing Activities:		
Securities purchases	($ 35)	($ 15)
Contributions	10	6
Repayment of long-term debt	(13)	0
Net cash from financing activities	($ 38)	($ 9)
Net increase (decrease) in cash and equivalents	$ 33	$ 13
Cash and equivalents, beginning of year	$ 41	$ 28
Cash and equivalents, end of year	$ 74	$ 41

When the three major sections are totaled, this is the result: a $96,000 – $25,000 – $38,000 = $33,000 net increase in cash (net cash inflow) during 2008. The bottom of Table 13.3 reconciles the 2008 net cash flow with the ending cash balance shown on the balance sheet. Park Ridge began 2008 with $41,000; experienced a cash inflow of $33,000 during the year; and ended the year with $41,000 + $33,000 = $74,000 in its cash and cash equivalents account, as verified by the value reported in Table 13.2.

Park Ridge's statement of cash flows shows nothing unusual or alarming. It does show that the business's operations are inherently profitable, at least in 2007 and 2008. Had the statement showed an operating cash drain, Lori would have had something to worry about; if it continued, such a drain could bleed the business to death.

The statement of cash flows also provides easily interpreted information about Park Ridge's financing and fixed-asset investing activities for the year. In essence, the business's cash flow from operations was used primarily to purchase new fixed assets, to invest in securities, and to pay off long-term debt. Such uses of operating cash flow do not raise any red flags regarding the business's financial actions.

Managers and investors must pay close attention to the statement of cash flows. Financial condition is driven by cash flows, and the statement gives a good picture of the annual cash flows generated by the business. An examination of Table 13.1—or, better yet, a series of such tables going back the last five years (if the business is that old) and projected five years into the future—would give managers and creditors an idea of whether or not the business's operations are self-sustaining.

Although the statement of cash flows is filled with valuable information, the bottom line tells little about the business's financial condition because operating losses can be covered by financing transactions, such as borrowing or selling new common stock (if investor-owned), at least in the short run.

(?) SELF-TEST QUESTIONS

1. What type of financial condition information is provided in the statement of cash flows?

2. Does the fact that its cash position has improved provide much insight into the business's financial condition?

3. What did Park Ridge's 2008 statement of cash flows tell us?

13.4 RATIO ANALYSIS

Now, let's turn our attention to interpreting the income statement and balance sheet. Although both of these statements contain a wealth of information, they yield raw data that do not help managers in making meaningful judgments about the business's financial condition. For example, a hospital may have $5,248,760 in long-term debt and interest charges of $419,900. The true burden of this debt, and the hospital's ability to pay the interest and principal due, cannot be easily determined without additional analysis.

Ratio analysis combines data to create single numbers that have easily interpreted significance (for our purposes, numbers that measure various

(!) CRITICAL CONCEPT
Ratio Analysis

Ratio analysis is a technique that helps interpret the data contained in a business's financial statements as well as in other contexts. By combining values (sometimes from different statements), analysts can gain a more complete view of the business's financial condition. The idea here is to create single values (ratios) from the raw data that have economic meaning and can be easily interpreted. For example, a business with $100,000 in debt and $250,000 in assets has a debt ratio of $100,000 / $250,000 = 0.040 = 40.0\%$, which tells us that it is financed with 40 percent debt and, by definition, 60 percent equity. Thus, this single value summarizes the business's financing situation (capital structure). Furthermore, it is easy to compare this value to industry averages or to other comparative values.

	2008	2007
Revenues:		
Net patient service revenue	$4,042	$2,687
Other operating revenue	27	32
Total revenues	$4,069	$ 2,719
Expenses:		
Salaries and benefits	$ 2,714	$ 1,835
Supplies and drugs	1,042	675
Insurance	90	83
Provision for bad debts	46	21
Depreciation	21	15
Interest	16	19
Total expenses	$3,929	$2,648
Operating income	$ 140	$ 71
Nonoperating income:		
Contributions	$ 10	$ 22
Investment income	13	6
Total nonoperating income	$ 23	$ 28
Net income (excess of revenues over expenses)	$ 163	$ 99

aspects of financial condition). An almost unlimited number of financial ratios can be constructed, and the choice of ratios depends in large part on the nature of the business being analyzed, the purpose of the analysis, and the availability of comparative data. Generally, ratios are grouped into categories to make them easier to interpret.

In the paragraphs that follow, we use the data presented in Tables 13.2 and 13.3 to calculate the 2008 financial ratios for Park Ridge Homecare. Then, we compare the calculated ratios with industry average ratios. Note that in a real analysis, many more ratios would be calculated and analyzed. Also, the specific ratios used in any analysis depend on the type of healthcare provider (in our case, it is a home health care business). Some ratios are meaningful for hospitals, some are for long-term care facilities, some are for group practices, and so on.

	2008	2007
ASSETS		
Current Assets:		
Cash and cash equivalents	$ 74	$ 41
Short-term investments	147	137
Accounts receivable, net	727	476
Inventories	27	22
Total current assets	$ 975	$ 676
Investments	$ 125	$ 100
Property and Equipment:		
Medical and office equipment	$ 56	$ 54
Vehicles	70	47
Total	$ 126	$ 101
Less: Accumulated depreciation	(45)	(24)
Net property and equipment	$ 81	$ 77
Total assets	$1,181	$ 853
LIABILITIES AND EQUITY		
Current Liabilities:		
Notes payable	$ 13	$ 13
Accounts payable	40	21
Accrued expenses	496	337
Total current liabilities	$ 549	$ 371
Long-term debt	154	167
Total liabilities	$ 703	$ 538
Equity (net assets)	$ 478	$ 315
Total liabilities and equity	$1,181	$ 853

TABLE 13.3
Park Ridge Homecare: Balance Sheets December 31, 2008 and 2007 (in thousands)

Finally, note that the data we present (both for Park Ridge and the industry averages) are purely fictitious and should not be used for other purposes. Also, for simplicity of presentation, the thousands (000s) in the calculations shown here have been omitted.

PROFITABILITY RATIOS

Profitability is the net result of a large number of managerial policies and decisions. As such, profitability ratios provide a measure of the aggregate financial condition of a business.

Margin Measures

Total (profit) margin
Net income divided by total revenues, which measures the amount of total profit per dollar of total revenues. Profit margin includes nonoperating activities. Also called total margin.

Margin measures focus on how much money a business earns on its revenues. The *total margin*, often called *profit margin*, is defined as net income (excess of revenues over expenses) divided by total revenues:

Total margin = Net income/Total revenues = $163/($4,096 + $23) = $163/$4,119
= 0.04 = 4.0%.
Industry average = 6.8%.

Park Ridge's total margin of 4.0 percent shows that the business makes 4.0 cents on every dollar of total revenues, including both operating and nonoperating revenues. The total margin measures the ability of a business to control its expenses. With all else the same, the higher the total margin, the lower the expenses relative to revenues.

Park Ridge's total margin is below the industry average of 6.8 percent, indicating that the business's expenses are higher than they should be or that revenues are too low for the expense structure of the business. Thus, low margins indicate a problem with expenses, revenues, or both. The industry data source also reports quartiles; for total margin, the upper quartile was 10.4 percent, meaning that 25 percent of the industry had total margins higher than 10.4 percent, while the lower quartile was 2.1 percent. Thus, although Park Ridge's total margin was below average, it did not fall in the lower quartile (lower 25 percent) of all home health care businesses.

The industry average is not a magic number that all businesses should strive to achieve. In fact, some well-managed businesses are above the average, while other good firms are below it. However, if a business's ratios are far removed from the average for the industry, its managers should be concerned about why this difference occurs. (Note that the industry data presented in this section were adjusted to account for Park Ridge's not-for-profit status.)

As mentioned, Park Ridge's relatively low total margin could mean that its reimbursement is relatively low, its costs are relatively high, or a combination of the two. A thorough examination of relevant operational data, such as average cost per home visit and average reimbursement per visit, would help pinpoint the cause or causes of this low total margin.

When data are available, another useful margin measure is the *operating margin*, defined as operating income divided by operating revenues:

Operating margin = Operating income/Operating revenues = $140/$4,069
                 = 0.034 = 3.4%.
Industry average = 5.5%.

Park Ridge's operating margin of 3.4 percent shows that the business makes 3.4 cents on every dollar of operating revenues. The advantage of this measure over the total margin is that it focuses on core business operations and hence removes the influence of nonoperating income, which often is transitory and unrelated to core operations. However, the format of many healthcare organizations' financial statements often makes this ratio difficult to determine without additional information.

Return Measures

Return measures focus on how much a business earns on its asset or equity investment. The ratio of net income to total assets measures the *return on total assets*, often just called *return on assets (ROA)*:

Return on assets = Net income/Total assets = $163/$1,181 = 0.138 = 13.8%.
Industry average = 9.5%.

Park Ridge's 13.8 percent ROA, which means that each dollar of assets generated 13.8 cents in profit, is above the 9.5 percent average for the home health care industry.

ROA tells managers the productivity, in a financial sense, of a business's total assets. The higher the ROA, the greater the net income for each dollar invested in assets and hence the more "productive" the assets. ROA measures a business's ability to control expenses (as expressed by the total margin) and ability to use its assets to generate revenue.

Another return measure is *return on equity (ROE)*, defined as the ratio of net income to total equity (net assets):

Return on equity = Net income/Total equity = $163/$478 = 0.341 = 34.1%.
Industry average = 26.3%.

Park Ridge's 34.1 percent ROE is above the 26.3 percent industry average. The business was able to generate 34.1 cents of income for each dollar of equity investment, while the average home health care business produced 26.3 cents.

ROE is especially meaningful for investor-owned businesses because owners are concerned with how well the business's managers are using owner-supplied capital, and ROE gives the answer to this question. For not-for-profit businesses, such as Park Ridge,

---

Operating margin
Net operating income divided by total operating revenues, which measures the amount of operating profit per dollar of operating revenues. Operating margin focuses on the core activities of the business.

Return on total assets (ROA)
Net income divided by the book value of total assets, which measures the amount of profit per dollar of investment in total assets. ROA indicates the financial productivity of a business's total assets.

Return on equity (ROE)
Net income divided by the book value of equity (net assets), which measures the dollars of earnings per dollar of equity investment. ROE indicates the financial productivity of a business's equity financing.

ROE tells its board of trustees and managers how well, in financial terms, its community-supplied capital is being managed.

Park Ridge's 2008 total margin was below the industry average, yet its returns on assets and equity were above the industry averages. As explained later in the section on Du Pont analysis, this seeming inconsistency is a result of the business's smaller asset base (and hence lower need for equity).

LIQUIDITY RATIOS

Liquidity
The ability of a business to meet its cash obligations as they become due.

One of the first concerns of managers, and the major concern of a firm's short-term creditors, is the business's *liquidity*, which means its ability to meet its cash obligations as they become due.

Park Ridge had obligations totaling $549,000 (its current liabilities) at the end of 2008 that must be paid off during 2009. Will the business be able to make these payments? A full liquidity analysis requires the use of tools that are beyond the scope of this text. However, by relating the amount of cash and other current assets to current obligations, ratio analysis provides a quick, easy-to-use, rough measure of liquidity.

The most basic liquidity measure is the *current ratio*, which is defined as total current assets divided by total current liabilities:

Current ratio
Total current assets divided by total current liabilities, which measures the number of dollars of current assets available to pay each dollar of current liabilities.

Current ratio = Current assets/Current liabilities = $975/$549 = 1.8, or 1.8 times.
Industry average = 2.0.

The current ratio tells managers that the liquidation of Park Ridge's current assets at book value would provide $1.80 of cash for every $1 of current liabilities. If a business is getting into financial difficulty, it will begin paying its accounts payable more slowly, building up short-term bank loans (notes payable), and so on. If these current liabilities rise faster than current assets, the current ratio will fall, and this could spell trouble. Because the current ratio is an indicator of the extent to which short-term obligations are covered by assets that are expected to be converted to cash in the near term, it is a commonly used measure of liquidity.

Park Ridge's current ratio is slightly below the average for the home health care industry. Because current assets should be converted to cash in the near future, these assets are highly likely to be liquidated at close to their stated values. With a current ratio of 1.8, the business could liquidate current assets at only 56 percent of book value and still pay off current creditors in full. (To obtain this value, divide 1 by the current ratio: 1/1.8 = 0.56 = 56%.)

The current ratio measures liquidity on the basis of balance sheet accounts, and hence it is a static measure of liquidity. However, the true measure of a business's liquidity is whether or not the business can meet its payments as they become due, so liquidity is more related to cash flows than to assets and liabilities.

The *days-cash-on-hand* ratio moves closer to those factors that truly determine liquidity:

$$\text{DCOH} = \frac{\text{Cash} + \text{Short-term investments}}{(\text{Expenses} - \text{Provision for bad debts} - \text{Depreciation})/365}$$

$$= \frac{\$74 + \$147}{(\$3,929 - \$46 - \$21) / 365} = \frac{\$221}{\$3,862 / 365} = \frac{\$221}{\$10.58} = 20.9 \text{ days.}$$

Industry average = 22.6 days.

The denominator of the equation estimates average daily cash expenses by stripping out noncash expenses from reported total expenses and then dividing by 365 days per year. The numerator is the cash and securities that are available to make those cash payments. Because Park Ridge's days cash on hand is slightly lower than the industry average, its liquidity position as measured by days cash on hand is a little less than that of the average home health care business.

For Park Ridge, the two measures of liquidity—current ratio and days cash on hand—give a picture of about-average liquidity. However, both of these measures are rough, so additional analysis is required to make a supportable judgment concerning Park Ridge's liquidity position. (The best measure of a business's liquidity is provided by a cash budget, which details the business's expected cash inflows and outflows. Cash budgeting is beyond the scope of this book.)

Days cash on hand
The number of days it would take to run out of cash if the business does not receive any additional revenues or financing.

DEBT MANAGEMENT (CAPITAL STRUCTURE) RATIOS

The degree to which a firm uses debt financing, or *financial leverage*, is an important measure of financial performance for several reasons. First, by raising funds through debt, owners of for-profits can maintain control of the firm with a limited investment. For not-for-profits, debt financing allows the organization to provide more services than it could if it were solely financed with contributed and earned capital.

Financial leverage
The use of fixed cost financing, primarily debt.

Second, creditors look to equity capital to provide a margin of safety; if the owners (or community) have provided only a small proportion of total financing, the risks of the enterprise are borne mainly by its creditors.

Third, if a firm earns more on investments financed with borrowed funds than it pays in interest, its return on equity capital is increased when debt financing is used.

Two types of ratios are used to assess debt management:

1. *Capitalization ratios.* These ratios use balance sheet data to determine the extent to which borrowed funds have been used to finance assets.

2. *Coverage ratios.* Here, income statement data are used to determine the extent to which fixed financial charges are covered by reported profits or cash flow.

The two sets of ratios are complementary, so most financial statement analyses examine both types.

Capitalization Ratios

Debt ratio

Total liabilities divided by total assets, which measures the proportion of debt in a business's total financing mix.

The ratio of total debt (total liabilities) to total assets (total liabilities and equity), generally called the *debt ratio*, is a capitalization ratio that measures the percentage of total capital provided by creditors and other capital suppliers that have fixed claims:

Debt ratio = Total liabilities/Total assets = $703/$1,181 = 0.595, or 59.5%.
Industry average = 63.0%.

For our purposes, we define debt as all debt, including current liabilities and long-term debt—that is, everything but equity. However, as illustrated by the next ratio discussed, capitalization ratios have many variations, many of which use different definitions of what constitutes debt financing.

Creditors prefer low debt ratios (low leverage) because the lower the ratio, the greater the cushion against creditors' losses in the event of bankruptcy and liquidation. Conversely, owners of for-profit firms may seek high leverage either to increase returns or to prevent giving up some degree of control when they sell new stock. In not-for-profit organizations, managers may seek high leverage to offer more services. However, as discussed in Chapter 8, the greater the amount of debt financing, the higher the interest rate on that debt and the greater the risk of bankruptcy.

Park Ridge's debt ratio is 59.5 percent. This means that its creditors (and other fixed claimants) have supplied about 60 percent of the business's total financing. Put another way, each dollar of assets was financed with roughly 60 cents of "debt," and consequently, 40 cents of equity. Because the average debt ratio for the home health care industry is more than 63 percent, Park Ridge uses a little less non-equity financing than the average home health care business. The slightly-lower-than-average debt ratio indicates that Park Ridge probably could borrow a limited amount of additional funds at a relatively reasonable rate.

Debt-to-capitalization ratio

Long-term debt divided by long-term capital (long-term debt plus equity), which measures the proportion of long-term debt in a business's permanent (long-term) financing mix.

The *debt-to-capitalization ratio* is another capitalization ratio. It is defined as long-term debt divided by long-term capital (long-term debt plus equity), and it focuses on the proportion of debt used in a business's permanent (long-term) capital structure. This ratio is also called the long-term-debt-to-capitalization ratio or just capitalization ratio.

Debt-to-capitalization ratio = Long-term debt/(Long-term debt + Equity)
= $154/($154 + $478) = $154/$632 = 0.244, or 24.4%.
Industry average = 28.6%.

Many analysts believe that the debt-to-capitalization ratio best reflects the capital structure of a business. This belief is based on the fact that most businesses use as much free credit (current liabilities less short-term bank loans) as they can get. Furthermore, short-term interest-bearing debt typically is used only to fund temporary current asset needs. Thus, the "true" capital structure of a business—the one that reflects its target structure—is best measured by the debt-to-capitalization ratio, which focuses on long-term (permanent) financing.

Park Ridge's debt-to-capitalization ratio is 24.4 percent, compared to the industry average of 28.6 percent. This low use of debt financing in the business's permanent capital mix confirms the conclusion we made earlier that the business has some unused debt capacity. That is, the business could easily obtain additional debt financing.

Another common capitalization ratio is the debt-to-equity ratio, which is defined as Total liabilities / Total equity. This ratio gives the number of dollars of debt financing per dollar of equity. The higher the ratio, the greater the use of financial leverage. In essence, the debt ratio and debt-to-equity ratio provide the same information, but in slightly different formats.

Coverage Ratios

The most basic coverage ratio is the *times interest earned (TIE)* ratio, which is defined as earnings before interest and taxes (EBIT) divided by interest charges. EBIT is used in the numerator because it represents the amount of income that is available to pay interest expense. For a not-for-profit business, which does not pay taxes, EBIT = Net income + Interest expense.

> TIE ratio = EBIT/Interest expense = ($163 + $16)/$16 = $179/$16 = 11.2 times.
> Industry average = 5.9.

The TIE ratio measures the number of dollars of accounting income (as opposed to cash flow) available to pay each dollar of interest expense. In essence, it is an indicator of the extent to which income can decline before it is less than annual interest costs. Failure to pay interest might trigger legal action by creditors, which could result in the firm's bankruptcy.

Park Ridge's interest is covered 11.2 times, so it has $11.20 of accounting income to pay each dollar of interest expense. Because the industry average TIE ratio is 5.9 times, the business is covering its interest charges by a relatively high margin of safety. Thus, the TIE ratio reinforces the previous conclusions based on capitalization ratios—namely, Park Ridge could expand its use of debt financing.

Coverage ratios often are better measures of a firm's debt utilization than capitalization ratios are because coverage ratios discriminate between low-interest rate debt and high-interest rate debt. For example, a large group practice might have $10 million of 4 percent debt on its balance sheet, while another might have $10 million of 8 percent debt. If both practices have the same income and assets, both would have the same debt

Times interest earned ratio (TIE)
Earnings before interest and taxes divided by interest charges, which measures the number of times that a business's interest expense is covered by the earnings available to pay that expense. This ratio indicates how much earnings could fall before the business has trouble meeting its interest payments.

Cash flow coverage ratio

A measure of the amount of cash flow generated by a business per dollar of fixed expense. Similar to the TIE ratio, but more inclusive.

ratio. However, the group that pays 4 percent interest would have lower interest charges and hence would be in better financial condition than the group that pays 8 percent. This difference in financial condition is captured by the TIE ratio.

Although the TIE ratio is easy to calculate, it has two major deficiencies:

1. The TIE ratio ignores lease payments, which, like debt payments, are contractual obligations. Also, many debt contracts require that principal payments be made over the life of the loan, rather than only at maturity. Thus, most businesses must meet fixed financial charges (lease and principal payments) other than interest.

2. The TIE ratio ignores the fact that accounting income, whether measured by EBIT or net income, does not reflect the actual cash flow available to meet a business's fixed payments.

These deficiencies are corrected in the *cash flow coverage (CFC) ratio*, which shows the amount by which cash flow covers fixed financial requirements. Here is Park Ridge's 2008 CFC ratio, assuming the business had $18,000 of lease payments and $13,000 of required debt principal repayments:

$$\text{CFC ratio} = (\text{EBIT} + \text{Lease payments} + \text{Depreciation expense})/(\text{Interest expense} + \text{Lease payments} + \text{Debt principal})$$
$$= (\$163 + \$16 + \$18 + \$21)/(\$16 + \$18 + \$13) = \$218/\$47 = 4.6 \text{ times.}$$
Industry average = 2.8.

Like its TIE ratio, Park Ridge's CFC ratio exceeds the industry standard, indicating that the business is better at covering total fixed payments with cash flow than is the average home health care business. This fact should be reassuring both to creditors and management, and it reinforces the view that Park Ridge has untapped debt capacity.

ASSET MANAGEMENT (ACTIVITY) RATIOS

Fixed assets turnover (utilization) ratio

Total revenues divided by net fixed assets, which measures the ability of a business's fixed assets to generate revenues.

The next group of ratios, the asset management ratios, is designed to measure how effectively a business's assets are being used. These ratios help to answer whether or not the amount of each type of asset as reported on the balance sheet seems reasonable, too high, or too low in view of current (or projected) operating levels. Park Ridge and all businesses must borrow or raise equity capital to acquire assets. If they have too many assets, then their capital costs will be too high and their profits will be depressed. Conversely, if the level of assets is too low, then volume may be lost or vital services not offered.

The *fixed assets turnover ratio*, also called the *fixed assets utilization ratio*, measures the utilization of plant and equipment, and it is the ratio of total revenues to net fixed assets (net property and equipment):

$$\text{Fixed assets turnover} = \text{Total revenues/Net fixed assets} = (\$4{,}069 + \$23)/\$81 = \$4{,}092/\$81$$
$$= 50.5 \text{ times.}$$
Industry average = 31.4.

Park Ridge's ratio of 50.5 indicates that each dollar of fixed assets generated $50.50 in revenue. This value compares favorably with the industry average of 31.4 times, indicating that Park Ridge is using its fixed assets much more productively than is the average home health care business. (The upper quartile value for the industry is 138.4; thus, Park Ridge is doing well, but not well enough to fall in the top 25 percent of the industry.)

The *total assets turnover ratio* measures the turnover, or utilization, of all of a business's assets. It is calculated by dividing total revenues by total assets:

Total assets turnover = Total revenues/Total assets = ($4,069 + $23)/$1,181
= $4,092/$1,181 = 3.5 times.
Industry average = 1.4.

Total assets turnover (utilization) ratio
Total revenues divided by total assets, which measures the amount of revenue generated by each dollar of total assets.

⚠ CRITICAL CONCEPT
Summary of Key Ratios

Ratio	Formula	Definition
Total (profit) margin	Net income divided by total revenues	Measures the ability to control expenses (dollars of income per dollar of revenue)
Operating margin	Net operating income divided by operating revenues	Measures the ability to control operating expenses (dollars of operating income per dollar of operating revenue)
Return on assets (ROA)	Net income divided by total assets	Measures the ability of a business's assets to generate profits (dollars of profitability per dollar of total assets)
Return on equity (ROE)	Net income divided by total equity	Measures the ability of a business's equity financing to generate profits (dollar of profitability per dollar of equity investment)
Current ratio	Current assets divided by current liabilities	Measures the dollars of current assets per dollar of current liabilities—a rough measure of liquidity
Days cash on hand	Cash and short-term investments divided by daily cash expenses	Measures the number of days that a business can continue to pay its bills without new revenue or financing
Debt ratio	Total liabilities divided by total assets	Measures the proportion of debt in a business's total financing
Capitalization ratio	Long-term debt divided by long-term capital (long-term debt and equity)	Measures the proportion of debt in a business's long-term financing
Times-interest-earned (TIE) ratio	Earnings before interest and taxes (EBIT) divided by interest expense	Measures the dollars of accounting income available to pay each dollar of interest expense
Cash flow coverage (CFC) ratio	Cash flow divided by fixed financial charges	Measures the dollars of cash flow available to pay each dollar of fixed financial charges
Fixed assets turnover ratio	Total revenues divided by net fixed assets	Measures the dollars of revenue per dollar of fixed assets
Total assets turnover ratio	Total revenues divided by total assets	Measures the dollars of revenue per dollar of total assets
Average collection period (days in patient accounts receivable)	Net accounts receivable divided by daily patient revenue	Measures the average number of days it takes to collect a business's receivables

Each dollar of total assets generated $3.50 in total revenue. Thus, both Park Ridge's fixed assets and total assets turnover ratios are above the industry averages. The bottom line here is that the business generates a relatively large amount of revenues for its asset base. That's good news!

Days in (patient) accounts receivable is used to measure effectiveness in managing receivables. This measure of financial performance, which is sometimes classified as a liquidity ratio rather than an asset management ratio, has many names, including average collection period (ACP) and days' sales outstanding (DSO). It is computed by dividing net accounts receivable by average daily patient revenue to find the number of days that it takes an organization, on average, to collect its receivables:

> **Days in (patient) accounts receivable**
> The average length of time it takes a provider to collect its receivables. Also called days' sales outstanding or average collection period.

Days in patient accounts receivable = Net patient accounts receivable/(Net patient service revenue/365) = $727/($4,042/365)= $727/11.07
                        = 65.7 days.
Industry average = 55.2 days.

Park Ridge is not doing as well as the industry average in collecting its receivables. Perhaps its payer mix is dominated by "slow" payers, or it is using manual rather than electronic billing. Still, the lower quartile value is 71.7 days, so a relatively large number of home health care businesses are doing worse. As discussed in Chapter 7, businesses must collect their receivables as soon as possible. Clearly, Park Ridge should strive to increase its performance in this key area.

OTHER RATIOS

Because of space constraints, and the fact that ratio analysis discussions can cause instant drowsiness, we have described only a few of the many financial ratios used in practice today. Remember that to gain the most value from a financial ratio analysis, an operational ratio analysis should also be conducted, which will help explain the financial condition assessed. (Operational analysis is introduced in Chapter 7.)

For a more comprehensive list of financial ratios, see the ratios appendix at ache.org/books/FinanceFundamentals.

? SELF-TEST QUESTIONS

1. What is the purpose of ratio analysis?

2. What are two ratios that measure profitability?

3. What are two ratios that measure liquidity?

4. What are two ratios that measure debt management?

5. What are two ratios that measure asset management?

13.5 COMPARATIVE AND TREND ANALYSIS

When conducting ratio analysis, the value of a particular ratio, in the absence of other information, reveals almost nothing about a business's financial condition. For example, if a nursing home management company has a current ratio of 2.5, it is virtually impossible to say whether this ratio is good or bad. Additional data are needed to help interpret the ratio.

In our discussion of Park Ridge Homecare's ratios, the focus was on **comparative analysis (benchmarking),** in which the business's ratios were compared with the industry average ratios. Another useful ratio analysis tool is trend analysis, in which the trend of a single ratio is analyzed over time. **Trend analysis** gives clues about whether a business's financial condition is improving, holding constant, or deteriorating.

> ### ⓘ CRITICAL CONCEPT
> Comparative (Benchmarking) and Trend Analyses
>
> A single ratio—say, a debt ratio of 60 percent—does not tell much about the business's financial condition. To help interpret the ratios, analysts use comparative and trend analyses. Comparative analysis (benchmarking) compares a business's ratios with established values, such as industry averages, leading companies in the industry, or primary competitors. For example, does the business use more or less debt financing than the industry average? Trend analysis focuses on changes in the business's ratios over time. For example, has the business's use of debt financing increased or decreased over the last five years? The calculation of the ratios is not a big deal; a spreadsheet can easily do that. What matters is the interpretation of the ratios, and comparative and trend analyses are vital to this process.

It is easy to combine comparative and trend analyses in a single graph, such as the one shown in Figure 13.1. Here, Park Ridge's ROE (the solid lines) and industry average ROE (the dashed lines) data are plotted for the past five years. The graph shows that the business's ROE has increased substantially since it opened in 2004. After three years of being below average, ROE was above the industry average for 2007 and 2008, but not so high as to be in the upper quartile. Although comparative and trend analyses are illustrated here with one ratio, other ratios can be analyzed similarly. Also, for presentation purposes, charts often are used, with the comparative data color coded for ease of recognition and interpretation.

All comparative analyses require comparative data. Such data are available from a number of sources, including commercial suppliers, federal and state governmental agencies, and various industry trade groups. Each of these data suppliers uses a somewhat different set of ratios designed to meet its own needs. Thus, the comparative data source selected dictates the ratios used in the analysis.

Also, there are minor, and sometimes major, differences in ratio definitions between data sources—for example, one source may use a 365-day year, while another may go by a 360-day year. Another source might use operating values as opposed to total values when constructing ratios.

Knowing the specific definitions used in the comparative data is imperative, because definitional differences between the ratios being calculated and the comparative ratios can lead to erroneous interpretations and conclusions. Thus, the first task in any ratio

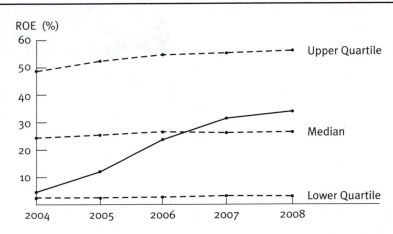

| Year | Park Ridge Homecare | Return on Equity (ROE) | | |
| | | Industry | | |
		Lower Quartile	Median	Upper Quartile
2004	4.5%	3.2%	24.6%	48.9%
2005	12.1	3.5	25.4	52.2
2006	23.7	3.9	26.4	54.9
2007	31.4	4.1%	26.1	55.1
2008	34.1	3.8	26.3	56.3

analysis is to identify the comparative data set and the ratios to be used. Then, make sure that the ratio definitions used in the analysis match those in the comparative data set.

Choosing the best available comparative data also is a must. For example, industry averages should reflect businesses of roughly the same size and operating in the same geographic area as the one being analyzed. Also, in general, not-for-profit businesses should be compared to one another and not to for-profit businesses.

(?) SELF-TEST QUESTIONS

1. How can comparative and trend analyses be used to help interpret a ratio?

2. Why is it important to be familiar with the comparative data set?

13.6 DU PONT ANALYSIS

Financial ratio analysis provides a great deal of information about a business's financial condition, but it does not provide an overview nor does it tie any of the ratios together.

Du Pont analysis provides an overview of a business's financial condition and helps managers and investors understand the relationships among several ratios.

Du Pont analysis, so named because managers at the Du Pont Company developed it, combines basic financial ratios in a way that provides valuable insights into a business's profitability. The analysis decomposes return on equity (ROE), perhaps the most important measure of profitability, into the product of three other ratios, each of which has an important economic interpretation. (Remember, ROE is defined as Net income/Total equity.) The result is the Du Pont equation:

ROE = Total margin × Total asset turnover ×
    Equity multiplier
   = Net income/Total revenue × Total
    revenue/Total assets × Total assets/Total equity.

> ### (!) CRITICAL CONCEPT
> #### Du Pont Analysis
>
> Du Pont analysis, which decomposes the profitability of a business into three components, uses this equation:
>
> ROE = Total margin x Total asset turnover x Equity multiplier.
>
> The idea here is that a business's profitability (as measured by ROE) is a function of these factors: (1) expense control, which is measured by total margin; (2) asset utilization, which is measured by total asset turnover; and (3) debt utilization, which is measured by the equity multiplier. By analyzing the Du Pont equation, managers can determine how each of these factors contributes to a business's profitability and hence can identify areas of strength and weakness.

Again, we use Park Ridge Homecare's 2008 data to illustrate the Du Pont equation. Also, we have included the industry average Du Pont equation for later comparison. (Note that the ratios used in the analysis are rounded to the nearest tenth of a percent, so the multiplication results are not exact.)

    Park Ridge Homecare: ROE = 34.1% = 4.0% × 3.5 × 2.5
    Industry average: ROE = 26.3% = 6.8% × 1.4 × 2.7

In the Du Pont equation, the product of the first two terms on the right side is return on assets (ROA), so the equation can also be written as ROE = ROA × Equity multiplier. Park Ridge's 2008 total margin was 4.0 percent, so the business made 4.0 cents profit on each dollar of total revenue. Furthermore, assets were turned over (or created revenues) 3.5 times during the year, so the business earned a return of 4.0% × 3.5 = 13.8% on its assets. This value for ROA is the same as was calculated previously in our ratio analysis discussion. (Again, there is a rounding difference because the Du Pont components are expressed to the nearest tenth percent.)

If the business used only equity financing, its 13.8 percent ROA would equal its ROE. However, creditors and other suppliers of liability capital provided 59.5 percent of Park Ridge's financing, while the equityholders (the community) supplied the rest.

Because the 13.8 percent ROA belongs exclusively to the suppliers of equity capital, which makes up only 40.5 percent of total capital, Park Ridge's ROE is higher than its 13.8 percent ROA.

Equity multiplier
The ratio of total assets to total equity, which indicates how many dollars of assets are supported by each dollar of equity financing.

Specifically, ROA must be multiplied by the *equity multiplier*, which shows the amount of assets working for each dollar of equity capital, to obtain the ROE of 34.1 percent. Of course, ROE can be calculated directly: ROE = Net income / Total equity = $163 / $478 = 0.341 = 34.1%. However, the Du Pont equation shows how total margin, which measures expense control; total asset turnover, which measures asset utilization; and financial leverage, which measures debt utilization, interact to determine ROE.

Lori uses the Du Pont equation to suggest how to improve Park Ridge's profitability (ROE) and hence financial condition. To influence the profit margin, Park Ridge must increase revenues and/or reduce costs. Thus, Lori can study the effects of raising charges to increase revenues, lowering charges to increase volume, moving into new services or markets with higher margins, entering into new contracts with managed care plans, and so on.

Furthermore, she can study the expense items and, working with clinical staff, seek ways to reduce costs. To boost total asset turnover, Lori can investigate ways of reducing investments in various types of assets. Finally, she can analyze alternative financing strategies to ensure that the optimal amount of debt financing is being used.

The Du Pont equation also provides a useful comparison between a business's performance as measured by ROE and the performance of an average home health care business. The Du Pont analysis tells managers and creditors that Park Ridge has a lower profit margin and thus needs to do a better job of controlling expenses and increasing revenues. However, the business is getting above-average utilization from its assets. Thus, in spite of its relatively low total margin, its superior asset utilization gives it a higher-than-average ROA. Finally, Park Ridge uses roughly the same amount of debt financing as the industry. The end result is that it gets a better return on its equity capital than does the average home health care business.

⑦ SELF-TEST QUESTIONS

1. Explain how the Du Pont equation combines several ratios to obtain an overview of a business's financial condition.

2. What role does asset and debt utilization play in a business's profitability as measured by return on equity?

(✱) INDUSTRY PRACTICE Some Hospital Ratios and How They Compare to Home Health Care

To gain a better understanding of ratio analysis, let's examine some financial ratios for the hospital industry to see how they compare to the home health care industry. Note that the data presented here for the home health care industry cover all businesses in that industry, while the comparative data used in the ratio analysis illustrations (presented earlier) are for businesses of roughly the same size as Park Ridge Homecare.

First, let's examine profitability:

	Home Health Care	Hospitals
Total margin	4.0%	4.1%
Return on assets	10.3	4.5
Return on equity	27.1	7.9

Here, we see that both the home health care and hospital industries have about the same total margin, so their ability to generate profits per dollar of revenue is quite similar. Thus, although the types of services the two providers offer are different, their cost structures per revenue dollar are similar.

However, the home health care industry has a significantly higher return on its asset investment and an even higher differential return on its equity investment. This means that the home health care industry (1) creates more revenues (but does not earn more on each dollar of revenue) per dollar of asset investment and (2) finances its assets with a higher proportion of debt. Let's look at a few more ratios to confirm these assertions.

Here's a look at asset productivity and capital structure:

	Home Health Care	Hospitals
Total asset turnover	2.6	1.1
Fixed asset turnover	26.6	2.5
Equity multiplier (assets/equity)	2.8	1.8

(Continued)

INDUSTRY PRACTICE Some Hospital Ratios and How They Compare to Home Health Care

These indicate that the assets of a typical home health care business are much more productive (in the financial sense) than hospital assets. For example, each dollar of home health care total assets (plant and equipment) generates $2.60 of revenues, while a dollar of hospital total assets generates only $1.10 in revenues. The underlying reason is that hospitals must have a large investment in land, buildings, and equipment to provide patient services, while home health care businesses can simply lease office space and start operations.

Also, note that home health care businesses, on average, use more debt financing. Thus, each dollar of equity financing in a home health care business supports $2.80 of assets, while that same dollar of equity in a hospital supports only $1.80 of assets. The net result is that the total margin of a home health care business is leveraged up by asset productivity and debt financing to a greater extent than in the hospital industry, which creates a higher return on equity.

Finally, let's examine liquidity:

	Home Health Care	Hospitals
Current ratio	1.6	2.1
Days cash on hand	21.9	25.8

On average, hospitals are more liquid than are home health care businesses. Of course, in general, hospitals are much larger in scale (assets and revenues) than are home health care businesses, and hence have higher levels of current assets and daily cash transactions. For these reasons, it makes sense that hospitals would want to maintain higher levels of liquidity than would home health care businesses.

The main point of this discussion is that basic differences exist in the financial and operational structures of different healthcare providers. Hospitals are inherently different from home health care businesses, which are inherently different from nursing homes, and so on. When performing financial condition analyses, the unique features of the industry must be recognized.

Note: This industry practice is based on data in (1) Risk Management Association (RMA). 2007. *Annual Statement Studies*, and (2) Ingenix. 2007. *Almanac of Hospital Financial and Operating Indicators*.

13.7 OTHER ANALYTICAL TECHNIQUES

Besides ratio and Du Pont analyses, two additional techniques are frequently used in financial statement analysis.

In *common size analysis*, all income statement items are divided by total revenues and all balance sheet items are divided by total assets. Thus, a common size income statement shows each item as a percentage of total revenues, and a common size balance sheet shows each account as a percentage of total assets. The advantage of common size statements is that they facilitate comparisons of income statements and balance sheets over time and across companies because they remove the influence of the scale (size) of the business. For an example of a common size analysis, see the Industry Practice box in Chapter 12.

In *percentage change analysis*, the percentage changes in the balance sheet accounts and income statement items from year to year are calculated and compared. In this format, it is easy to see what accounts and items are growing faster or slower than others and thus to identify which are under control and which are out of control.

To illustrate, Park Ridge Homecare's operating revenues grew from $2,719,000 to $4,069,000 during 2008, or by $1,350,000. This dollar increase in revenues translates to a $1,350 / $2,719 = 0.497 = 49.7% increase. Over the same period, inventories increased by only ($27 − $22) / $22 = 0.227 = 22.7 percent. Thus, percentage change analysis reveals that revenues increased at more than twice the rate of inventories during 2008. Because inventories require both initial expenditures and carrying costs, the ability to grow revenues faster than inventories has a positive impact on profitability and hence financial condition.

The conclusions reached in common size and percentage change analyses generally parallel those derived from ratio analysis. However, occasionally a serious deficiency is highlighted by only one of the three analytical techniques, while the other two techniques fail to bring the deficiency to light. Thus, a thorough financial statement analysis usually consists of a Du Pont analysis to provide an overview and then includes several different techniques such as ratio, common size, and percentage change analyses.

Common size analysis
A financial statement analysis technique that uses percentages instead of dollars for income statement items and balance sheet accounts. Common size analysis is especially useful when comparing one firm's financial statements to another (or to the industry).

Percentage change analysis
A financial statement analysis technique that expresses year-to-year changes in income statement items and balance accounts as percentages. Percentage change analysis shows which items and accounts are growing faster (or slower) than others.

? SELF-TEST QUESTIONS

1. How are common size statements created?

2. What advantage do common size statements have over regular statements when conducting a financial statement analysis?

3. What is percentage change analysis, and why is it useful?

4. Which analytical techniques should be used in a complete financial statement analysis?

13.8 LIMITATIONS OF FINANCIAL STATEMENT ANALYSIS

While financial statement analysis can provide a great deal of useful information regarding a business's financial condition, such analyses have limitations that necessitate care and judgment. In this section, some of the problem areas are highlighted.

First, many large healthcare businesses operate a number of divisions in different lines of business, which makes developing meaningful comparative data difficult. This problem tends to make financial statement analyses more useful for providers with single service lines than for large, multiservice companies.

Second, generalizing about whether or not a particular value is good or bad can be complicated. For example, a high current ratio may show a strong liquidity position (which is good) or an excessive amount of current assets (which is bad). Similarly, a high total asset turnover ratio may denote either a business that uses its assets efficiently or one that is undercapitalized and simply cannot afford to buy enough assets. In addition, firms often have some ratios that look good and others that look bad, which makes the firm's financial position, strong or weak, difficult to determine. For this reason, significant judgment is required when analyzing financial condition.

Third, varying accounting practices can distort financial statement comparisons. For example, businesses can use different accounting (fiscal) years. If a business is highly seasonal, such as a walk-in clinic in a ski resort, financial statement ratios in December can look dissimilar from those in July. In addition, firms can use different accounting conventions to value inventories, which can lead to ratio distortions. Other accounting practices, such as those related to leases, can also create distortions.

Finally, inflation effects can distort a firm's financial statements. Recall that most asset values listed on the balance sheet reflect historical costs rather than current values. Inflation and depreciation have caused the values of many assets that were purchased in the past to be seriously understated. Therefore, if an old hospital that had acquired much of its plant and equipment years ago is compared to a new hospital with the same physical capacity, the old hospital, because of a lower book value of fixed assets, would report a higher turnover ratio. This difference in fixed-asset turnover is more reflective of the inability of financial statements to deal with inflation than of any inefficiency on the part of the new hospital's managers.

⟨?⟩ SELF-TEST QUESTION

1. Briefly describe some of the problems encountered when performing financial statement analyses.

THEME WRAP-UP   TECHNIQUES FOR EVALUATING FINANCIAL STATEMENTS

After a cursory ratio analysis, we (as well as Lori) know that Park Ridge Homecare is on a sound financial footing. Its return on equity is above the industry average, as is its ability to use its asset base to generate revenues. However, Park Ridge's expense control needs improvement. Also, it could use a little more debt financing.

However, when all relevant factors are considered, Park Ridge's business model is financially sustainable. Given the right competitive environment, Lori should be able to start a second location without placing Park Ridge in financial jeopardy. She could probably take funds out of the short-term and long-term investment accounts and, with a moderate amount of new debt financing, acquire sufficient assets to start the new enterprise. If she applies the Park Ridge model to this second business, the new office is likely to quickly become operationally self-supporting. But Lori has to watch the expenses.

Let's wish Lori lots of luck!

KEY CONCEPTS

This chapter presents the methods used by managers and investors to assess a business's financial condition as reflected by data in its financial statements. Here are the key concepts:

➤ *Financial statement analysis* uses data found in a business's financial statements to assess financial condition. *Operational analysis*, which uses data typically not found in financial statements, provides insights into why a firm is in a given financial condition.

➤ *Ratio analysis* is one technique designed to help interpret the data contained in financial statements, as well as other data. In essence, two data elements are combined to create a single value whose economic meaning can be easily interpreted.

➤ *Profitability ratios* show the combined effects of liquidity, asset management, and debt management on operating results. Profitability ratios are subdivided into *margin* measures and *return* measures.

➤ *Liquidity ratios* indicate the business's ability to meet its short-term cash obligations.

➤ *Asset management ratios* measure how effectively managers are using the business's assets.

➤ *Debt management ratios* reveal the extent to which the firm is financed with debt. These ratios are further categorized as *capitalization* ratios and *coverage* ratios.

➤ Ratios are analyzed using *comparative analysis* or *benchmarking* (in which a firm's ratios are compared with industry averages or other benchmarks) and *trend analysis* (in which a firm's ratios are examined over time).

➤ The *Du Pont equation*, which provides a good overview of the factors that affect profitability, shows how the total margin, total asset turnover, and amount of debt financing interact to influence a business's return on equity.

➤ In a *common size analysis,* a business's income statement and balance sheet are expressed in percentages. This facilitates comparisons between firms of different sizes and a single firm that grows over time.

➤ In *percentage change analysis,* the differences in income statement items and balance sheet accounts from one year to the next are expressed in percentages. In this way, it is easy to identify items and accounts that are growing appreciably faster or slower than average.

➤ Financial condition analysis is hampered by some serious problems, including *development of comparative data*, *interpretation of results*, and *inflation effects*.

Financial condition analysis has its limitations, but if used with care and judgment, it can provide managers with a good picture of a business's financial condition as well as identify those operational factors that contributed to that condition.

END-OF-CHAPTER QUESTIONS

13.1 a. What is the primary difference between financial statement analysis and operational analysis?

b. Why are both types of analyses useful to healthcare managers and investors?

13.2 Should financial statement analyses be conducted only on historical data? Explain your answer.

13.3 One asset management ratio, the inventory turnover ratio, is defined as revenues divided by inventories. Would this ratio be more important for a medical device manufacturer or a hospital management company?

13.4 a. Assume that Old Gatorland and Badger Manor, two operators of nursing homes, have fiscal years that end at different times—say, one in June and one in December. Would this fact cause any problems when comparing ratios between the two businesses?

b. Assume that two companies that operate walk-in clinics both have the same December year end, but one (a winter resort) is based in Aspen, while the other (a summer resort) operates on Nantucket Island. Would this lead to problems in a comparative analysis?

13.5 a. How does inflation distort ratio analysis comparisons, both for one company over time and when different companies are compared?

b. Are only balance sheet accounts or both balance sheet accounts and income statement items affected by inflation?

13.6 a. What is the difference between trend analysis and comparative analysis?

b. Which one is more important?

13.7 Assume that a large group practice has a low return on equity (ROE). How could Du Pont analysis be used to identify possible actions to help boost profitability?

13.8 Regardless of the specific line of business, should all healthcare businesses use the same set of ratios when conducting a financial statement analysis? Explain your answer.

13.1 a. General Hospital has a current ratio of 0.5. Which of the following actions would improve (increase) this ratio? (Hint: Create a simple balance sheet that has a current ratio of 0.5. Then, judge how the transactions below would affect the balance sheet.)

    1. Use cash to pay off current liabilities.

    2. Collect some of the current accounts receivable.

    3. Use cash to pay off some long-term debt.

    4. Purchase additional inventory on credit (i.e., accounts payable).

    5. Sell some of the existing inventory at cost (book value).

  b. Now assume that General Hospital has a current ratio of 1.2. In this situation, which of the above actions would improve this ratio?

13.2 Southwest Physicians, a medical group practice in Oklahoma City, is just being formed. It will need $2 million of total assets to generate $3 million in revenues. Furthermore, the group expects to have a total margin of 5 percent. The group is considering two financing alternatives. First, it can use all-equity financing by requiring each physician to contribute his or her pro rata share. Second, the practice can finance up to 50 percent of its assets with a bank loan. Assuming that the debt alternative has no impact on the expected total margin, what is the difference between the expected return on equity (ROE) if the group finances with 50 percent debt versus the expected ROE if it finances entirely with equity capital?

13.3 Park Ridge Homecare's financial statements are presented in Tables 13.1, 13.2, and 13.3. In the chapter, we calculated selected ratios for 2008.

  a. Calculate the business's financial ratios for 2007. Assume that Park Ridge had $18,000 in lease payments in 2007. (Use the ratio analysis discussion to identify the applicable ratios.)

  b. Interpret the ratios. For the analysis, assume that the industry average data presented in the ratio analysis section is valid for 2007.

13.4 Consider the following financial statements for BestCare HMO, a not-for-profit managed care plan:

BestCare HMO

Statement of Operations and Change in Net Assets

Year Ended June 30, 2008

(in thousands)

Revenue:

Premiums earned	$26,682
Coinsurance	1,689
Interest and other income	242
Total revenue	$28,613

Expenses:

Salaries and benefits	$ 15,154
Medical supplies and drugs	7,507
Insurance	3,963
Provision for bad debts	19
Depreciation	367
Interest	385
Total expenses	$27,395
Net income	$ 1,218
Net assets, beginning of year	$ 900
Net assets, end of year	$ 2,118

BestCare HMO

Balance Sheet

June 30, 2008

(in thousands)

Assets

Cash and cash equivalents	$ 2,737
Net premiums receivable	821
Supplies	387
Total current assets	$ 3,945

Net property and equipment	$ 5,924
Total assets	$ 9,869

Liabilities and Net Assets

Accounts payable—medical services	$ 2,145
Accrued expenses	929
Notes payable	141
Current portion of long-term debt	241
Total current liabilities	$ 3,456
Long-term debt	$ 4,295
Total liabilities	$ 7,751
Net assets (equity)	$ 2,118
Total liabilities and net assets	$ 9,869

a. Perform a Du Pont analysis on BestCare. Assume that the industry average ratios are as follows:

Total margin	3.8%
Total asset turnover	2.1
Equity multiplier	3.2
Return on equity	25.5%

b. Calculate and interpret the following ratios for BestCare:

	Industry Average
Return on assets	8.0%
Current ratio	1.3
Days cash on hand	41 days
Average collection period	7 days
Debt ratio	69%
Debt-to-equity ratio	2.2
Times interest earned ratio	2.8
Fixed asset turnover ratio	5.2

13.5 Consider the following financial statements for Green Valley Nursing Home, Inc., a for-profit, long-term care facility:

Green Valley Nursing Home, Inc.

Statement of Income and Retained Earnings

Year Ended December 31, 2008

Revenue:	
Net patient service revenue	$3,163,258
Other revenue	106,146
Total revenues	$3,269,404
Expenses:	
Salaries and benefits	$ 1,515,438
Medical supplies and drugs	966,781
Insurance and other	296,357
Provision for bad debts	110,000
Depreciation	85,000
Interest	206,780
Total expenses	$3,180,356
Operating income	$ 89,048
Provision for income taxes	31,167
Net income	$ 57,881
Retained earnings, beginning of year	$ 199,961
Retained earnings, end of year	$ 257,842

Green Valley Nursing Home, Inc.

Balance Sheet

December 31, 2008

Assets

Current Assets:	
Cash	$ 105,737
Short-term securities	200,000
Net patient accounts receivable	215,600
Supplies	87,655
Total current assets	$ 608,992

Property and equipment	$2,250,000
Less accumulated depreciation	356,000
Net property and equipment	$1,894,000
Total assets	$2,502,992

Liabilities and Shareholders' Equity

Current Liabilities:

Accounts payable	$ 72,250
Accrued expenses	192,900
Notes payable	100,000
Current portion of long-term debt	80,000
Total current liabilities	$ 445,150
Long-term debt	$ 1,700,000

Shareholders' Equity:

Common stock, $10 par value	$ 100,000
Retained earnings	257,842
Total shareholders' equity	$ 357,842
Total liabilities and shareholders' equity	$2,502,992

a. Perform a Du Pont analysis on Green Valley. Assume that the industry average ratios are as follows:

Total margin	3.5%
Total asset turnover	1.5
Equity multiplier	2.5
Return on equity	13.1%

b. Calculate and interpret the following ratios:

	Industry Average
Return on assets	5.2%
Current ratio	2.0
Days cash on hand	22 days
Average collection period	19 days
Debt ratio	71%

Debt-to-equity ratio	2.5
Times interest earned ratio	0.6
Fixed asset turnover ratio	1.4

13.6 Examine the industry average ratios given in Problems 13.4 and 13.5 above. Explain why the ratios are different between the managed care and nursing home industries.

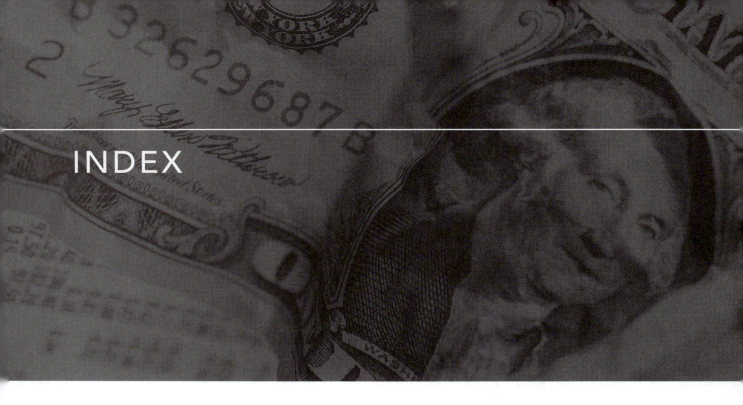

INDEX

ABOUT THE AUTHOR

Louis C. Gapenski, PhD, is a professor in both health services administration and finance at the University of Florida. He received a BS degree from the Virginia Military Institute; an MS degree from the US Naval Postgraduate School; and MBA and PhD degrees from the University of Florida, the latter two in finance. In addition to teaching at the University of Florida, he was on the national faculty of the University of Wisconsin's Program in Administrative Medicine and has taught in programs at numerous other universities.

Dr. Gapenski is the author or coauthor of more than 20 textbooks on corporate and healthcare finance. His books are used worldwide, with Canadian and international editions as well as translations into Russian, Bulgarian, Chinese, Indonesian, Italian, Polish, Portuguese, and Spanish. In addition, he has published more than 40 journal articles related to corporate and healthcare finance and has authored a self-study program in healthcare finance for the American College of Healthcare Executives.

Dr. Gapenski is a member of the Association of University Programs in Health Administration, the American College of Healthcare Executives, the Medical Group Management Association, and the Healthcare Financial Management Association. He has acted as academic advisor, chaired sessions, and presented papers at numerous national meetings. Additionally, Dr. Gapenski has been an editorial board member and reviewer for many academic and professional journals.